Therapeutic Targets for Diabetic Retinopathy

Therapeutic Targets for Diabetic Retinopathy
A Translational Approach

Weiye Li

Professor emeritus of Ophthalmology,
Drexel University College of Medicine,
Philadelphia, Pennsylvania

Jingfa Zhang

Senior Scientist and Attending Physician,
Department of Ophthalmology,
Shanghai General Hospital (Shanghai First People's Hospital),
Shanghai

ELSEVIER

Therapeutic Targets for Diabetic Retinopathy   ISBN: 978-0-323-93064-2

Publisher: Sarah E. Barth
Acquisitions Editor: Kayla Wolfe
Editorial Project Manager: Sam Young
Production Project Manager: Kiruthika Govindaraju
Cover Designer: Mark Rogers

3251 Riverport Lane
St. Louis, Missouri 63043

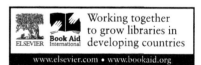

For Dr. Samuel Zigler

Contents

About the authors

Weiye Li, MD, PhD

Dr. Weiye Li, Professor Emeritus, Retina Surgeon, and Researcher of Drexel University, College of Medicine, an internationally renowned expert in the study of diabetic retinopathy and age-related macular degeneration, shares his practice, experience, and insight in this book.

Jingfa Zhang, MD, PhD

Dr. Jingfa Zhang, Senior Scientist and Attending Physician at the Department of Ophthalmology, Shanghai General Hospital (Shanghai First People's Hospital), Shanghai Jiao Tong University, Shanghai, P.R. China, is a physician-scientist focusing on diabetic retinopathy and age-related macular degeneration.

Preface

Diabetic retinopathy (DR) is the leading cause of vision loss among working age population worldwide. Due to numerous advances in the modern medicine, substantial progress has been made in the treatment of DR. The central role of vascular endothelial growth factor (VEGF) in the pathogenesis of DR was validated by the finding that the higher concentrations of VEGF-A in vitreous correlate positively with the more advanced stages of DR and diabetic macular edema (DME).[1] The studies on diabetic animal models and clinical practice demonstrated that the VEGF-A blockade is effective to treat proliferative diabetic retinopathy (PDR) and DME and even to halt the progression or reverse the stages of moderate-to-severe non−proliferative diabetic retinopathy (NPDR).[2] Hence, ophthalmologists learnt from oncologists and adapted anti-VEGF therapy to counterattack VEGF-driven etiology of DR. The anti-VEGF therapy has revolutionized DR treatment. However, a significant subset of patients with DME and PDR failed to respond to anti-VEGF therapy.[3] Nevertheless, the strategies for prevention and management of early DR are still lacking. Therefore, there is an urgent need for the discovery of new therapeutic targets for managing DR.

This book tries to update the basic understanding of aberrant metabolisms induced by diabetes mellitus, by which the homeostasis of retinal neurovascular unit (NVU) is disturbed in DR. The diabetes-induced disturbed retinal neurovascular coupling among neurons, glia, and vascular cells results in key pathogenic events of DR. These pathogenic events include hyperglycemia-induced oxidative stress, apoptosis, microinflammation, blood−retinal barrier breakdown, and pathological angiogenesis.

Based on the new understanding of these pathogenic mechanisms, the aim of this book is to explore how these research achievements can be translated into current and future clinical applications from physician's and researcher's perspective. This book emphasizes how several novel pathobiological concepts of DR have been translated into potential therapeutic targets. First of all, DR is a complication of diabetes. Most advances in systemic treatment of diabetes have been related to secondary prevention of DR. Second, DR is defined as a disease of NVU, comprising both neurodegeneration and microangiopathy. The interplay between these two components in retinal NVU determines that the therapeutic strategy must cover both. Third, the development and progression of DR are disease stage specific.[4] The anatomically regressive stage of DR, such as dynamic nonperfused retina, is due to vascular and neuronal apoptosis. In this stage antiapoptotic, protective therapy is essential, while the proliferative stage of DR is based on pathologic angiogenesis. Therefore, targeting VEGF and non-VEGF pathways to suppress angiogenesis is imperative. Fourth, DR refers to a disease of microinflammation. Abnormal activation of glia and inflammatory cells and the imbalance of pro- and antiinflammatory cytokines contribute to and aggravate different stages of DR. Thereby, antiinflammatory therapy is gaining ground in treating DR, particularly for DME in years to come. Fifth, this book tries to point out how the advances of multimodal imaging techniques and artificial intelligence-directed medicine have been translated from bench to bedside. Lastly, we expect that the rapidly improving retinal microsurgery will bring promise for patients with late stage of PDR. Although this book has emphasized the translational approach, the current evidence-based DR management is still introduced in the highest priority, followed by therapies in pipeline for DR. In a sequential order, the potential mechanism-based therapies are discussed at the end of each chapter.

The study of "therapeutic targets for DR" from molecule to system is far ranging, which is beyond the scope of this book. We humbly present this book to readers, to make some initial remarks to set the ball rolling for future breakthroughs.

Weiye Li and Jingfa Zhang

References

1. Aiello LP, Avery RL, Arrigg PG, et al. Vascular endothelial growth factor in ocular fluid of patients with diabetic retinopathy and other retinal disorders. *N Engl J Med.* 1994; 331(22):1480−1487. https://doi.org/10.1056/NEJM199412013312203.
2. Brown DM, Wykoff CC, Boyer D, et al. Evaluation of intravitreal aflibercept for the treatment of severe nonproliferative diabetic retinopathy: results from the PANORAMA randomized clinical trial. *JAMA Ophthalmol.* 2021;139(9):946. https://doi.org/10.1001/jamaophthalmol.2021.2809.
3. Tan Y, Fukutomi A, Sun MT, Durkin S, Gilhotra J, Chan WO. Anti-VEGF crunch syndrome in proliferative diabetic retinopathy: a review. *Surv Ophthalmol.* 2021;66(6): 926−932. https://doi.org/10.1016/j.survophthal.2021.03.001.
4. Wilkinson CP, Ferris FL, Klein RE, et al. Proposed international clinical diabetic retinopathy and diabetic macular edema disease severity scales. *Ophthalmology.* 2003;110(9): 1677−1682. https://doi.org/10.1016/S0161-6420(03)00475-5.

Acknowledgments

The authors carried out their clinical and basic research on diabetic retinopathy in collaboration with the laboratories of Dr. John H. Rockey, Dr. Gustavo D. Aquirre, and Dr. Guo-Tong Xu at different periods in the past 40 years. The authors are grateful for all their consistent support and intellectual inspirations.

August 2022

Introduction of diabetic retinopathy and principles of treatment

Epidemiology of diabetes mellitus and diabetic retinopathy

Diabetes mellitus (diabetes or DM) is a chronic metabolic disease that is characterized by a prolonged period of hyperglycemia, that is, elevated glucose in the blood.[1] The elevated glucose occurs either when the pancreas does not produce enough insulin or when the body cannot effectively use the insulin it produces. There are three main types of diabetes, which are type 1, type 2, and gestational diabetes.[2] The most common type is type 2 diabetes (T2DM) that comprises about 90% cases. T2DM usually occurs in adults when the body becomes resistant to insulin. As the disease progresses, a lack of insulin may also develop. Type 1 diabetes (T1DM) accounts for 5% to 10% of the total cases of diabetes worldwide.[3] T1DM, once known as juvenile diabetes or insulin-dependent diabetes, is a chronic condition in which the pancreas produces little or no insulin. The cause of T1DM is believed to be an environmentally triggered autoimmune destruction of pancreatic beta cells among patients with genetic susceptibility.[4] Gestational diabetes is a hyperglycemic condition developed in pregnancy. Notably, T2DM has become one of the most serious health challenges of the 21st century worldwide. The number of patients with diabetes aged 20−79 years old is predicted to rise to 642 million by 2040.[5] Based on the world health organization database, the number of people with diabetes rose from 108 million in 1980 to 422 million in 2014.[1] The number could rise to 700 million in 2045.[6] In other words, in 2014, 8.5% of adults aged 18 years and older had diabetes globally. In the past 3 decades, the prevalence of diabetes has risen more dramatically in developing countries than in developed countries.[1] Diabetes is a risk factor for cardiovascular events and mortality in mid-aged adults.[7] Recent studies also demonstrated significantly higher mortality rates in subgroups, either diabetic people aged ≥70 years or young-onset T2DM patients aged <40 years, as compared to those without diabetes.[8,9] In 2019, an estimated 1.5 million deaths were directly caused by diabetes worldwide.[1]

Because of the high rates of diabetes-related mortality, hospitalization, and comorbidities, the socioeconomic burden of diabetes is huge. The epidemiologic data also documented that diabetes is a major cause of blindness, kidney failure, heart attacks, stroke, and lower limb amputation.[1] Diabetic retinopathy (DR) is a leading cause of blindness of the working-age population. Despite advances in optimal control of blood glucose, blood pressure, and lipids and the use of anti-vascular endothelial growth factor agents, the prevalence of DR remains high in people with diabetes.

In 2012, a pooled analysis from population-based studies around the world was conducted.[10] This study provided epidemiologic analysis of vision-threatening diabetic retinopathy (VTDR), proliferative diabetic retinopathy (PDR), and diabetic macular edema (DME). Pooled prevalence estimates were age-standardized to the 2010 World Diabetes Population aged 20−79 years old. Based on this dataset, 52% were female, 44.4% were Caucasian, 30.9% were Asian, 13.9% were Hispanic, and 8.9% were African American. The mean age was 58.1 years, median diabetes duration was 7.9 years (range 3−16), and median hemoglobin A_{1c} (HbA$_{1c}$) was 8.0% (6.7%−9.9%). The overall DR prevalence in diabetic patients is 35%. Among them PDR was 6.96%, DME was 6.8%, and VTDR was 10.2%. The authors estimated that 92.6 million (91.2−94.0) adults had some forms of DR, 17.2 million (16.6−17.7) had PDR, 20.6 million (19.6−21.6) had DME, and 28.4 million (27.6−29.2) had VTDR. These data demonstrate that DR is a major cause of visual impairment and blindness worldwide.[10]

The Wisconsin Epidemiologic Study of Diabetic Retinopathy (WESDR) is a classical population-based study, in which patients diagnosed as diabetes at age 30 years or older were examined to determine the prevalence and severity of DR and associated risk factors. The prevalence of DR varied from 28.8% in persons who had diabetes for less than 5 years to 77.8% in persons who had diabetes for 15 or more years. The duration of DR is also associated with severity of retinopathy. For instance, the rate of PDR varied from 2.0% in persons who had diabetes for less than 5 years to 15.5% in persons who had diabetes for 15 or more years. Based on the same dataset, Cox regression model was used to analyze the significance of variables that may affect the severity of retinopathy. Among these variables, the duration of diabetes is strongly associated with the severity of retinopathy.[11]

Since the prevalence of diabetes in the United States has increased in recent decades, the investigation of DR prevalence was revisited in US adults with diabetes aged 40 years or older using the data collected through National Health and Nutrition Examination Survey (NHNES) in 2005−2008.[12] In this survey, severity of DR was graded in all studies by color fundus photography reading centers. Grading was performed using the Early Treatment of Diabetic Retinopathy Study (ETDRS) interim or final scale.[13] The prevalence of any DR and VTDR was 28.5% and 4.4%, respectively, among US adults with diabetes. Notably, the subjects who participated in the DR prevalence studies are mainly White people. The global prevalence and risk factors of DR cannot be simply extrapolated from these data. Meanwhile, fewer studies have addressed the variation of frequency of retinopathy by race/ethnicity. Non-Hispanic black individuals had a higher prevalence than non-Hispanic White individuals of DR (38.8% vs. 26.4%; $P = .01$) and VTDR (9.3% vs. 3.2%; $P = .01$). Overall, in a multiethnic cohort study in the United States, both African Americans and Hispanics have a higher prevalence of retinopathy than Caucasians.[14–16] In one dataset of an epidemiologic study on DR in Chinese Americans, the prevalence among the Chinese patients (25.7%) was similar to Whites (24.8%), which is in agreement with the findings on a cohort of Chinese patients with T2DM visiting a Beijing Hospital (27.3%). The epidemiologic features of Chinese populations with DR in China were summarized in a recent publication.[17–19]

Based on NHNES dataset from 2005–2008, established risk factors of DR included higher HbA_{1c} level (odds ratio (OR), 1.45), longer duration of diabetes (OR, 1.06 per year duration), and higher systolic blood pressure (OR, 1.03 per mmHg), each being independently associated with the presence of DR.[12] In the study of risk factors of DR, racial disparity among different race/ethnic groups is particularly important. This is because the racial disparity in DR prevalence involves a complex interaction between genetic susceptibility and environmental risk factors. Understanding the underlying mechanisms of this racial disparity is essential for screening and treatment of DR. For example, a prospective cohort study of diabetic adults participating in the Multi-Ethnic Study of Atherosclerosis was analyzed. The racial differences in the prevalence of any DR and VTDR were no longer significant when adjustment was made with other established risk predictors.[19] Thus, this study suggests that race is not an independent predictor of DR. Even though race/ethnicity was considered as a complex, independent risk factor for DR based on a major review of DR prevalence in various ethnic groups, this study will argue that race/ethnicity complex should be approached through a paradigm with biological, social, and economic dimensions shifting with environmental variations in both time and space.[20] First of all, all ethnic groups are susceptible to the established risk factors of DR as described above, such as the level of HbA_{1c}, duration of hyperglycemia, and hypertension. Therefore, the racial/ethnic factors may not be independent risk factors after adjustment with the established risk factors.[19] On the other hand, the ethnic-specific risk factors may influence the prevalence rates of DR independently, because they present differential susceptibility to conventional risk factors, such as insulin resistance, truncal obesity, urbanization, genetic susceptibility, and variations in access to health-care systems.[20] It is notable that in current health-care systems worldwide, the control of the established risk factors, so-called modifiable risk factors, varies among different ethnic groups. Data from National Health Interview Survey also suggest that non-Hispanic black individuals and Hispanics are less likely to use eye care services in the United States.[21] In a broader view, data from the Medical Expenditure Panel Survey demonstrated that Whites had consistently higher dilated eye examination rates than minority populations across an 8-year period (2002–2009).[22] The different rates in eye examinations for patients with diabetes may have been attributed in part to racial/ethnic differences in other established risk factors of DR.[22,23]

In addition, the prevalence rate of DR in different populations is dynamic.[24] It has been reported that the prevalence of all stages of DR has been declining since 1980 in populations with improved diabetes control.[25] On the other hand, the prevalence of visual impairment caused by DR increased substantially between 1990 and

2015 according to the report of the Vision Loss Expert Group of the Global Burden of Disease Study, largely because of the predominantly increased prevalence of T2DM in low-income and middle-income countries.[26] All these findings suggest that improved screening and glycemic control could change the perspective of DR prevention and management. The rapid change of the landscape of DR prevalence in recent decades indicates that the influence of environmental/socioeconomic factors exceeds that of genetic susceptibility of different ethnic groups. Therefore, the ethnic-specific risk factors merit further identification and study.

Taken together, the epidemiologic findings on the prevalence of DR may be outlined as follows: First, there is a global increase in the prevalence of diabetes. Second, the epidemic of diabetes is mainly attributable to T2DM, which represents about 90% of all diabetic cases. Third, DME is the most common cause of vision loss, overriding PDR, among diabetic patients, because of an increasing prevalence of the global epidemic in T2DM. Fourth, prevalence of PDR is higher in T1DM than in people with T2DM. Fifth, a decline in the incidence of blindness due to DR has been found in developed countries due to improved glycemic control in recent decades.[10] Sixth, overall, DR is a major cause of visual impairment and blindness worldwide. Seventh, hyperglycemia remains the most consistent risk factor for DR in patients with T1DM or T2DM.[27] Eighth, blood pressure is an important risk factor for DR in T2DM (see Chapter 10). Ninth, DR awareness remains patchy and low in most populations. Tenth, DR prevention in low-resource countries requires different models from that developed in high-resource countries.[28] Eleventh, the racial/ethnic disparity in prevalence rates of DR demands the development of more sophisticate ethnic-specific guidelines in health-care systems worldwide. These epidemiologic findings highlight the disease burden and pathogenicity of DR. These epidemiologic trends should be further translated into preventive efforts for reduction of DR prevalence.

Classification, staging, and severity of DR

DME and PDR are blinding complications of DR.[29] DME is the most common cause of vision loss in patients with DR followed by PDR. DR is present in approximately 35% of persons with diabetes. DME has a prevalence of 6.8% among people with diabetes. Macular edema can occur in any stage of DR, either nonproliferative diabetic retinopathy (NPDR) or PDR. DME mainly results from breakdown of the blood–retinal barrier (BRB). In diabetic retina, fluid by extravasation from retinal vessels and leakage of outer BRB accumulates as intraretinal or subretinal fluid. In addition, DME may be associated with hard exudates, which are precipitates of plasma lipoproteins (Fig. 1.1).[30]

DME prevalence depends on the type of diabetes and the duration of the disease. Based on population-based WESDR and other cross-sectional studies, the prevalence of DME is estimated to be higher in T2DM than that in T1DM patients. In contrast, the prevalence of PDR is higher in T1DM than that in T2DM

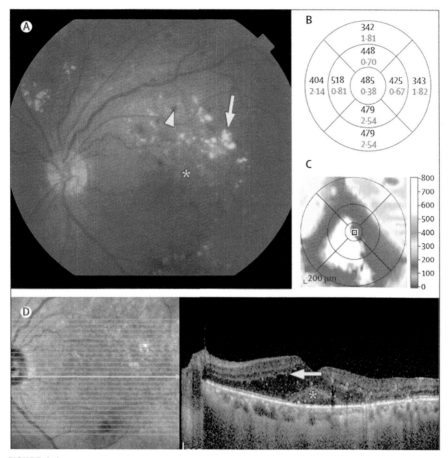

FIGURE 1.1

Clinical and OCT features of center-involved diabetic macular edema (CI-DME). (A) Color fundus photography of macula (*left eye*) to identify retinal thickening, hard exudates (*arrow*), microaneurysms (*asterisk*), and dot/blot hemorrhages (*arrow head*). Quantitative assessment with OCT: (B) quantitative average retinal thickness in μm (*black*) and retinal volume map of the macula in mm^3 (*red*); (C) overall topography of the macula; (D) horizontal cross-sectional images of the macula showing intraretinal thickening (*arrow*), subretinal fluid (*asterisk*) and multiple intraretinal hyperreflective foci in CI-DME.

Modified from Tan et al.[30]

patients.[31,32] Since the majority of diabetic patients have T2DM, the increasing prevalence of DME links to the global epidemic in T2DM. After 30 year duration, both types 1 and 2 were found to be associated with increasing prevalence of DME, but the increase still tended to be higher in T2DM than in T1DM.[33] The pathophysiology of DME starts with decreased retinal oxygen tension. The reduced oxygen tension of diabetic retina manifests as capillary hyperpermeability and increased intravascular pressure, which are mediated by vascular endothelial growth factor (VEGF) and retinal vascular autoregulation, respectively. Spectral-domain optical coherence tomography (SD-OCT) is the cornerstone of clinical assessment of DME. The foundation of treatment is metabolic control of hyperglycemia and blood pressure. Specific ophthalmic treatments include intravitreal anti-VEGF drug injections, intravitreal corticosteroid injections, focal laser photocoagulation, and vitrectomy. However, a substantial fraction of eyes respond incompletely to all of these modalities resulting in visual loss and disordered structure and vasculature visible on SD-OCT and OCT angiography (OCTA). Currently, therapeutic efforts to close the gap between the results of interventions within randomized clinical trials and in real-world contexts and to reduce the cost of care occupy innovation in the social organization of ophthalmic care of DME. Pharmacologic research is exploring other biochemical pathways involved in retinal vascular homeostasis that may provide new points of intervention effective in those cases unresponsive to current treatments.[32] In addition to duration of diabetes, systemic risk factors associated with DME include higher systolic blood pressure and higher HbA_{1c}. The main ocular risk factor of DME is the severity of DR, as increasing severity is associated with increasing prevalence of DME, although DME can be present in any severity level of DR.[34,35]

All these data raise several fundamental questions in understanding and managing of DME. First, does the type of diabetes matter in the DME etiology and therapy?[32] Second, how does longer duration of diabetes, associated with numerous metabolic abnormalities such as hyperglycemia and high HbA_{1c}, turn into systemic risk factors of DME? Third, how does hypertension become a pathogenic factor of DME? Fourth, how is the prevalence of DME depending upon the severity of DR? In order to answer these questions in the following chapters, the classification of DME needs to be updated in the era of OCT and OCTA. The ETDRS, the first prospective randomized clinical trial of photocoagulation in diabetic patients with non—high-risk PDR, established a guideline for managing DME by color fundus photography.[36] It defined clinically significant macular edema (CSME) into three categories as the indication for focal laser photocoagulation. The three categories of CSME include: (1) retinal thickening within 500 μm of the center of the macula; (2) hard exudate within 500 μm of the center of macula, if associated with retinal thickening, the thickening itself may be outside the 500 μm; (3) retinal thickening one disc area (1500 μm) or larger, any part of which is within the disc diameter of the center of macula. Since the algorithm of DME treatment evolved rapidly, intravitreal injection of anti-VEGF drugs has supplanted the macular laser therapy as the first-line therapy. This classification of DME has been updated based on OCT testing. DME is now defined as center-involved DME (CI-DME) or non-center-involved form (non-CI-DME). In CI-DME, the central retinal subfield is thickened on OCT scan, and the central visual acuity is impaired. Visual acuity testing is a subjective widely employed method based on the resolution ability of the fovea. However, visual acuity does not reflect all alterations affecting central vision, such as perifoveal scotoma or reading speed reduction. In addition to central vision loss, usually experienced as a relative central scotoma affecting far- and near-vision, patients with CI-DME often also complain of metamorphopsia, reading difficulties, impaired stereopsis, or disturbed color vision.[37,38] The newly defined CI-DME or non-CI-DME paradigm allows better quantitative interpretation of the correlation between macular structure damage and functional abnormalities both for clinical management and as a validated clinical research endpoint (Fig. 1.1).

Consensus on the classification of staging and severity of DR was reached by the ETDRS in early 1990s[39] and detailed in a 2017 position statement from the American Diabetes Association.[40] In clinical practice, DR is categorized into NPDR and PDR. NPDR is staged into no DR, very mild DR, mild NPDR, moderate NPDR, severe NPDR, and very severe NPDR based on the presentation of microaneurysms, dot/blot hemorrhage, hard exudates, venous beading, and intraretinal microvascular abnormalities (IRMAs) (Table 1.1). PDR is staged into mild-moderate PDR, high-risk PDR, and advanced diabetic eye disease. The advanced diabetic eye disease is characterized by tractional retinal detachment, significant persistent vitreous hemorrhage, and neovascular glaucoma. DME develops as a result of increased permeability of retinal vessels and from microaneurysms, as well as dysfunction of Müller glial cells, leading to the accumulation of extracellular and intracellular fluid and thickening of macular tissue. As the severity of DR increases, the risk of developing DME similarly increases.[35] Loss of vision from DME is correlated with the location and extent of retinal thickening on OCT scans and also correlates with retinal blood vessel leakage and perfusion. It is important to know that CI-DME has a nearly tenfold higher risk of moderate vision loss as compared to thickening without center involvement.[36] The current management of different stages of DR and different types of DME is briefly summarized in Table 1.1.

As DR progresses, it has been postulated that over one-quarter of the retina must be nonperfused due to capillary damage before development of retinal neovascularization. Although with ultrawide field fluorescein angiography (UWF-FA), it is clear that retinal new vessels may arise anywhere in the retina including peripheral retina; they are most commonly seen at the posterior pole.[42] Clinical examination shows different type and location of new vessels in PDR. New vessels at the disc (NVD) are defined as neovascularization on or within one disc diameter of the optic nerve head. New vessels elsewhere (NVE) are neovascularization further away from the disc (Fig. 1.2).

Long-standing NVD/NVE may be associated with increasing growth of fibrosis. Fibrous tissue that is initially fine gradually enlarges in association with the increment of new vessels. New vessels on the iris, known as rubeosis iridis, carry a high risk of progression to neovascular glaucoma. Vascular leakage is one of the important pathologic characteristics of PDR. By using OCTA, the vascular changes of DR including microaneurysms, retinal nonperfusion, IRMA, and neovascularization can be clearly visualized. Despite these advantages, imaging with OCTA can only provide a limited view of the peripheral retina and is unable to demonstrate leakage, staining, or pooling. However, neovascular leakage, that is, NVD and NVE can be easily distinguished by UWF-FA (Fig. 1.3).[43]

Table 1.1 Modified ETDRS classification/staging/severity of DR.

Category description	Presence of macular edema	Follow-up schedule
NPDR		
No DR	No	12 months
Mild NPDR	No	12 months
Any or all of microaneurysms, hemorrhage, exudates, CWS	Non-CI-DME	4–6 months
	CI-DME	1 month
Moderate NPDR	No	6–12 months
Severe hemorrhage, significant venous beading no more than 1 Q, commonly CWS	Non-CI-DME	3–6 months
	CI-DME	1 month
Severe NPDR	No	4 months
The 4:2:1 rule: severe hemorrhage in all 4 Q; significant venous beading in 2 or more Q; moderate IRMA in 1 Q	Non-CI-DME	2–4 months
	CI-DME	1 month
PDR		
Non–high-risk PDR	No	4 months
NVD or NVE, but extent insufficient to meet high-risk criteria	Non-CI-DME	2–4 months
	CI-DME	1 month
High-risk PDR	No	4 months
NVD ≥1/3 disc area; any NVD with vitreous hemorrhage; NVE ≥1/2 disc area with vitreous hemorrhage	Non-CI-DME	4 months
	CI-DME	1 month
Involuted PDR	No	6–12 months
	Non-CI-DME	4 months
	CI-DME	1 month
Advanced diabetic eye disease Significant persistent vitreous hemorrhage; tractional retinal detachment; neovascular glaucoma	Consider pars plana vitrectomy and combined surgery	

Abbreviations: CI-DME, center-involved diabetic macular edema; CWSs, cotton wool spot; DR, diabetic retinopathy; ETDRS, the early treatment of diabetic retinopathy study; Non-CI-DME, non-center-involved diabetic macular edema; NPDR, nonproliferative diabetic retinopathy; NVD, neovascularization on the disc; NVE, neovascularization elsewhere; PDR, proliferative diabetic retinopathy; Q, quadrant.
Modified from AAO Retina and Vitreous 2019–20 BCSC.[41]

Current management and its limitations for DR, DME, and PDR

Control of systemic risk factors

Diabetes affects multiple organs. Diabetic macroangiopathy includes cerebrovascular disease, coronary artery disease, and peripheral artery disease, whereas microangiopathy comprises retinopathy, nephropathy, and peripheral neuropathy. DR is secondary to a combination of multiple metabolic insults and disorders. Large

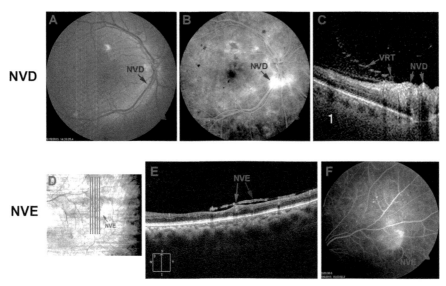

FIGURE 1.2

Neovascularization on disc (NVD in the *upper row*) and neovascularization elsewhere (NVE at the *bottom row*) of diabetic eyes with PDR are viewed by multimodal imaging techniques. *Upper row*, NVD as seen by color fundus photograph (A), NVD leakage is only detected by fluorescein angiography (B), NVD and vitreoretinal traction (VRT) are viewed by SD-OCT (C). *Bottom row*, NVE is seen by red-free image and SD-OCT in (A and B). The leaky vessels are demonstrated by fluorescein angiography (C).

Data from W. Li.

prospective randomized studies have documented that the duration of diabetes and inadequacy of glycemic control are two of the major systemic contributors to the onset and development of DR.[10] Epidemiological, clinical, and laboratory studies have further increased our understanding of the pathophysiology of DR. Particularly, hyperglycemia, hypertension, and dyslipidemia combined with the duration of diabetes contribute to the onset of DR. Thereby, control of these systemic risk factors is a fundamental strategy for the prevention and treatment of early DR. In fact, patients with chronically higher hyperglycemia have substantially more severe retinopathy than those with lower blood glucose levels. On the other hand, intensive blood glucose control has been demonstrated to reduce the risk of progression of DR in large, well-designed randomized controlled trials. The Diabetes Control and Complications Trial (DCCT) showed that intensive glycemic control in T1DM reduced the risk of developing retinopathy by 76% and slowed its progression in a group with mild retinopathy at baseline, that is, reduced the risk of three-step progression by 54%, and also reduced the risk of proliferative disease and the need for laser treatment.[44] The Epidemiology of Diabetes Interventions and Complications study and observational follow-up of T1DM participants in DCCT over 30 years showed

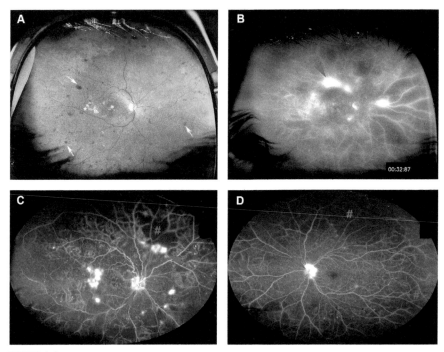

FIGURE 1.3

Ultrawide field photography and ultrawide field fluorescein angiography (UWF-FA) clearly demonstrate peripheral retina and leakage by NVD and NVE in PDR. (A) Hemorrhages (*white arrows*) and hard exudate (*) are seen in color ultrawide field photography. (B) UWF-FA shows the distribution of nonperfused (#) and neovascularized (*red arrow*) retinal lesions at the posterior pole as well as the midperipheral zone and far-peripheral zone. (C) The nonperfusion (#) is prominent at the far-peripheral zone. The majority of dye leakage at A-V phase indicating neovascularization (*red arrow*) is concentrated at the areas between far- and midperipheral zone. (D) Neovascularization on optic disc (*red arrow*) and nonperfusion (#) was indicated. *A-V*, arterial-venous; *NVD*, neovascularization on disc; *NVE*, neovascularization elsewhere; *PDR*, proliferative diabetic retinopathy.

Data from W. Li.

persistent benefits of slowing development of DR with intensive glycemic control as compared to conventional glycemic therapy. For patients with T2DM, the UK Prospective Diabetes Study (UKPDS) showed that intensive diabetic control can reduce the risk of needing retinal photocoagulation and the risk of progressing to diabetic blindness of one eye.[45] However, it should be noted that the worsening of DR is associated with the initiation of effective treatment of hyperglycemia in some patients with diabetes, in which the large and rapid reductions in blood glucose levels are associated with early worsening of DR (EWDR).[46] EWDR has been described during intensive treatment in patients with uncontrolled T1DM or T2DM. The disturbance of VEGF signaling after glycemic fluctuation has been proposed as an underlying mechanism of EWDR. In the ischemic retina, expression of VEGF is blunted when glucose concentrations are high, but it will increase after normalization of glucose levels. Other theories include the perturbed somatotropic axis and angiogenic growth factors. However, these hypothetical risk factors have not been studied in an EWDR-specific context.[47] In order to minimize the adverse effects of EWDR, identification and control of risk factors after intensive treatment are essential. Feldman-Billard et al.[47] recommended an applicable algorithm for monitoring and treating EWDR, which is introduced in Fig. 1.4.

Blood pressure levels have been claimed to influence retinopathy development and progression. The UKPDS examined the effect of intensive blood pressure control with captopril or atenolol on microvascular complications in 1148 hypertensive patients with T2DM.[48] The results showed that tight blood pressure control in patients with hypertension and T2DM achieves a clinically important reduction in the risk of complications related to diabetes, progression of DR, and deterioration in visual acuity. However, other multiple controlled clinical trials of antihypertensive agents in diabetic subjects have produced only weak evidence of benefit from blood pressure lowering on the incidence and progression of DR.

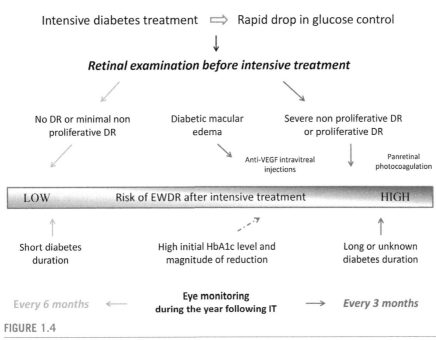

FIGURE 1.4

Eye monitoring and treatment algorithm associated with intensive diabetes treatment. *DR*, diabetic retinopathy; *EWDR*, early worsening diabetic retinopathy; *VEGF*, vascular endothelial growth factor; *IT*, intensive treatment.

Modified from Feldman-Billard et al.[47]

Increased blood lipids, or dyslipidemia, seems to play a role in the progression of retinopathy, and two trials of fenofibrate have shown benefit in preventing retinopathy progression. The Action to Control Cardiovascular Risk in Diabetes (ACCORD) Eye Study showed a 40% reduction in relative risk of retinopathy progression with the addition of fenofibrate to simvastatin.[49] Thus, intensive glycemic control and intensive combination treatment of dyslipidemia seem to reduce the rate of progression of DR.

In addition to the modifiable systemic risk factors as described above, genetic factors that play a major role in etiology of diabetes have long been appreciated.[50] However, the genetic pathogenicity of DR has not been fully clarified.[51,52] In Chapter 10, the future of genetic study on DR is discussed.

Anti-VEGF therapy

Vitreous VEGF-A levels are considerably higher in patients with DME than those without DME. In other words, the severity of leakage in DME is correlating with the level of VEGF-A.[53] Clinical trials of anti-VEGF agents for DME have demonstrated significant benefits. Currently, anti-VEGF therapy is the first-line treatment of CI-DME, supplanting focal photocoagulation. Ranibizumab was the first medication approved by the United States Food and Drug Administration (FDA) for the treatment of DME. Ranibizumab consists of a humanized monoclonal antibody fragment that binds to all isoforms of VEGF-A. RISE (NCT00473330) and RIDE (NCT00473382) were two major randomized controlled trials that in phase three compared monthly ranibizumab with sham injections in DME patients. The percentage of patients with ≥15 ETDRS letters gain at both 2- and 3-year end points was approximately double in patients receiving ranibizumab (40%) compared with the sham group (20%).[54,55] The Diabetic Retinopathy Clinical Research Network (DRCR.net) Protocol I was another phase three trial with four treatment arms. The four treatments are as follows: ranibizumab with immediate focal/grid laser, ranibizumab with macular laser given only for persistent DME after 6 months, intraocular triamcinolone plus immediate macular laser, and macular laser with sham injections. This study yielded similar vision improvements as seen in RISE and RIDE in patients treated with ranibizumab versus sham injection or when comparing with intravitreal triamcinolone (Protocol I at Chapter 9). Additionally, at five-year follow-up for these patients, it was found that the initial visual acuity gains at one year of treatment were maintained, with a progressively decreasing frequency of retreatment as needed.[56]

Bevacizumab is a full-length humanized monoclonal antibody to VEGF-A. Bevacizumab is originally approved by FDA for the treatment of metastatic colorectal cancer in combination with chemotherapy. Off-label intravitreal use of bevacizumab was pioneered by Rosenfeld et al.[57] Currently, off-label use of bevacizumab is widespread for wet age-related macular degeneration and DME in real clinical settings. A two-year randomized controlled trial (BLOT) comparing intravitreal bevacizumab with laser therapy showed that the bevacizumab arm had a mean gain of +8.6 letters, compared with a mean loss of −0.5 letters in the laser arm.[58]

Aflibercept is a soluble fusion protein and VEGF receptor analog consisting of the extracellular domains of VEGF receptors fused with the Fc fragment of human immunoglobulin G1. The VIVID (NCT01331681) and VISTA (NCT01363440) studies were the major studies that investigated the use of aflibercept in DME. The arms of the study consisted of aflibercept given every 4 weeks, aflibercept given every 8 weeks after 5 initial monthly doses, or laser photocoagulation. Both studies found an improvement in gains of visual acuity in those treated with aflibercept versus laser control. VISTA showed gains of +10.4 letters with monthly aflibercept as compared with +1.4 letters in laser. VIVID presented similar gains, +10.3 letters versus +1.6 letters. Additionally, the percentage of patients with a greater than 15 letters gain from baseline was higher after treatment with aflibercept in both studies, compared with laser photocoagulation alone.[59] Based on these impressive clinical benefits, the FDA approved aflibercept for treatment of DME. Regarding the comparison between different anti-VEGF agents and their comparable effects on DME, the most comprehensive data comes from the DRCR.net Protocol T. This study evaluated visual outcomes in patients with macular edema treated with ranibizumab, bevacizumab, or aflibercept up to every 4 weeks, with additional focal laser if indicated at or after 6 months. For initial visual acuities of 20/40 or better, there was no statistically significant difference among the three agents. For patients presenting with visual acuities of 20/50 or worse, after one year of treatment, aflibercept had statistically significantly greater gains in visual acuity compared with ranibizumab and bevacizumab. There were no statistically significant differences between ranibizumab and bevacizumab.[60] After two years of follow-up, in eyes with initial acuity of 20/50 or worse, the superior visual acuity gains of aflibercept compared with ranibizumab were not maintained, although both aflibercept and ranibizumab maintained greater outcomes than bevacizumab in this group.[61] Some have interpreted these results to suggest that aflibercept should be the first-line treatment for DME when visual acuity has declined to 20/50 or worse.[62]

In Table 1.2, the current anti-VEGF drugs are characterized based on molecular structure, molecular weight, binding affinity, targeted VEGF molecules, and origin of production.

When compared with laser photocoagulation, the prior standard of care, the benefit of anti-VEGF therapy in the treatment of DME is clearly demonstrated. However, there has been a recognition that many patients are incomplete or nonresponders to anti-VEGF therapy and are being underserved by the current paradigm of anti-VEGF injections alone.[63] In subanalysis of the DRCR.net Protocol I data, based on whether a 20% reduction in central subfoveal thickness was achieved by ranibizumab, approximately 50% of the patients received inconsistent benefit.[64] In another subanalysis of the DRCR.net Protocol I data, based on distribution of visual acuity gains at 12 weeks after the first three ranibizumab injections, 37.1% of eyes had a greater than 10 letters visual gain, with 23.2% having a five to nine letters gain, and 39.7% of eyes having less than five letters gain. These data demonstrated that the visual acuity gain of DME patients who received anti-VEGF therapy reached a plateau, suggesting that initial visual acuity response after three anti-VEGF

Table 1.2 The anti-VEGF drugs for the treatment of retinal vascular diseases.

Brand name	Macugen	Avastin	Lucentis	Beovu	Eylea	Lumitin
Molecular name	Pegatanib	Bevacizumab	Ranibizumab	Brolucizumab	Aflibercept	Conbercept
Molecular structure	Polyethylene glycol aptamer	Humanized monocolonal antibody	Humanized fab	scFv	Fusion protein	Fusion protein
Molecular weight (kDa)	50	149	48	26	115	143
Production	Chemically synthesized	CHO	E. coli	E. coli	CHO	CHO
VEGF165 kD (pM)	50	58–1100	46–192	28.4	0.5	0.5
Targets	VEGF165	VEGF-A	VEGF-A	VEGF-A	VEGF-A, VEGF-B, PIGF	VEGF-A, VEGF-B, PIGF
Concentration (mg/mL)	3.33	25	10	120	40	10
Dose (mg)	0.3	1.25	0.5	6	2	0.5
Relative moles	/	2.4	3	66	5	1
$t_{1/2}$ (days)	3.9 (monkey)	6.7–10	7.1	2.4	7.1	/
Plasma $t_{1/2}$ (days)	10	21	0.25	1.9	18	4–5 (monkey)

Abbreviations: CHO, Chinese hamster ovary; E. coli, Escherichia coli; Fab, antigen-binding fragment antibody; PlGF, placental growth factor; scFv, single chain fragment variable; VEGF, vascular endothelial growth factor.

injections is predictive of long-term response to anti-VEGF treatment for DME. The underlying mechanisms for the variability in response to anti-VEGF treatment are not completely understood.[65] In addition, identification of other factors that could be targeted as DME therapies requires further studies.[38]

Gross and coauthors reported the 5-year result of a multicenter randomized clinical trial comparing prompt panretinal photocoagulation (PRP) to the long-term intravitreal ranibizumab (IVR) for the treatment of PDR. This study is a continuation of the two-year report of Protocol S study conducted by DRCR.net.[66] The current data showed that both treatments are safe with few serious complications such as neovascular glaucoma. There is no significant difference of visual acuity outcome between the two treatment groups. It is very interesting that the greater peripheral visual field loss from baseline in the PRP group than that of ranibizumab group at the two-year Protocol S report diminished in a five-year subgroup analysis, suggesting that anti-VEGF treatment leads to more rapid visual field loss from years two through five. The five-year follow-up revealed a critical point that PRP and anti-VEGF are comparable therapies for PDR patients. Intravitreal anti-VEGF therapy is an alternative to PRP in treating patients with PDR.[67] We generally understand that PRP leads to more permanent therapeutic outcome than anti-VEGF for PDR. It would be meaningful to revisit information of this study about the visual outcome of the patients who dropped from the current five-year study in both groups (39%, 74 out of 191 in IVR group and 39%, 80 out of 203 in PRP group). Is the discontinuation of a long-term anti-VEGF more risky to worsen visual outcome than that of PRP?[66]

Recently, the DRCR.net Protocol W randomized clinical trial using aflibercept for treating moderate to severe NPDR patients was conducted. Moderate to severe NPDR is considered as the high-risk group to progress to PDR and CI-DME with vision loss. This study has compared the two-year cumulative probability of DR progression with versus without anti-VEGF therapy.[68] The two-year cumulative probability of developing PDR was 13.5% in the aflibercept group versus 33.2% in the sham group, and the probability of developing CI-DME with vision loss was 4.1% in the aflibercept group versus 14.8% in the sham group. However, proof of a long-term functional benefit of using aflibercept as a preventive strategy in moderate or severe NPDR cohort awaits more data. It must be noted that despite all eyes in the aflibercept group receiving a mean of 8 anti-VEGF injections through two years, 16.3% of aflibercept group eyes developed PDR or CI-DME with visual loss in 2-year follow-up. This finding shows that anti-VEGF treatment does not guarantee the prevention of vision-threatening complications in this high-risk cohort.[68] On the other hand, the recent PANORAMA study, a double-masked, randomized, phase 3 trial compared two different treatment regimens of aflibercept with sham injections in patients with moderately severe to severe NPDR. In this study, intravitreal aflibercept injection 2 mg q 16 weeks (2q16) and aflibercept injection 2 mg q8 weeks (2q8) or sham were performed. Through week 52, 9% and 15% of 2q16 and 2q8 eyes, respectively, versus <1% of sham eyes had a ≥3-step improvement in Diabetic Retinopathy Severity Scale score.[69] Additionally, through week 100,

18%, 21%, versus 58% of patients in the three groups, respectively, developed vision-threatening complications (i.e., PDR, anterior segment neovascularization, or CI-DME).[59] These findings demonstrated that aflibercept injection reduces the risk of vision-threatening complications in patients with moderate to severe NPDR and may even reverse disease progression in these patients.

The challenges that we are facing with the current and emerging anti-VEGF therapies are still enormous. We must understand the burden of disease for individuals affected by DR and CI-DME. We should differentiate the usage of current and emerging anti-VEGF therapies based on their safety, efficacy, durability, administration, and dosing for alignment of decision-making with current guidelines. In particular, the appropriate combination of anti-VEGF and other antiangiogenic therapies and the emerging antiinflammatory therapies needs to be explored further.[70] This discussion continues in later chapters.

Corticosteroid therapy

DME comprises vasogenic and cytotoxic edema. The vasogenic edema, known as extracellular edema, results from breakdown of the BRB. Cytotoxic edema, so called intracellular edema, is caused by altered cellular ionic exchanges, resulting in elevated $[Na^+]$ inside retinal neurons and glial cells.[71] Retina consists of microglia and two types of macroglia, that is, Müller cells and astrocytes.[72] Activated retinal glial cells release proinflammatory cytokines responsible for the recruitment of leukocytes,[65] and vasogenic factors such as VEGF, leading to low-grade inflammation and retinal edema, respectively. Cytotoxic edema is initially not a true edema but only a redistribution of water into the cell from its normal extracellular location, consequently causing cell swelling and release of more vasogenic factors.[65,72] Increasing evidence shows that vasogenic and inflammatory factors act interdependently during the development of DME.[73] Therefore, the pharmacologic targets of DME are blockage of vasogenic factors such as VEGF and inhibition of inflammatory factors. Notably, dysfunction of Müller cells is responsible for cytotoxic, vasogenic, and inflammatory-based edema. Müller cells are the central players in DME formation.[74] Ultimately, DME can be characterized as an inflammatory disease.[73]

Glucocorticoids are potent drugs with unsurpassed antiinflammatory effects for central nervous system and retinal edema.[75] As mentioned above, DME comprises both cytotoxic and vasogenic edema. The cytotoxic (intracellular) edema not only precedes vasogenic (extracellular) edema in the disease progression but also can lead to retinal neuron death in the early stage of DME. Steroids could effectively prevent neuronal death in the retina.[76,77] Given that in the retina, glucocorticoid receptors (GRs) are expressed almost exclusively in Müller cells, corticosteroids are able to maintain the central homeostatic balance in diabetic retinas by regulating Müller cell GR signaling.[78] That is to say, the efficacy of glucocorticoid for DME involves suppression of proinflammatory chemokines and leukostasis, as well as inhibition of VEGF and protection of neurons. The DRCR Protocol I trial has shown the efficacy of intravitreal triamcinolone in DME.[79] There was visual improvement and reduction in central subfield thickness with triamcinolone, similar to that of ranibizumab up to 24 weeks, but after that period, the effectiveness of triamcinolone was hindered due to side effects such as high rates of cataract formation and elevation of intraocular pressure (IOP). In clinical practice, steroid treatment is the second-line therapy for DME at present time.

The dexamethasone implant (Ozurdex 0.7 mg) is a biodegradable copolymer that releases dexamethasone over a 6-month period. The safety and efficacy of the implant have been evaluated in multiple phase II studies, which found that the implant is effective in improving vision and in decreasing vascular leakage. The implant is approved by the FDA for DME treatment. In the MEAD study (NCT00168337 and NCT00168389), Ozurdex intravitreal implant resulted in visual improvement of >15 letters in 22% of patients compared with 12% in the sham group.[80] Cataract formation was seen in up to 68% of treated patients. Increases in IOP could be managed with medication. The FDA recently approved fluocinolone acetonide implant (Iluvien) containing 190 µg of drug, with release of 0.2 µg of drug per day. In the randomized Fluocinolone Acetonide for Macular Edema study, there was significant vision improvement in DME patients.[81] Thus, how to optimize steroid therapy for DME in combination with anti-VEGF is a critical question.

Laser photocoagulation

Laser photocoagulation causes denaturation of proteins and coagulative necrosis of the tissues. When targeting tissue, laser energy converts into thermal energy, raising the tissue temperature above 65°C. Laser energy is absorbed by posterior segment tissues such as retinal pigment epithelium (RPE), choroid and retino-choroidal vasculature, which contain melanin, xanthophyll, or hemoglobin. Melanin absorbs green, yellow, red, and infrared wavelengths. Macular xanthophyll readily absorbs blue but minimally absorbs yellow and red. Hemoglobin absorbs blue, green, and yellow but minimally absorbs red wavelengths. Based on the absorption characteristics, green light is the most popular laser for PRP because green laser is absorbed well by melanin and hemoglobin and less by xanthophyll. Since undesirable short wavelengths such as blue light are absent in green laser, the green laser has replaced the blue-green laser for treatment of retinal vascular abnormalities and choroidal neovascularization. The red laser penetrates through moderate vitreous hemorrhage better than those of other wavelength. Since the yellow laser has advantages including low xanthophyll absorption and little photochemical effects, it is safer for treating retinal and choroidal neovascular lesions adjacent to fovea. Overall, the coagulative nature of laser treatment determines that laser photocoagulation is a destructive treatment. However, laser photocoagulation remains one of the mainstays of ophthalmic therapy for vision-threatening complications of DR because of its remarkable efficacy in the prevention of visual loss if undertaken in a timely manner and with appropriate laser types. There are two types of laser therapies for DR, that is, PRP for PDR and macular (focal or grid) laser photocoagulation for DME.[82]

The procedure of PRP is to place laser burns over the entire retina, sparing the central macula to promote regression and arrest progression of retinal neovascularization. Because the laser is designed to destroy ischemic retina, growth factors such as VEGF from the ischemic retina may be suppressed. In addition, laser-induced necrosis of the outer retina brings the ischemic inner retina closer to the high oxygen level of the choriocapillaris. Death of photoreceptor cells after laser treatment, the major consumers of oxygen, allows more oxygen to reach the inner retina. The goal of PRP is to improve the oxygen saturation of retina and reduce the levels of ischemia-induced VEGF and other angiogenic factors.[83] Both Diabetic Retinopathy Study (DRS) and ETRDS established PRP as the primary treatment for PDR, in reducing the risk of severe visual loss (visual acuity $\leq$5/200 patients) by 50% over five years.[84,85] On the other hand, the destructive nature of PRP is associated with significant ocular side effects, which normally cannot be reversed. The side effects of PRP include difficulty with light-dark adaptation, a small decrease in visual acuity, and peripheral visual loss, which could impair night vision and affect driving. Other side effects of PRP, for example, worsening of macular edema, have been reported.[66] Based on DRCR net Protocol S, and despite the clinical side effects of PRP, ranibizumab is not suggested in real-world practice through two years for the treatment of PDR relative to PRP, unless DME was simultaneously present.[86] However, post hoc analysis based on Protocol S and recent CLARITY trials, the overall superiority of anti-VEGF therapy over PRP for PDR, following a long period, may establish a position as reasonable alternative to PRP for PDR in future.[87]

In ETDRS, macular laser reduced the risk of moderate visual loss from CSME by 50%. More recently, DRCR.net showed that about 30% of patients given macular laser gained better vision ($\geq$10 letters) over a two-year period.[88] In the past decade, new approaches in pharmaco-therapeutic management of DME have overshadowed developments in macular laser therapy. However, macular laser therapy continues to evolve. First of all, DRCR.net in 2007 illustrated the "less intense laser techniques" for the management of DME.[89] The purpose of the "mild laser" is to stimulate target tissue such as RPE instead of destroying it. To date, a newer mode of laser therapy, termed subthreshold or nonphotocoagulative laser, has been developed.[90] The laser spots stimulate outer retinal tissues, primarily RPE, to either increase production of metabolites that inhibit neovascularization such as pigment epithelium-derived factor or to downregulate mediators that increase vascular permeability and neovascularization.[91,92]

Currently, the therapeutic role of laser therapy in PDR and DME remains critical because it is able to improve or reverse the ischemic stress of diabetic retina. Most importantly, the efficacy of laser therapy is not only substantial but also sustainable. It is hoped that newer generations of subthreshold laser are developed for both PRP and macular laser, which are non- or less destructive, while keeping many of the benefits of conventional lasers.

Diabetic vitrectomy

Vitrectomy via pars plana (PPV) is an effective surgical technique for late stage of PDR and for posterior segment lesions. In 1970, Robert Machemer performed the first vitrectomy for a diabetic patient, creating the new era of surgical treatment for DR. His techniques are still the most commonly performed procedure in vitreoretinal surgery today. The purpose of PPV in patients with DR is to remove vitreous opacity, relieve vitreoretinal traction, restore the normal anatomical relationship of the neuroretina and RPE, and to access the subretinal space. The essential effect of diabetic vitrectomy itself, increasing retinal oxygenation, is the same as laser photocoagulation. It allows oxygen and other nutrients to be transported in water currents in the vitreous cavity from well oxygenated to ischemic areas of the retina. The improved retinal oxygenation can block hypoxia-induced VEGF signaling, thereby suppressing retinal neovascularization in PDR. A pilot study showed that PPV improves oxygen saturation in retinal veins but not in arteries.[93] A report from the same group further demonstrated that after vitrectomy, there is no increase in oxygen saturation but a slight decrease in vascular diameter (approximately 5%) in diabetic eyes in comparison to 2.5% among nondiabetic patients.[94] The reduced vascular diameter of the diabetic retina may be the consequence of the improved oxygenation of retinal tissues after vitrectomy. More studies are needed in this field for a comprehensive understanding. Diabetic vitrectomy also increases intraocular cytokine turnover and removes mechanical barriers to the egress of fluid and metabolites, as well as removing impediments to the intraretinal penetration of intravitreally administered medications.[95,96]

In the past 4 decades, diabetic vitrectomy has improved therapeutic results in several scenarios. These include nonclearing vitreous hemorrhage, tractional or tractional/rhegmatogenous retinal detachment (TRD/RRD) in PDR, and vitreoretinal interface abnormalities impeding macular edema resolution. In addition to the removal of the majority of the vitreous body along with the hyaloid membrane, PPV is particularly useful and effective in TRD/RRD in diabetic eyes. In this scenario, the current PPV is able to accomplish the following: removal any vitreous hemorrhage to gain visibility, alleviation of anterior—posterior traction, dissection and segmentation of fibrovascular proliferation (FVP) causing tangential traction, delamination of FVP with single or bimanual technique, peeling internal limiting membrane in selected cases, possible retinotomy/retinectomy, scleral buckling, endolaser treatment, using tamponade agents, intraoperative anti-VEGF agents, and steroid implants. Thus, PPV can provide access for various procedures targeting retinal and subretinal lesions such as laser photocoagulation, delivery of pharmacologic agents to the posterior segment, and other options in the vitrectomy armamentarium. The multimodal treatments via vitrectomy have made PPV a powerful surgery for late stages of PDR and intractable DME.[93] The current diabetic vitrectomy is at a transitional stage because intrinsic limitations of human surgeons' perception and dexterity during surgery have been realized. The future perspectives for vitrectomy will be discussed in Chapter 9.

References

1. WHO. *About Diabetes*. World Health Organization; 2021. Retrieved April 4, 2021. *Newsletter*. Accessed April 15, 2021.
2. Tao Z, Shi A, Zhao J. Epidemiological perspectives of diabetes. *Cell Biochem Biophys*. 2015;73(1):181−185. https://doi.org/10.1007/s12013-015-0598-4.
3. American Diabetes Association. Diagnosis and classification of diabetes mellitus. *Diabetes Care*. 2013;36(Suppl 1):S67−S74. https://doi.org/10.2337/dc13-S067.
4. Maahs DM, West NA, Lawrence JM, Mayer-Davis EJ. Epidemiology of type 1 diabetes. *Endocrinol Metab Clin N Am*. 2010;39(3):481−497. https://doi.org/10.1016/j.ecl.2010.05.011.
5. Chatterjee S, Khunti K, Davies MJ. Type 2 diabetes. *Lancet*. 2017;389(10085):2239−2251. https://doi.org/10.1016/S0140-6736(17)30058-2.
6. Teo ZL, Tham YC, Yu M, et al. Global prevalence of diabetic retinopathy and projection of burden through 2045: systematic review and meta-analysis. *Ophthalmology*. 2021;128(11):1580−1591. https://doi.org/10.1016/j.ophtha.2021.04.027.
7. Schneider ALC, Kalyani RR, Golden S, et al. Diabetes and prediabetes and risk of hospitalization: the atherosclerosis risk in communities (ARIC) study. *Diabetes Care*. 2016;39(5):772−779. https://doi.org/10.2337/dc15-1335.
8. Forbes A. Reducing the burden of mortality in older people with diabetes: a review of current research. *Front Endocrinol*. 2020;11:133. https://doi.org/10.3389/fendo.2020.00133.
9. Magliano DJ, Sacre JW, Harding JL, Gregg EW, Zimmet PZ, Shaw JE. Young-onset type 2 diabetes mellitus—implications for morbidity and mortality. *Nat Rev Endocrinol*. 2020;16(6):321−331. https://doi.org/10.1038/s41574-020-0334-z.
10. Yau JWY, Rogers SL, Kawasaki R, et al. Global prevalence and major risk factors of diabetic retinopathy. *Diabetes Care*. 2012;35(3):556−564. https://doi.org/10.2337/dc11-1909.
11. Klein R, Klein BE, Moss SE, Davis MD, DeMets DL. The Wisconsin epidemiologic study of diabetic retinopathy. III. Prevalence and risk of diabetic retinopathy when age at diagnosis is 30 or more years. *Arch Ophthalmol*. 1984;102(4):527−532. https://doi.org/10.1001/archopht.1984.01040030405011.
12. Zhang X, Saaddine JB, Chou CF, et al. Prevalence of diabetic retinopathy in the United States, 2005−2008. *JAMA*. 2010;304(6):649−656. https://doi.org/10.1001/jama.2010.1111.
13. Kempen JH, O'Colmain BJ, Leske MC, et al. The prevalence of diabetic retinopathy among adults in the United States. *Arch Ophthalmol*. 2004;122(4):552−563. https://doi.org/10.1001/archopht.122.4.552.
14. Klein R, Sharrett AR, Klein BEK, et al. The association of atherosclerosis, vascular risk factors, and retinopathy in adults with diabetes: the atherosclerosis risk in communities study. *Ophthalmology*. 2002;109(7):1225−1234. https://doi.org/10.1016/s0161-6420(02)01074-6.
15. Harris MI, Klein R, Cowie CC, Rowland M, Byrd-Holt DD. Is the risk of diabetic retinopathy greater in non-Hispanic blacks and Mexican Americans than in non-Hispanic whites with type 2 diabetes? A U.S. population study. *Diabetes Care*. 1998;21(8):1230−1235. https://doi.org/10.2337/diacare.21.8.1230.

16. Haffner SM, Hazuda HP, Stern MP, Patterson JK, Van Heuven WA, Fong D. Effects of socioeconomic status on hyperglycemia and retinopathy levels in Mexican Americans with NIDDM. *Diabetes Care*. 1989;12(2):128−134. https://doi.org/10.2337/diacare.12.2.128.

17. 李维业, 黎晓新, 徐国彤. 糖尿病视网膜病变 = *Diabetic Retinopathy*. 人民卫生出版社; 2018.

18. Liu DP, Molyneaux L, Chua E, et al. Retinopathy in a Chinese population with type 2 diabetes: factors affecting the presence of this complication at diagnosis of diabetes. *Diabetes Res Clin Pract*. 2002;56(2):125−131. https://doi.org/10.1016/S0168-8227(01)00349-7.

19. Wong TY, Klein R, Islam FMA, et al. Diabetic retinopathy in a multi-ethnic cohort in the United States. *Am J Ophthalmol*. 2006;141(3):446−455.e1. https://doi.org/10.1016/j.ajo.2005.08.063.

20. Sivaprasad S, Gupta B, Crosby-Nwaobi R, Evans J. Prevalence of diabetic retinopathy in various ethnic groups: a worldwide perspective. *Surv Ophthalmol*. 2012;57(4):347−370. https://doi.org/10.1016/j.survophthal.2012.01.004.

21. Zhang X, Saaddine JB, Lee PP, et al. Eye care in the United States: do we deliver to high-risk people who can benefit most from it? *Arch Ophthalmol*. 2007;125(3):411−418. https://doi.org/10.1001/archopht.125.3.411.

22. Shi Q, Zhao Y, Fonseca V, Krousel-Wood M, Shi L. Racial disparity of eye examinations among the U.S. Working-age population with diabetes: 2002−2009. *Diabetes Care*. 2014;37(5):1321−1328. https://doi.org/10.2337/dc13-1038.

23. Chiang PPC, Lamoureux EL, Cheung CY, et al. Racial differences in the prevalence of diabetes but not diabetic retinopathy in a multi-ethnic Asian population. *Invest Ophthalmol Vis Sci*. 2011;52(10):7586. https://doi.org/10.1167/iovs.11-7698.

24. Vujosevic S, Aldington SJ, Silva P, et al. Screening for diabetic retinopathy: new perspectives and challenges. *Lancet Diabetes Endocrinol*. 2020;8(4):337−347. https://doi.org/10.1016/S2213-8587(19)30411-5.

25. Wong TY, Mwamburi M, Klein R, et al. Rates of progression in diabetic retinopathy during different time periods: a systematic review and meta-analysis. *Diabetes Care*. 2009;32(12):2307−2313. https://doi.org/10.2337/dc09-0615.

26. Flaxman SR, Bourne RRA, Resnikoff S, et al. Global causes of blindness and distance vision impairment 1990−2020: a systematic review and meta-analysis. *Lancet Glob Health*. 2017;5(12):e1221−e1234. https://doi.org/10.1016/S2214-109X(17)30393-5.

27. Laakso M, Kuusisto J. Insulin resistance and hyperglycaemia in cardiovascular disease development. *Nat Rev Endocrinol*. 2014;10(5):293−302. https://doi.org/10.1038/nrendo.2014.29.

28. Sabanayagam C, Yip W, Ting DSW, Tan G, Wong TY. Ten emerging trends in the epidemiology of diabetic retinopathy. *Ophthalmic Epidemiol*. 2016;23(4):209−222. https://doi.org/10.1080/09286586.2016.1193618.

29. Klein R, Lee KE, Knudtson MD, Gangnon RE, Klein BEK. Changes in visual impairment prevalence by period of diagnosis of diabetes: the Wisconsin epidemiologic study of diabetic retinopathy. *Ophthalmology*. 2009;116(10):1937−1942. https://doi.org/10.1016/j.ophtha.2009.03.012.

30. Tan GS, Cheung N, Simó R, Cheung GCM, Wong TY. Diabetic macular oedema. *Lancet Diabetes Endocrinol*. 2017;5(2):143−155. https://doi.org/10.1016/S2213-8587(16)30052-3.

31. Klein R, Klein BE, Moss SE. Epidemiology of proliferative diabetic retinopathy. *Diabetes Care*. 1992;15(12):1875−1891. https://doi.org/10.2337/diacare.15.12.1875.
32. Zander E, Herfurth S, Bohl B, et al. Maculopathy in patients with diabetes mellitus type 1 and type 2: associations with risk factors. *Br J Ophthalmol*. 2000;84(8):871−876. https://doi.org/10.1136/bjo.84.8.871.
33. Browning DJ, Stewart MW, Lee C. Diabetic macular edema: evidence-based management. *Indian J Ophthalmol*. 2018;66(12):1736−1750. https://doi.org/10.4103/ijo.IJO_1240_18.
34. Browning DJ, Fraser CM, Clark S. The relationship of macular thickness to clinically graded diabetic retinopathy severity in eyes without clinically detected diabetic macular edema. *Ophthalmology*. 2008;115(3):533−539.e2. https://doi.org/10.1016/j.ophtha.2007.06.042.
35. Klein R, Knudtson MD, Lee KE, Gangnon R, Klein BEK. The Wisconsin epidemiologic study of diabetic retinopathy: XXII the twenty-five-year progression of retinopathy in persons with type 1 diabetes. *Ophthalmology*. 2008;115(11):1859−1868. https://doi.org/10.1016/j.ophtha.2008.08.023.
36. Photocoagulation for diabetic macular edema. Early treatment diabetic retinopathy study report number 1. Early treatment diabetic retinopathy study research group. *Arch Ophthalmol*. 1985;103(12):1796−1806.
37. Daruich A, Matet A, Moulin A, et al. Mechanisms of macular edema: beyond the surface. *Prog Retin Eye Res*. 2018;63:20−68. https://doi.org/10.1016/j.preteyeres.2017.10.006.
38. Urias EA, Urias GA, Monickaraj F, McGuire P, Das A. Novel therapeutic targets in diabetic macular edema: beyond VEGF. *Vision Res*. 2017;139:221−227. https://doi.org/10.1016/j.visres.2017.06.015.
39. Early Treatment Diabetic Retinopathy Study Research Group. Grading diabetic retinopathy from stereoscopic color fundus photographs—an extension of the modified Airlie House classification. ETDRS report number 10. *Ophthalmology*. 1991;98(5 Suppl):786−806.
40. Solomon SD, Chew E, Duh EJ, et al. Diabetic retinopathy: a position statement by the American diabetes association. *Diabetes Care*. 2017;40(3):412−418. https://doi.org/10.2337/dc16-2641.
41. American Association of Ophthalmology. Retina and vitreous. In: *Basic and Clinical Science Course*. 2019.
42. Lange J, Hadziahmetovic M, Zhang J, Li W. Region-specific ischemia, neovascularization and macular oedema in treatment-naïve proliferative diabetic retinopathy. *Clin Exp Ophthalmol*. 2018;46(7):757−766. https://doi.org/10.1111/ceo.13168.
43. Duh EJ, Sun JK, Stitt AW. Diabetic retinopathy: current understanding, mechanisms, and treatment strategies. *JCI Insight*. 2017;2(14). https://doi.org/10.1172/jci.insight.93751.
44. Diabetes Control and Complications Trial Research Group, Nathan DM, Genuth S, et al. The effect of intensive treatment of diabetes on the development and progression of long-term complications in insulin-dependent diabetes mellitus. *N Engl J Med*. 1993;329(14):977−986. https://doi.org/10.1056/NEJM199309303291401.
45. UK Prospective Diabetes Study (UKPDS) Group. Intensive blood-glucose control with sulphonylureas or insulin compared with conventional treatment and risk of complications in patients with type 2 diabetes (UKPDS 33). *Lancet*. 1998;352(9131):837−853.
46. Bain SC, Klufas MA, Ho A, Matthews DR. Worsening of diabetic retinopathy with rapid improvement in systemic glucose control: a review. *Diabetes Obes Metabol*. 2019;21(3):454−466. https://doi.org/10.1111/dom.13538.

47. Feldman-Billard S, Larger É, Massin P. Standards for screening and surveillance of ocular complications in people with diabetes SFD study group. Early worsening of diabetic retinopathy after rapid improvement of blood glucose control in patients with diabetes. *Diabetes Metab.* 2018;44(1):4—14. https://doi.org/10.1016/j.diabet.2017.10.014.

48. UK Prospective Diabetes Study Group. Tight blood pressure control and risk of macrovascular and microvascular complications in type 2 diabetes: UKPDS 38. *BMJ.* 1998;317(7160):703—713.

49. ACCORD Study Group, ACCORD Eye Study Group, Chew EY, et al. Effects of medical therapies on retinopathy progression in type 2 diabetes. *N Engl J Med.* 2010;363(3):233—244. https://doi.org/10.1056/NEJMoa1001288.

50. Kuo JZ, Wong TY, Rotter JI. Challenges in elucidating the genetics of diabetic retinopathy. *JAMA Ophthalmol.* 2014;132(1):96—107. https://doi.org/10.1001/jamaophthalmol.2013.5024.

51. Billings LK, Florez JC. The genetics of type 2 diabetes: what have we learned from GWAS? *Ann N Y Acad Sci.* 2010;1212:59—77. https://doi.org/10.1111/j.1749-6632.2010.05838.x.

52. Han J, Lando L, Skowronska-Krawczyk D, Chao DL. Genetics of diabetic retinopathy. *Curr Diabetes Rep.* 2019;19(9):67. https://doi.org/10.1007/s11892-019-1186-6.

53. Funatsu H, Yamashita H, Sakata K, et al. Vitreous levels of vascular endothelial growth factor and intercellular adhesion molecule 1 are related to diabetic macular edema. *Ophthalmology.* 2005;112(5):806—816. https://doi.org/10.1016/j.ophtha.2004.11.045.

54. Brown DM, Nguyen QD, Marcus DM, et al. Long-term outcomes of ranibizumab therapy for diabetic macular edema: the 36-month results from two phase III trials: RISE and RIDE. *Ophthalmology.* 2013;120(10):2013—2022. https://doi.org/10.1016/j.ophtha.2013.02.034.

55. Boyer DS, Nguyen QD, Brown DM, Basu K, Ehrlich JS, RIDE and RISE Research Group. Outcomes with as-needed ranibizumab after initial monthly therapy: long-term outcomes of the phase III RIDE and RISE trials. *Ophthalmology.* 2015;122(12):2504—2513.e1. https://doi.org/10.1016/j.ophtha.2015.08.006.

56. Elman MJ, Ayala A, Bressler NM, et al. Intravitreal ranibizumab for diabetic macular edema with prompt versus deferred laser treatment: 5-year randomized trial results. *Ophthalmology.* 2015;122(2):375—381. https://doi.org/10.1016/j.ophtha.2014.08.047.

57. Rosenfeld PJ, Fung AE, Puliafito CA. Optical coherence tomography findings after an intravitreal injection of bevacizumab (avastin) for macular edema from central retinal vein occlusion. *Ophthalmic Surg Laser Imag.* 2005;36(4):336—339.

58. Rajendram R, Fraser-Bell S, Kaines A, et al. A 2-year prospective randomized controlled trial of intravitreal bevacizumab or laser therapy (BOLT) in the management of diabetic macular edema: 24-month data: report 3. *Arch Ophthalmol.* 2012;130(8):972—979. https://doi.org/10.1001/archophthalmol.2012.393.

59. Jennifer IL. Intravitreal aflibercept injection for nonproliferative diabetic retinopathy: year 2 results from the PANORAMA study. In: *ARVO Meeting Abstract.* 2020.

60. Diabetic Retinopathy Clinical Research Network, Wells JA, Glassman AR, et al. Aflibercept, bevacizumab, or ranibizumab for diabetic macular edema. *N Engl J Med.* 2015;372(13):1193—1203. https://doi.org/10.1056/NEJMoa1414264.

61. Wells JA, Glassman AR, Ayala AR, et al. Aflibercept, bevacizumab, or ranibizumab for diabetic macular edema: two-year results from a comparative effectiveness randomized

clinical trial. *Ophthalmology.* 2016;123(6):1351−1359. https://doi.org/10.1016/j.ophtha.2016.02.022.

62. Vaziri K, Schwartz SG, Relhan N, Kishor KS, Flynn HW. New therapeutic approaches in diabetic retinopathy. *Rev Diabet Stud.* 2015;12(1−2):196−210. https://doi.org/10.1900/RDS.2015.12.196.

63. Jampol LM, Bressler NM, Glassman AR. Revolution to a new standard treatment of diabetic macular edema. *JAMA.* 2014;311(22):2269−2270. https://doi.org/10.1001/jama.2014.2536.

64. Bressler SB. Factors associated with changes in visual acuity and central subfield thickness at 1 year after treatment for diabetic macular edema with ranibizumab. *Arch Ophthalmol.* 2012;130(9):1153. https://doi.org/10.1001/archophthalmol.2012.1107.

65. Miller K, Fortun JA. Diabetic macular edema: current understanding, pharmacologic treatment options, and developing therapies. *Asia Pac J Ophthalmol (Phila).* 2018;7(1):28−35. https://doi.org/10.22608/APO.2017529.

66. Gross JG, Glassman AR, Liu D, et al. Five-year outcomes of panretinal photocoagulation vs intravitreous ranibizumab for proliferative diabetic retinopathy: a randomized clinical trial. *JAMA Ophthalmol.* 2018;136(10):1138. https://doi.org/10.1001/jamaophthalmol.2018.3255.

67. Glassman AR. Results of a randomized clinical trial of aflibercept vs panretinal photocoagulation for proliferative diabetic retinopathy: is it time to retire your laser? *JAMA Ophthalmol.* 2017;135(7):685. https://doi.org/10.1001/jamaophthalmol.2017.1652.

68. Maturi RK, Glassman AR, Josic K, et al. Effect of intravitreous anti-vascular endothelial growth factor vs sham treatment for prevention of vision-threatening complications of diabetic retinopathy: the Protocol W randomized clinical trial. *JAMA Ophthalmol.* 2021;30. https://doi.org/10.1001/jamaophthalmol.2021.0606. Published online March.

69. Wilkinson CP, Ferris FL, Klein RE, et al. Proposed international clinical diabetic retinopathy and diabetic macular edema disease severity scales. *Ophthalmology.* 2003;110(9):1677−1682. https://doi.org/10.1016/S0161-6420(03)00475-5.

70. Sun JK, Jampol LM. The diabetic retinopathy clinical research Network (DRCR.net) and its contributions to the treatment of diabetic retinopathy. *Ophthalmic Res.* 2019;62(4):225−230. https://doi.org/10.1159/000502779.

71. Cunha-Vaz J. Diabetic macular edema. *Eur J Ophthalmol.* 1998;8(3):127−130.

72. Omri S, Behar-Cohen F, de Kozak Y, et al. Microglia/macrophages migrate through retinal epithelium barrier by a transcellular route in diabetic retinopathy: role of PKCζ in the Goto Kakizaki rat model. *Am J Pathol.* 2011;179(2):942−953. https://doi.org/10.1016/j.ajpath.2011.04.018.

73. Romero-Aroca P, Baget-Bernaldiz M, Pareja-Rios A, Lopez-Galvez M, Navarro-Gil R, Verges R. Diabetic macular edema pathophysiology: vasogenic versus inflammatory. *J Diabetes Res.* 2016;2016:2156273. https://doi.org/10.1155/2016/2156273.

74. Reichenbach A, Wurm A, Pannicke T, Iandiev I, Wiedemann P, Bringmann A. Müller cells as players in retinal degeneration and edema. *Graefes Arch Clin Exp Ophthalmol.* 2007;245(5):627−636. https://doi.org/10.1007/s00417-006-0516-y.

75. Michinaga S, Koyama Y. Pathogenesis of brain edema and investigation into anti-edema drugs. *Int J Mol Sci.* 2015;16(5):9949−9975. https://doi.org/10.3390/ijms16059949.

76. Raffaele N, Marchese A, Ghigo D. Compared antioxidant activity among corticosteroids on cultured retinal pigment epithelial cells. *Graefes Arch Clin Exp Ophthalmol.* 2016;254(12):2411−2416. https://doi.org/10.1007/s00417-016-3519-3.

77. Marquioni-Ramella MD, Cubilla MA, Bermúdez V, Tate PS, Marazita MC, Suburo AM. Glucocorticoid and progesterone mechanisms in photoreceptor survival. *Exp Eye Res.* 2020;190:107854. https://doi.org/10.1016/j.exer.2019.107854.

78. Ghaseminejad F, Kaplan L, Pfaller AM, Hauck SM, Grosche A. The role of Müller cell glucocorticoid signaling in diabetic retinopathy. *Graefes Arch Clin Exp Ophthalmol.* 2020;258(2):221−230. https://doi.org/10.1007/s00417-019-04521-w.

79. Diabetic Retinopathy Clinical Research Network, Elman MJ, Aiello LP, et al. Randomized trial evaluating ranibizumab plus prompt or deferred laser or triamcinolone plus prompt laser for diabetic macular edema. *Ophthalmology.* 2010;117(6):1064−1077.e35. https://doi.org/10.1016/j.ophtha.2010.02.031.

80. Boyer DS, Yoon YH, Belfort R, et al. Three-year, randomized, sham-controlled trial of dexamethasone intravitreal implant in patients with diabetic macular edema. *Ophthalmology.* 2014;121(10):1904−1914. https://doi.org/10.1016/j.ophtha.2014.04.024.

81. Campochiaro PA, Brown DM, Pearson A, et al. Long-term benefit of sustained-delivery fluocinolone acetonide vitreous inserts for diabetic macular edema. *Ophthalmology.* 2011;118(4):626−635.e2. https://doi.org/10.1016/j.ophtha.2010.12.028.

82. Cheung N, Mitchell P, Wong TY. Diabetic retinopathy. *Lancet.* 2010;376(9735):124−136. https://doi.org/10.1016/S0140-6736(09)62124-3.

83. Aiello LP. Angiogenic pathways in diabetic retinopathy. *N Engl J Med.* 2005;353(8):839−841. https://doi.org/10.1056/NEJMe058142.

84. The Diabetic Retinopathy Study Research Group. Photocoagulation treatment of proliferative diabetic retinopathy. Clinical application of diabetic retinopathy study (DRS) findings, DRS report number 8. *Ophthalmology.* 1981;88(7):583−600.

85. Early Treatment Diabetic Retinopathy Study Research Group. Focal photocoagulation treatment of diabetic macular edema. Relationship of treatment effect to fluorescein angiographic and other retinal characteristics at baseline: ETDRS report no. 19. *Arch Ophthalmol.* 1995;113(9):1144−1155.

86. Bressler SB, Beaulieu WT, Glassman AR, et al. Photocoagulation versus ranibizumab for proliferative diabetic retinopathy: should baseline characteristics affect choice of treatment? *Retina.* 2019;39(9):1646−1654. https://doi.org/10.1097/IAE.0000000000002377.

87. Chatziralli I, Loewenstein A. Intravitreal anti-vascular endothelial growth factor agents for the treatment of diabetic retinopathy: a review of the literature. *Pharmaceutics.* 2021;13(8):1137. https://doi.org/10.3390/pharmaceutics13081137.

88. Diabetic Retinopathy Clinical Research Network. A randomized trial comparing intravitreal triamcinolone acetonide and focal/grid photocoagulation for diabetic macular edema. *Ophthalmology.* 2008;115(9):1447−1449. https://doi.org/10.1016/j.ophtha.2008.06.015, 1449.e1−10.

89. Comparison of the modified early treatment diabetic retinopathy study and mild macular grid laser photocoagulation strategies for diabetic macular edema. *Arch Ophthalmol.* 2007;125(4):469. https://doi.org/10.1001/archopht.125.4.469.

90. Mansour SE, Browning DJ, Wong K, Flynn HW, Bhavsar AR. The evolving treatment of diabetic retinopathy. *Clin Ophthalmol.* 2020;14:653−678. https://doi.org/10.2147/OPTH.S236637.

91. Akduman L, Olk RJ. Subthreshold (invisible) modified grid diode laser photocoagulation in diffuse diabetic macular edema (DDME). *Ophthalmic Surg Laser.* 1999;30(9):706−714.

92. Laursen ML, Moeller F, Sander B, Sjoelie AK. Subthreshold micropulse diode laser treatment in diabetic macular oedema. *Br J Ophthalmol.* 2004;88(9):1173−1179. https://doi.org/10.1136/bjo.2003.040949.

93. Sín M, Sínová I, Chrapek O, et al. The effect of pars plan vitrectomy on oxygen saturation in retinal vessels—a pilot study. *Acta Ophthalmol.* 2014;92(4):328−331. https://doi.org/10.1111/aos.12238.

94. Šín M, Chrapek O, Karhanová M, et al. The effect of pars plana vitrectomy and nuclear cataract on oxygen saturation in retinal vessels, diabetic and non-diabetic patients compared. *Acta Ophthalmol.* 2016;94(1):41−47. https://doi.org/10.1111/aos.12828.

95. Mason JO, Colagross CT, Vail R. Diabetic vitrectomy: risks, prognosis, future trends. *Curr Opin Ophthalmol.* 2006;17(3):281−285. https://doi.org/10.1097/01.icu.0000193098.28798.18.

96. Stefánsson E. The therapeutic effects of retinal laser treatment and vitrectomy. A theory based on oxygen and vascular physiology. *Acta Ophthalmol Scand.* 2001;79(5):435−440. https://doi.org/10.1034/j.1600-0420.2001.790502.x.

Diabetes-induced metabolic disorders of diabetic retinopathy

Hyperglycemia-induced metabolic pathways and therapeutic targets for diabetic retinopathy

The chronic hyperglycemia present in diabetes often activates multiple biochemical pathways. These pathways are interconnected and implicated in diabetic retinopathy (DR). They include the activation of the polyol pathway (Polyol), hexosamine biosynthetic pathway (HBP), and protein kinase C (PKC), increased advanced glycation end products (AGEs) formation, activation of renin−angiotensin−aldosterone system (RAAS), and low-grade inflammation, etc. These activated biochemical pathways cause increased oxidative stress and poly(ADP-ribose) polymerase (PARP) activation leading to disturbance of retinal tissues; therefore, these disturbed biochemical pathways and the resultant oxidative stress are potential targets in treating DR (Fig. 2.1).

The diverse hyperglycemia-induced biochemical events are interconnected. In other words, each abnormal pathway contributes to the activation of several other pathways. When acting together, these pathways give rise to increased levels of reactive oxygen species (ROS) and decreased levels of endogenous antioxidants, thus further aggravating oxidative stress. They also inhibit the activity of glyceraldehyde-3-phosphate dehydrogenase (GAPDH), which catalyzes the sixth step of glycolysis, breaking down glucose for energy and carbon molecules. Increased oxidative stress damages deoxyribonucleic acid (DNA), which activates the PARP family of nuclear enzymes. PARP enzymes, especially PARP-1, are involved in the DNA damage response, acting as a first responder by detecting DNA strand breaks and contributing to DNA repair. PARP activation depletes its own substrate, nicotinamide adenine dinucleotide (+) (NAD^+), slowing the rate of glycolysis, electron transport, and adenosine triphosphate (ATP) formation. Additionally, PARP inhibits GAPDH by direct poly(ADP-ribosy)lation of GAPDH using NAD^+. The inhibition of GAPDH blocks or slows glucose metabolisms through the glycolytic pathway, and thus further increases the flux of glucose into the biochemical pathways (Fig. 2.1). These biochemical disturbances affect all cellular components in the retinal neurovascular unit, resulting in neurodegeneration and microangiopathy in DR. Targeting the specific cells and molecules and normalizing the abnormal

Therapeutic Targets for Diabetic Retinopathy. https://doi.org/10.1016/B978-0-323-93064-2.00009-3

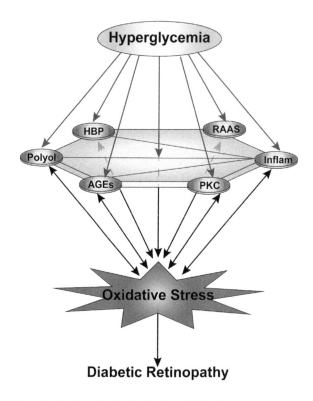

FIGURE 2.1

Hyperglycemia-induced biochemical perturbations include activation of the polyol pathway (Polyol), hexosamine biosynthetic pathway (HBP), advanced glycation end products (AGEs), protein kinase C (PKC) pathway, renin—angiotensin—aldosterone system (RAAS), and low-grade inflammation. The disturbed biochemical pathways increase oxidative stress and activate poly(ADP-ribose) polymerase (PARP), disrupting retinal neurovascular coupling and resulting in neurodegeneration, glial activation, and microangiopathy in diabetic retinopathy.

biochemical pathways have been proposed as the general strategy for treating DR. We discuss the link between hyperglycemia and hyperglycemia-induced pathogenicity of diabetic retina in the following sections.

Polyol pathway activation

Increased glucose flux to the polyol pathway plays a pivotal role in potential cellular toxicity of retinal tissues under hyperglycemic condition (Fig. 2.2).[1,2,3] The polyol pathway is a two-step metabolic pathway in which glucose is reduced to sorbitol, then converted to fructose. The rate-limiting enzyme for the polyol pathway is aldose reductase (AR, ALR2, EC 1.1.1.21), which converts the excess glucose to sorbitol, using the reduced form of nicotinamide adenine dinucleotide phosphate

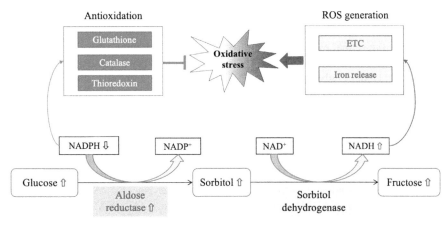

FIGURE 2.2

Aldose reductase (ALR) and the polyol pathway. Aldose reductase reduces glucose to sorbitol, using NADPH as a cofactor. Sorbitol is further converted to fructose by sorbitol dehydrogenase, using NAD$^+$ as a cofactor. The depletion of NADPH and NAD$^+$ results in oxidative stress. NADPH potentiates cellular antioxidation capability by acting as a substrate for glutathione reductase to reduce GSSG (oxidized form of glutathione) to GSH (reduced form of glutathione). GSH is required for the activities of glutathione peroxidase and glutathione-S-transferases. NADPH can also increase antioxidation capacity by activating catalase and promoting thioredoxin reductase mediated regeneration of thioredoxin. NADH can increase reactive oxygen species (ROS) generation by the electron transport chain (ETC) or by inducing iron release from ferritin. Thus, decreased NAPDH and increased NADH/NAD$^+$ decreases the antioxidant capacity of the retina, which eventually results in oxidative stress.

Modified from Kang and Yang[1] and Singh et al.[2]

(NADPH) as a cofactor. Sequentially, the sorbitol is further oxidized to fructose by sorbitol dehydrogenase. During hyperglycemia, sorbitol is formed more rapidly than it is converted to fructose due to the differing affinities and capacities of aldose reductase and sorbitol dehydrogenase. More importantly, the polarity of sorbitol hinders an easy penetration through membranes and subsequent removal from tissues by diffusion, resulting in accumulation of intracellular sorbitol and elevated intracellular osmolarity. The increased osmolarity in turn can lead to an influx of fluid and disruption of tissue osmotic homeostasis. Although fructose can be phosphorylated to fructose-6-phosphate and enter the glycolysis pathway, under chronic hyperglycemia, the glycolysis pathway is already saturated, thus the activated polyol pathway results in the increased production and accumulation of sorbitol. The polyol pathway consumes lots of cofactors, including NADPH and NAD$^+$ for sorbitol and fructose production. NADPH plays an important role in cellular antioxidation by promoting glutathione regeneration, activating catalase, and promoting generation of thioredoxin, while nicotinamide adenine diphosphate hydride (NADH) can increase ROS generation by the electron transport chain (ETC) or by inducing iron release from ferritin. Thus, the concurrent depletion of NADPH and the imbalance of the $NADH/NAD^+$ ratio via activation of the polyol pathway decrease the antioxidation capacity of the retina, eventually leading to increased oxidative stress (Fig. 2.2).

Normally, aldose reductase has a lower substrate affinity for glucose than does hexokinase. Under euglycemic conditions, glucose is preferentially phosphorylated with ATP by hexokinase in glycolytic pathway, thus the conversion of glucose to sorbitol by aldose reductase through the polyol pathway is nonsignificant. However, under hyperglycemic conditions, hexokinase is rapidly saturated and the polyol pathway becomes activated with a large production of intracellular sorbitol and fructose. Detrimental effects of the hyperglycemia-induced increase in glucose flux through the polyol pathway in DR could be explained by a number of mechanisms including sorbitol-induced osmotic stress, decreased Na^+-K^+ ATPase activity, decreased cytosolic NADPH, and increased cytosolic $NADH/NAD^+$. In DR, the increased amount and enhanced activity of aldose reductase lead to the overproduction of sorbitol and fructose through polyol pathway. Increased sorbitol leads to the osmotic stress on retinal cells. Excess sorbitol and fructose inside the retinal cells cause the apoptosis of endothelial cells, neurons, and astrocytes.[4,5] Further, excess fructose is phosphorylated to fructose-3-phosphate, which in turn is broken down to 3-deoxyglucosone, promoting the formation of AGEs. Fructose and its metabolites are almost 10 times more potent for nonenzymatic AGEs production than glucose. The increased glucose flux to the polyol pathway results in the depletion of cellular NADPH and also NAD^+ (Fig. 2.2), thus causing substantially decreased ratios of $NADPH/NADP^+$ and $NAD^+/NADH$. This induces a state of pseudohypoxia inside the cell, contributing to the onset of hyperglycemia-induced oxidative stress through the accumulation of ROS.[6,7] ROS, in turn, triggers the activation of a broad range of other major pathways (indicated in Fig. 2.1), including PKC, PARP, mitogen-activated protein kinases (MAPKs), and the inflammatory cascade. The depletion of cytosolic NADPH also affects the production of reduced glutathione and nitric oxide (NO), thereby resulting in antioxidant imbalance and causing oxidative stress, and further aggravating the polyol pathway. Besides the above biochemical alterations, genetic analysis shows that an aldose reductase gene polymorphism (*AKR1B1*) could play a role in the development of diabetic complications, producing decreased nerve function in an adolescent diabetic cohort after 7-year longitudinal follow-up.[8] In a separate metaanalysis, a genetic association was found between an aldose reductase polymorphism (*ALR* C106T) and the risk of DR of type 1 diabetes mellitus (DM) patients.[9]

Since aldose reductase is the rate-limiting enzyme of the polyol pathway, targeting aldose reductase represents an effective strategy to prevent or delay the progression and the severity of DR. The retinal ganglion cells (RGCs), Müller glia, pericytes, and endothelial cells abundantly express aldose reductase, and thus are the primary sites where the polyol pathway is involved in the pathogenesis of DR.[10] Aldose reductase (ALR2) is a small (36 kDa), cytosolic, monomeric enzyme, which belongs to the aldo-keto reductase (AKR) superfamily. It catalyzes the NADPH-dependent reduction of a wide variety of aldehydes to their corresponding alcohols, showing a broad substrate specificity. Another member of the AKR super-family is aldehyde reductase (ALR1, EC 1.1.1.2). ALR1 is present in all tissues and is responsible for the reduction of toxic aldehydes. ALR1 and ALR2 are similar in amino acid sequence and share structural homology. Approximately, 65% of the amino acid sequences are identical. The co-inhibition by these two enzymes may result in undesired side effects.[11] Thus, development of specific and selective aldose reductase inhibitors (ARIs) targeting ALR2, but not ALR1, is of great importance.

In rodent diabetic animal models, the ARIs sorbinil and beta-glucogallin can prevent DR progression. Diabetic mice with aldose reductase knockout were protected from diabetes-induced visual function loss.[12] To date, several ARIs have been studied in clinical trials, but none have received the United States Food and Drug Administration (FDA) approval. One of the main reasons is their poor selectivity for ALR2 over ALR1, which leads to toxic effects. For example, tolrestat and zopolrestat displayed severe liver toxicity, and sorbinil showed hypersensitivity reactions related to the presence of the hydantoin ring. A long-term trial demonstrated that sorbinil did not prevent the worsening of DR in spite it slightly slowed the progression rate of microaneurysm count.[13] Although an initial clinical trial using the ARI, epalrestat prevented the progression of diabetic complications, such as neuropathy, retinopathy, and nephropathy,[14] the results of a major follow-up clinical trial were disappointing.

In recent years, a number of ARIs have been developed from natural products and plant extracts or from synthetic molecules (carboxylic acid based—inhibitors and noncarboxylic acid based—inhibitors),[15] as well as indole-based bifunctional ARIs/antioxidants[16] that show a promising preclinical ability to address both diabetic complications and inflammatory diseases. Aldose reductase differential inhibitors (ARDIs) from synthetic origin may be able to target diabetic complications and inflammatory diseases while leaving unaltered the detoxifying role of the enzyme. ARDIs have the promising potential to overcome the existing limits of ARIs and minimize their side effects.

Increased accumulation of AGEs

AGEs have been implicated in the pathogenesis of various diseases, including diabetic complications, neurodegenerative disorders, inflammatory disorders, and age-related diseases. There is strong evidence linking AGEs accumulation in vivo to diabetes (Fig. 2.1). Glycation of biomacromolecules derived from exogenous or endogenous sources results in lifelong accumulation of AGEs in multiple tissues.[17] AGEs are formed by spontaneous posttranslational modification in which a carbonyl group on reducing sugars is covalently coupled to proteins, lipids, or nucleic acids. D-glucose per se is an aldehyde with carbonyl group that participates in such nonenzymatic glycosylation.[18] AGEs are a complex and heterogeneous group of compounds, which are the products of nonenzymatic glycoxidation and glycation of various biomolecules and sugar metabolites. In diabetes, pathways leading to the formation of AGEs largely involve sugars and glycolytic intermediates. Some of

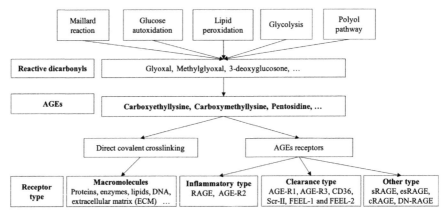

FIGURE 2.3

Production and accumulation of AGEs, their effects, and receptors. Endogenous glycation is produced by complex nonenzymatic reactions between glucose, ribose, fructose, amino acids, and lipids. Various biochemical pathways, including the Maillard reaction, glucose autoxidation, lipid peroxidation, glycolysis, polyol pathway, etc., lead to reactive dicarbonyl intermediates, such as glyoxal, methylglyoxal, and 3-deoxyglucosone. These reactive dicarbonyls result in the formation of AGEs, such as carboxyethyllysine, carboxymethyllysine, and pentosidine. AGEs exert their effects via two important mechanisms, that is, direct covalent crosslinking and interaction with their receptors. Abbreviations: AGEs, advanced glycation end products; AGE-R1/OST-48, oligosaccharyl transferase-48; AGE-R2, 80K-H phosphoprotein; AGE-R3, galectin-3; CD36, cluster of differentiation 36; cRAGE, proteolytic cleavage RAGE; DN-RAGE, dominant negative RAGE; esRAGE, endogenous secretory RAGE; FEEL-1/2, fasciclin, EGF-like, laminin-type EGF-like, and link domain-containing scavenger receptor-1/2; RAGEs, the receptor for advanced glycation end products; sRAGE, decoys soluble RAGE.

Modified from Ruiz et al.[19] and Sourris et al.[20]

the best chemically characterized AGEs are carboxyethyllysine (CEL), carboxyme-thyllysine (CML), and pentosidine (Fig. 2.3). Endogenous AGEs cause oxidative stress and activation of inflammatory signaling pathways via their specific receptors (Fig. 2.3). Studies have shown that AGEs are localized in retinal blood vessels in diabetic patients and correlate with the degree of retinopathy,[21] suggesting the contributory role of AGEs in the pathogenesis of DR (Fig. 2.1).

In diabetes-related complications and age-related diseases, AGEs gradually in-crease and accumulate inside the tissues, further increasing the glycation rate of long-lived proteins.[22] AGEs participate in diabetic disorders via two important mechanisms, that is, direct covalent crosslinking and interaction with receptors. AGEs can direct covalently crosslink serum proteins, enzymes, lipids, DNA, extra-cellular matrix (ECM) proteins, and alter their biological functions.[22,23] Glycation of proteins disrupts normal functions of proteins by altering molecular conformation and enzymatic activity, and interfering with receptor function. Chronic hyperglyce-mia induces structural and functional changes of many proteins, such as albumin, globulins, fibrinogen, collagens, etc. Glycation causes posttranslational crosslinking of elastin and ECM proteins decreasing viscoelasticity and resulting in stiffening of the skin and vascular systems.[24] Glycation of lens α-crystallin induces crosslinking of the water-soluble protein and contributes to reduction in lens transparency and increases in light scattering in diabetic cataracts.[25]

Furthermore, AGEs evoke intensive intracellular signaling cascades through binding to the receptor for advanced glycation end products (RAGE). RAGE, an immunoglobulin-family transmembrane protein, is the most-studied AGEs−receptor interaction, which is commonly referred to as the AGEs−RAGE axis. RAGE is a pattern-recognizing multiligand receptor with different isoforms expressed in tissues, including brain and retina, and in different types of cells including endothelial cells, pericytes, RPE cells, astrocytes, macrophages/monocytes, neutrophils, and lymphocytes.[26] Besides RAGE, many other AGEs receptors are generally identified as either inflammatory (RAGE and AGE-R2) or clearance type receptors (AGE-R1, AGE-R3, CD36, Scr-II, FEEL-1, and FEEL-2).[20] Due to the structural specificity of the RAGE V domain, not all AGEs possess the same affinity for RAGE.[27] For example, methylglyoxal-derived AGEs have strong affinity for RAGE,[28] while CML-modified proteins are unable to bind to RAGE to activate inflammatory signaling pathways (Fig. 2.3).[29] In addition to binding AGEs, RAGE also binds to other extracellular ligands such as high mobility group box 1, the S100 family of calcium-binding proteins, beta-amyloid peptides, etc.

In vivo, exogenous and endogenous AGEs are partially detoxified by glyoxalase-1 (Glo-1) before interacting with RAGE. Other AGE receptors are also involved in preventing AGEs from interacting with the complete RAGE receptor, thereby protecting cells from damage. These receptor isoforms include, but are not limited to, decoy receptors, soluble RAGE (sRAGE), endogenous secretory RAGE, proteolytic cleavage RAGE, dominant negative RAGE, etc. (Fig. 2.3), which are proteolytically cleaved from the complete transmembrane full-length RAGE or spliced from the RAGE gene.

Although many AGEs and different RAGE isoforms have been identified, AGEs−RAGE signaling is mostly investigated by using AGEs-modified albumin, CML, CEL, and pentosidine. The signaling events involved in the AGEs−RAGE axis are complex because of the diversity of RAGE ligands and their effects in different cell types. AGEs−RAGE signaling activation alters the intracellular signaling and gene expression. In DR, AGEs/RAGE-activated retinal cells release proinflammatory cytokines, proangiogenic factors, and free radicals, causing sustained inflammation, neurodegeneration, and retinal microvascular dysfunction. Molecular mechanisms of the interaction of AGEs with their receptors are fairly well defined from animal models. Recent studies highlight the role of AGEs as damage-associated molecular patterns, which trigger innate immunity defenses and sterile inflammation. Extracellular AGEs-activated RAGE signaling leads to the activation of its downstream signaling pathways, such as Ras/MAPK/NF-κB, JAK/STAT, and Rac1/Cdc42. The activation of the AGEs−RAGE signaling pathway promotes ROS production via NADPH oxidase (Nox) and increases the expression of proinflammatory cytokines (e.g., IL-6, TNF-α) and proangiogenic factors (e.g., VEGF-A, ICAM-1). Thus, in DR, the AGEs—RAGE signaling pathway activation leads to oxidative stress, inflammation, leukostasis, breakdown of the blood—retinal barrier (BRB), and angiogenesis.[30]

Both intracellular and extracellular formation of AGEs could produce detrimental events in DR since they alter protein biochemistry and distort their structures. Intracellular AGEs accumulation generated from glucose-derived dicarbonyl precursors plays important roles as stimuli in activating intracellular signaling pathways as well as modifying the function of intracellular proteins.[31] During diabetes, AGEs induce intracellular ROS production through mitochondrial dysfunction, activation of NADPH oxidases, or the redox crosstalk between these two ROS-producing mechanisms. Oxidative stress has also been shown to accelerate the formation of AGEs. Generation of ROS further induces endoplasmic reticulum stress through stimulation of the unfolded protein response, leading to cell apoptosis induced by CCAAT/enhancer-binding proteins homologous protein (CHOP). The modifications of AGEs on mitochondrial enzymes cause permanent dysfunction of the mitochondria, leading to "metabolic memory," a distinct phenomenon in diabetes.

AGEs are elevated in ocular tissues of patients with diabetes compared with patients without diabetes.[21] In patients with proliferative DR (PDR), the vitreous AGEs levels are significantly elevated in patients with uncontrolled hyperglycemia and are positively correlated with blood hemoglobin A_{1c} level.[32] AGEs accumulation in retinal pigment epithelial (RPE) cells impairs the ubiquitin proteolysis system, leading to accumulation of undigested photoreceptor outer segments, resulting in lipofuscin accumulation, an additional source of glyoxal and methylglyoxal.[33] In diabetes, the modification of skin collagen, such as collagen CML and pentosidine, is enhanced via the Maillard reaction.[34] In addition, ECM components are subject to modification by AGEs, resulting in reduced proliferation of pericytes, while increased proliferation of endothelial cells in vitro.[35] Glycation of ECM proteins is an important contributor to the thickening of basement membranes of vascular endothelial cells observed in diabetic complications.[36] The crosslinking of ECM proteins by AGEs increases vascular stiffness, altering vascular structure and function.[37] Inhibition of AGEs formation by pyridoxamine was reported to reduce capillary dropout and decrease CML level in the retinal vasculature of diabetic rats.[38]

Targeting the AGEs—RAGE signaling pathway to modulate the AGEs—RAGE axis might offer opportunities for the treatment of DR and age-related diseases. There are several pharmacological strategies to target the AGEs—RAGE axis, that is, (1) AGEs inhibitors to block the formation or effect of reactive precursors and/or AGEs; (2) AGEs crosslink breakers; and (3) RAGE antagonists.[17] A number of AGEs-lowering therapies, including direct targeting (e.g., aminoguanidine, benfotiamine, and pyridoxamine) or indirect targeting (metformin and aspirin) agents, have been tested in diabetes.[20] It has been found that AGEs inhibitors can only limit AGEs or AGEs crosslink formation, but fail to act on crosslinks already created due to lifelong exposure of long-lived proteins. The success of aminoguanidine was demonstrated in animal studies but not in clinical trials.[39] Clinical results showed unwanted adverse effects of aminoguanidine, resulting in cessation of further human clinical trials. Recent human clinical trials showed that AGEs inhibitors, such as quercetin and L-carnosine, reduce serum AGEs and/or their precursors. Other AGEs inhibitors, such as atorvastatin, hydroxytyrosol, coenzyme Q10, and myoinositol hexaphosphate, all demonstrated promising results in AGEs reduction.[17] The AGEs crosslink breakers are intended to reverse AGEs-induced crosslinking of long-lived proteins. But their real effects are unlikely to be the result of cleavage or reversal of existing crosslinks. They may have other effects on AGEs action, such as antioxidation and chelation, or their reaction with α-dicarbonyl intermediates.[40] Agents that split AGEs crosslinks in tissue proteins include thiazolium derivatives such as alagebrium and N-phenacylthiazolium bromide, and pyridinium derivatives such as TRC4149 and TRC4186. Despite some positive results reported for the AGEs crosslink breakers such as alagebrium, no strong evidence of beneficial effects was demonstrated in clinical studies.[39] RAGE antagonists include anti-RAGE antibodies, sRAGE, and RAGE inhibitors (e.g., azeliragon and TTP4000).[17,39] TTP4000 inactivates RAGE by causing the ligand to bind with itself instead of the receptor, while azeliragon blocks the ligand from binding to RAGE. A Phase I clinical trial for TTP4000 was completed in 2013, but results have not yet been released. A clinical trial of azeliragon for treating patients with Alzheimer's disease was discontinued due to the failure to demonstrate significant cognitive or functional improvements in a Phase III trial.

In other strategies, aspirin was shown to scavenge free carbonyl groups and decrease AGEs levels by targeting preformed intermediates via chelation of copper and other transition metals which can contribute to ROS production. Pyridoxamine prevents the formation of AGEs from Amadori intermediates and cleaves 3-deoxyglucosone reactive carbonyl intermediates. Glo-1 is a naturally occurring detoxicant which reduces α-dicarbonyl levels, especially methylglyoxal; overexpression of Glo-1 was associated with reduced methylglyoxal production and end-organ protection. Enzymatic detoxication by Glo-1 reduces oxidative stress. A combination of transresveratrol and hesperetin increased Glo-1 expression and improved metabolic and vascular health in overweight and obese human subjects in a Phase I clinical trial.[41] This effect was achieved via the activation of nuclear factor (erythroid-derived 2)-like 2 (Nrf2). Despite the efforts of laborious clinical trials, only metformin has successfully completed a Phase IV trial in intercepting the AGEs−RAGE axis. Metformin, an insulin-sensitizing antidiabetic drug, is found to reduce AGEs deposition by preventing DNA methylation, thereby ameliorating fundamental aging factors that underlie multiple age-related conditions.[17] The drug successfully completed Phase IV of the Metformin in Longevity Study (MILES) clinical trial in May 2018 (NCT02432287). The results suggested that metformin is associated with improvement in learning/memory and attention. In one randomized clinical trial, metformin was as effective as pioglitazone in reducing AGEs accumulation in type 2 diabetic patients.[42] The modulation of the AGEs−RAGE axis as a means of delaying or preventing the progression of DR should be investigated further.

Hexosamine biosynthetic pathway activation

Hyperglycemia has been shown to increase flux through HBP resulting in glucose metabolism-related toxic effects. HBP is a relatively minor branch of glycolysis in which fructose-6-phosphate is converted to glucosamine-6-phosphate (Fig. 2.4). The major endpoint of the HBP is the formation of uridine 5′-diphospho-N-acetyl-D-glucosamine (UDP-GlcNAc), the donor for protein O-linked-N-acetylglucosaminylation (O-GlcNAcylation) and complex extracellular glycosylation.

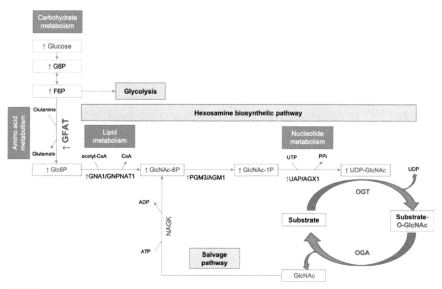

FIGURE 2.4

The complexity of the hexosamine biosynthetic pathway (HBP). Increased glucose is rapidly phosphorylated to G6P (glucose-6-phosphate) and undergoes conversion to F6P (fructose-6-phosphate). F6P is converted to Glc6P (glucosamine-6-phosphate) by the enzyme GFAT (glutamine:fructose-6-phosphate amidotransferase), utilizing glutamine that is involved in amino acid metabolism. GNA1/GNPNAT1 (glucosamine-6-phosphate N-acetyltransferase) converts Glc6P into GlcNAc-6P (N-acetyl-glucosamine-6-Phosphate), also utilizing acetyl-CoA that is made from fatty acid metabolism. This is then converted to GlcNAc-1P (N-acetylglucosamine 1-phosphate) by PGM3/AGM1 (phosphoglucomutase) and further to UDP-GlcNAc (uridine 5′-diphospho-N-acetyl-D-glucosamine) by UAP/AGX1 (UDP-N-acetylhexosamine pyrophosphorylase), utilizing UTP from the nucleotide metabolism pathway. O-GlcNAc transferase (OGT) catalyzes the transfer of GlcNAc moiety onto the serine or threonine site on the protein substrates, while O-GlcNAcase (OGA) is able to remove the GlcNAc. Free GlcNAc removed by OGA can reenter the HBP via the salvage pathway, in which GlcNAc is converted into GlcNAc-6P by N-acetylglucosamine kinase (GlcNAc kinase, NAGK). The biosynthesis of UDP-GlcNAc in HBP requires precursors from almost every metabolic pathway including amino acid metabolism, fatty acid metabolism, nucleotide metabolism, and carbohydrate metabolism.

Modified from Gurel and Sheibani[43] and Campbell et al.[44]

UDP-GlcNAc serves as a precursor for the synthesis of glycoproteins, glycolipids, and proteoglycans. HBP integrates four metabolic pathways, that is, carbohydrate (glucose), amino acid (glutamine), lipid (Acetyl-CoA), and nucleotide (UTP) (Fig. 2.4). Normally, glucose becomes fructose-6-phosphate through the initial two steps shared by the HBP and glycolysis pathway. Only 2%−3% of fructose-6-phosphate enters the HBP. Glutamine:fructose-6-phosphate amidotransferase (GFAT) is the key enzyme in the hexosamine pathway that produces UDP-GlcNAc, linking energy metabolism with posttranslational protein glycosylation (Fig. 2.4). During diabetes, chronic hyperglycemia increases glucose flux via HBP, thus increasing the production of UDP-GlcNAc, the donor substrate for O-GlcNAc transferase (OGT). Increased UDP-GlcNAc results in the increased O-GlcNAc modifications. Several studies demonstrated that O-GlcNAcylation is abnormally and globally increased in the cells and tissues of diabetic animals and humans, causing dysregulation of signaling cascades and transcription.[45]

The HBP is regulated by the first and rate-limiting enzyme, GFAT. Normally glucose is rapidly phosphorylated to glucose-6-phosphate, which is isomerized to fructose-6-phosphate during glycolysis after entering the cell. Chronic hyperglycemia leads to an enhanced influx through the HBP (Fig. 2.4). In HBP, fructose-6-phosphate is converted to N-acetylglucosamine-6-phosphate by GFAT. N-acetylglucosamine-6-phosphate is converted to N-acetylglucosamine-1, 6-phosphate, and UDP-GlcNAc. UDP-GlcNAc is then used for N-linked and O-linked glycosylation in the endoplasmic reticulum and Golgi and for O-GlcNAc modification of nuclear and cytoplasmic proteins. O-GlcNAcylation is a type of glycosylation, in which OGT catalyzes the transfer of the O-GlcNAc moiety onto serine or threonine sites on nuclear or cytoplasmic proteins and which can be reversibly removed by O-GlcNAcase (OGA) and returned to the HBP pool for recycling through the salvage pathway, where GlcNAc is converted into GlcNAc-6P by N-acetylglucosamine kinase (GlcNAc kinase, NAGK) (Fig. 2.4).[44,46]

Diabetes promotes the posttranslational modification of proteins by O-linked addition of GlcNAc (O-GlcNAcylation) to serine/threonine (Ser/Thr) residues of proteins and thereby contributes to diabetic complications. In vitro and in vivo studies revealed that the increased flux of glucose via the HBP has been implicated in insulin resistance, diabetic vascular complications, and stimulation of the synthesis of growth factors. Chronic hyperglycemia increases O-GlcNAcylation in diabetic retinal tissues.[45] The increased glucose flux via HBP may directly trigger retinal neurons to undergo apoptosis in a bimodal fashion,[47] that is, via altered glycosylation of proteins (increased UDP-N-acetylhexosamines) and via perturbation of the neuroprotective effect of insulin mediated by protein kinase B (also known as Akt). All of these biochemical events indicate that HBP is involved in retinal neurodegeneration in diabetes. Additionally, retinal pericytes exhibit increased O-GlcNAcylation in high blood glucose levels and manifest an increase in apoptosis and decrease in cell proliferation.[48] In an experimental mouse model, using click-it chemistry and liquid chromatography-mass spectrometry analysis, the increased O-GlcNAc modification of p53 was found, which may contribute to pericyte loss during diabetes.[48] Therefore, HBP is also involved in the development of retinal microangiopathy in diabetes. O-GlcNAcylation links the processes of nutrient sensing, metabolism, signal transduction, and transcription. O-GlcNAcylation has been shown to have major roles in nearly all aspects of transcription. Most RNA polymerase II transcription factors, as well as the catalytic subunit of RNA polymerase are extensively modified by O-GlcNAc. Specificity protein 1 (Sp1), a so-called housekeeping transcription factor that is dysfunctional in diabetes is highly O-GlcNAcylated.[45] O-GlcNAcylation of Sp1 has been shown to increase its stability, nuclear localization, and transcriptional activity and is thought to affect promoter specificity. For example, Sp1 has been implicated in diabetic nephropathy via the upregulation of transforming growth factor β1 (TGF-β1) and SERPINE1 (PAI-1). The VEGF-A promoter is also responsive to Sp1. The increased O-GlcNAcylation on Sp1 could directly increase binding to the VEGF-A promoter and upregulation of VEGF-A expression.[49]

Cumulative studies have indicated that O-GlcNAcylation affects the functions of protein substrates in a number of ways, including protein cellular localization, protein stability, and protein/protein interaction. Particularly, O-GlcNAcylation has been shown to have intricate crosstalk with phosphorylation as they both modify serine or threonine residues. Aberrant O-GlcNAcylation on various protein substrates has been implicated in many diseases, including neurodegenerative diseases, diabetes, and cancers.[45] The O-GlcNAc modification has been implicated in the etiology of microvascular complications and neurovascular dysfunction in DR. For example, O-GlcNAcylation of Forkhead box O1 (FoxO1), a transcription factor, upregulates the expression of angiopoietin-2 (Ang-2), which destabilizes blood vessels and initiates vascular regression. In streptozotocin-induced diabetic mice, O-GlcNAcylation of the p65 subunit of NF-κB has been shown to be responsible for hyperglycemia-induced activation of NF-κB and RGCs death, linking the involvement of imbalanced O-GlcNAc modification to the etiology of the microvascular abnormalities in DR. Increased protein O-GlcNAcylation was observed during mouse postnatal retinal vascularization and aging. This increase of protein O-GlcNAcylation was also found in the retinas of diabetic Ins2[Akita] mouse and in the retinas during the neovascularization phase of oxygen-induced mouse ischemic retinopathy. The migration of retinal pericytes, but not retinal endothelial cells, is attenuated by increased O-GlcNAc modification.[50] The increased O-GlcNAc modification under hyperglycemia and/or ischemia suggests its contribution to the pathogenesis of the DR and retinal neovascularization. In diabetic models, diabetes-induced O-GlcNAcylation alters the selection of mRNAs for translation and elevates 4E-BP1/2, a mitochondrial protein, thus promoting oxidative stress in retina.[51] O-GlcNAcylation enhances cellular respiration and promotes mitochondrial superoxide levels in cells, which is dependent on 4E-BP1/2. On the other hand, 4E-BP1/2 deletion prevents O-GlcNAcylation-induced mitochondrial superoxide in mouse embryonic fibroblasts and in mouse retinas.[51] A recent study showed that angiotensin-(1−7) inhibits retinal protein O-GlcNAcylation to protect retina from diabetic insults,[52] demonstrating the impact of the renin-angiotensin system on retinal protein O-GlcNAcylation. Angiotensin-(1−7) represses OGT activity by elevating production of cyclic AMP (cAMP), activating exchange protein activated by cAMP, and increasing GTP loading of the small GTPase Ras-associated protein 1 (Rap1). Therefore, angiotensin-(1−7) downregulates retinal protein O-GlcNAcylation. The regulation/inhibition of GFAT (GFAT) in the diabetic retina has been studied. Total levels of O-GlcNAc-modified proteins in retinal pericytes cultured with high glucose concentrations were decreased by addition of the GFAT inhibitor, deoxynorleucine.[50] Use of an inhibitor of OGT to decrease O-GlcNAc modification was unsatisfactory. A uridine analog, alloxan, was also used to inhibit OGT in cells,[53] producing nonspecific effects by interfering with many enzymes that utilize uridine nucleotides.[54] In addition, increased HBP activity decreases the $NADPH/NADP^+$ ratio due to the inhibition of glucose-6-phosphate dehydrogenase and induces oxidative stress by two mechanisms, that is, decreasing the bioavailability of GSH and decreasing the enzymatic activity of catalase.[55]

Overall, a translational gap remains between understanding of hyperglycemia-induced increase in flux through HBP and an efficacious strategy to regulate altered O-GlcNAc signaling in the development of diabetic complications.

PKC activation

Chronic hyperglycemia activates PKC isoforms (Figs. 2.1 and 2.5). Among the various PKC isoforms, the beta- and delta-isoforms appear to be activated preferentially in the vasculatures of diabetic animals, although other PKC isoforms are also

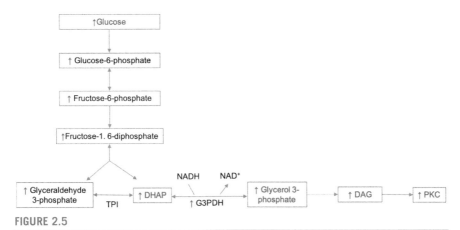

FIGURE 2.5

Activation of protein kinase C (PKC) pathway by hyperglycemia. Under hyperglycemic or diabetic conditions, diacylglycerol (DAG) level is elevated chronically due to an increase in the glycolytic intermediate dihydroxyacetone phosphate (DHAP). This intermediate is reduced to glycerol-3-phosphate by glycerol 3-phosphate dehydrogenase (G3PDH). Increased glycerol-3-phosphate subsequently increases de novo synthesis of DAG, which activates PKC. TPI: Triose-phosphate isomerase.

increased in the renal glomeruli and retina. PKC consists of a family of multifunctional serine/threonine kinases, which are involved in the control of protein functions. So far, at least 12 PKC isoforms have been identified and can be subdivided into three groups, that is, classical/conventional (PKC-α, $\beta1$, $\beta2$, and γ), novel (PKC-δ, -θ, -η, and -ε), and atypical (PKC-ζ and -ι/λ). The conventional PKCs are activated by phosphatidylserine, calcium, diacylglycerol (DAG), or phorbol esters. The novel PKCs are activated by phosphatidylserine, DAG, or phorbol 12-myristate 13-acetate (PMA), while the atypical PKCs (aPKCs) are not activated by either calcium, DAG, or PMA. The activation of PKC regulates various vascular functions by modulating enzymatic activities such as cytosolic phospholipase A2 and Na^+-K^+-ATPase. It also regulates gene expression including ECM components and contractile proteins. Among the various isoforms of PKC, the beta isoforms are predominantly activated in cultured vascular cells exposed to high glucose and in vascular tissues isolated from animal models of diabetes. Activation of PKC is associated with vascular alterations such as increases in permeability, contractility, ECM synthesis, cell growth and apoptosis, angiogenesis, leukocyte adhesion, and cytokine activation and inhibition. These perturbations in vascular cell homeostasis are caused by different PKC isoforms and are linked to the development of macrovascular and microvascular complications of diabetes.[56]

Hyperglycemia-induced PKC activation is closely associated with various pathophysiological processes, including retinal hemodynamics, endothelial permeability, the enhanced activation and adhesion of leukocytes (leukostasis), and expression of VEGF, etc.[57] Hyperglycemia activates the DAG-PKC pathway and then activates NADPH oxidase (Nox), resulting in increased ROS production, which is referred to the "dangerous metabolic route in diabetes."[58] Nox can promote ROS production in many vascular cells including endothelial cells, smooth muscle cells, and pericytes.[59] In DR, chronic hyperglycemia persistently elevates DAG, which activates its downstream classical PKCs (PKC-α, -$\beta1/2$, and PKC-δ), causing the damage and dysfunction of the neurovascular unit in retina. These activated PKCs affect the retinal vascular cells through regulation of vascular permeability, ECM production, cell growth, angiogenesis, increased cytokine production, as well as the leukocyte adhesions. Numerous studies have demonstrated the contribution of PKC activation in decreasing retinal blood flow. Activation of the PKC pathway could cause vasoconstriction and decrease retinal blood flow through increasing the expressions of endothelin A (ET-A) and VEGF. ET-A further aggravates the hypoxic conditions in the retina, whereas VEGF increases vascular permeability. ET-A and VEGF together cause breakdown of BRB and the formation of microaneurysms. In diabetic rats, intravitreal injection of an ET-A receptor antagonist prevents the decreased retinal blood flow and ameliorates the retinal hypoxia, further confirming the causal effect of ET-A in the pathogenesis of DR. PKCδ and p38 MAPK activation increase the expression of Src homology 2 domain-containing phosphatase-1 (SHP-1), a protein tyrosine phosphatase, which dephosphorylates the platelet-derived growth factor (PDGF) receptor β (PDGF-β) and induces pericyte apoptosis.[60] In addition, hyperglycemia activates PKC isoforms indirectly through the AGEs—RAGE signaling and polyol pathway by increasing ROS. In a recent study, the effects of hyperglycemia and oxidative stress on aldose reductase and PKC as well as the signaling molecules such as NF-κB, inhibitor kappa B-alpha (IkB-α), c-Jun, and stress-activated protein kinases/Jun amino-terminal kinases were evaluated in human retinal pigment epithelial cells-19 (ARPE-19).[61] The data showed that aldose reductase, PKC protein levels, and the related signaling molecules are increased under the conditions of hyperglycemia and oxidative stress. The ARI sorbinil decreases PKC expression and activity, while upregulation of aldose reductase expression increased PKC expression and activity. In other words, PKC activation is influenced by aldose reductase activity during diabetes. In experimental DR, both VEGF and TNF-α are required to induce changes in retinal vascular permeability and inflammation, while treatment with an aPKC inhibitor prevents VEGF/TNF-α-induced permeability.[62] In a genetically engineered mouse model, either a kinase-dead aPKC transgene was expressed or a small molecule inhibitor (ethyl 2-amino-4-(3,4-dimethoxyphenyl)-3-thiophenecarboxylate) for aPKC was used to establish a model of aPKC inhibition. Lin et al. demonstrated that PKC inhibition represses vascular permeability and retinal edema in ischemia/reperfusion injury and in VEGF/TNF-α—mediated BRB breakdown. Furthermore, aPKC inhibition decreased the retinal innate immune response to ischemia/reperfusion and reduced immune cell infiltration and inflammatory gene expression.[62] This study contributes to the mechanistic understanding of sterile inflammation-mediated vascular permeability and demonstrates that small-molecule aPKC inhibitors have therapeutic potential in inflammatory ocular disease.

Studies focusing on PKC agonists or antagonists have revealed decreased or increased retinal blood flow, respectively. Introduction of phorbol esters, an agonist of PKC into the retina, reduces retinal blood flow; this decreased blood flow can be reversed by PKC inhibitors. Natural products derived from plants, animals, microorganisms, and marine organisms have been used as medicine from prehistoric times. Recently, several compounds derived from plants have been found to modulate PKC activities through competitive binding with ATP and other allosteric regions of PKC.[63] The natural products and their derivatives including curcumin, rottlerin, quercetin, ellagic acid, epigallocatechin-3 gallate, ingenol 3 angelate, resveratrol, bryostatin, staurosporine, and midostaurin play regulatory roles in PKC activity during various diseases. However, extensive research is needed to circumvent the challenge of isoform specific regulation of PKC by natural products. In future studies, adopting selective inhibitors or regulator for different PKC isoforms might benefit the treatment of DR.

A recent study showed that the antiamyotrophic lateral sclerosis drug, riluzole, attenuates monocyte chemotactic protein-1 (MCP-1, also known as CCL-2) in cultured retinal pericytes as well as in diabetic rats via targeting PKCβ pathway. For instance, Ruboxistaurin, an oral PKCβ inhibitor, showed a potential use for the treatment of DR.[64] The efficacy of ruboxistaurin in reducing vision loss in patients with DR was demonstrated in the PKC DRS2 trial. Patients with diabetic macular edema appear to respond to ruboxistaurin with both anatomic and functional benefits. Although studies have indicated that the treatment of diabetic patients with ruboxistaurin may reduce vision loss in diabetic patients, the overall benefit seems to be small.[65]

Renin—angiotensin—aldosterone system activation

The RAAS is vital as it maintains plasma sodium concentration, arterial blood pressure, and extracellular volume (Fig. 2.6).[67] RAAS is characterized as a paracrine system and found to be present in many organs and tissues, including the eye,[68] brain, vessels, adrenal gland, etc. The classical RAAS begins with the synthesis of preprorenin in juxtaglomerular cells of the kidney, which is then cleaved to prorenin and released as either prorenin or renin. The precursor of renin (prorenin) is a 406 amino acid-long protein, which can be proteolytically activated in the kidney by neuroendocrine convertase 1 (proprotein convertase 1) or cathepsin B, and nonproteolytically activated in many tissues by the renin/prorenin receptor (PRR). Renin (angiotensinogenase), an enzyme with 340 amino acids, is also considered to be a hormone for its signaling roles. Renin hydrolyzes the liver-secreted α-2-globulin protein angiotensinogen (about 118 amino acid) to angiotensin I (Ang I), by acting on the bond between leucine and valine. Ang I further undergoes cleavage by the endothelial-bound angiotensin-converting enzyme (ACE, EC 3.5.15.1). The enzyme ACE, also known as kininase II, peptidyl-dipeptidase A, or CD143, is a carboxypeptidase, and it converts Ang I into angiotensin II (Ang II), by removing two C-terminal amino acids (Fig. 2.6).

RAAS is pivotal in regulating vascular pressure, as well as ionic and pH homeostasis[67] via its two main effectors, Ang II and aldosterone. Ang II acts upon two main receptors, the angiotensin type 1 receptor (AT1R) and the angiotensin type 2 receptor (AT2R). The engagement of Ang II with the AT1R results in vasoconstrictor and

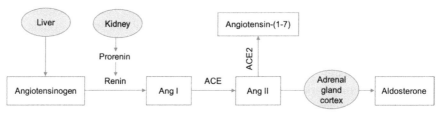

FIGURE 2.6

The renin—angiotensin—aldosterone system (RAAS). In RAAS, the precursor of renin (prorenin) is secreted by the kidney granular cells, which is processed to be the enzyme renin. Renin hydrolyzes the liver-secreted angiotensinogen to form angiotensin I (Ang I). Ang I further undergoes cleavage by angiotensin-converting enzyme (ACE) into angiotensin II (Ang II). Ang II stimulates the adrenal cortex to secrete aldosterone. Alternatively, Ang II can be further cleaved by an angiotensin-converting enzyme 2 (ACE2) into angiotensin-(1—7).

Modified from Wilkinson-Berka et al.[66]

pathological actions of Ang II. Furthermore, Ang II stimulates the release of aldosterone from zona glomerulosa cells of the adrenal glands. Aldosterone maintains sodium-potassium homeostasis by stimulating kidney proximal tubules to increase sodium reabsorption, hence, retaining sodium and losing potassium via the mineralocorticoid receptor (MR).

The RAAS also possesses a counterregulatory arm through the AT2R and Mas receptor (MasR). Binding of Ang II to AT2R has an opposing effect to AT1R, leading to vasodilation and decreasing fibrosis and inflammation. Ang II can be further cleaved by an ACE homologue (angiotensin-converting enzyme 2, ACE2) producing angiotensin-(1−7). Angiotensin-(1−7) acts on the AT2R and MasR to partially antagonize the effects of AT1R.[69] This protective ACE2/angiotensin-(1−7)/MasR axis may be upregulated during disease to reduce the availability and damaging actions of Ang II.[70] The components of RAAS exert their effects via binding to the corresponding receptors (in Table 2.1).

The negative impact of RAAS perturbation can be both local and systemic, as exemplified by DR and cardiovascular disease, respectively. Controlling this system is theoretically therapeutic for maintaining homeostasis of the body and treating organ-specific diseases. The components of RAAS, Ang II and aldosterone, are the two most powerful biologically active products of the RAAS (Fig. 2.6), exhibiting vasoconstriction, sodium retention, tissue remodeling, and proinflammatory and profibrotic effects.[71] There is considerable evidence that a local RAAS exists within the retina.[72] The components of RAAS are reported to be detected in various intraocular samples, including normal ocular tissues, and various human retinal cell lines such as RPE cells. In DR, RAAS was reported to increase vascular permeability causing BRB breakdown. Both Ang II and aldosterone influence vascular function

Table 2.1 The receptors, localization, ligand, and function in RAAS.

Receptors	Localization	Ligand	Function
PRR	Membrane	Prorenin, renin	Neovascularization, vascular leakage, inflammation
AT1R	Membrane	Ang II	Vasoconstriction, inflammation, neovascularization, vascular leakage, pericyte migration, endothelial degeneration, microaneurysm formation
AT2R	Membrane	Ang II, angiotensin-(1−7)	Antiangiogenesis, antiinflammation
MasR	Membrane	Angiotensin-(1−7)	Antiangiogenesis, antiinflammation
MR	Cytoplasm and nucleus	Aldosterone	Neovascularization, vascular leakage, inflammation

Abbreviations: Ang II, angiotensin II; AT1R, angiotensin type 1 receptor; AT2R, angiotensin type 2 receptor; MasR, Mas receptor; MR, mineralocorticoid receptor; PRR, prorenin receptor.
Modified from Wilkinson-Berka et al.[66]

and inflammation in DR, central serous chorioretinopathy, retinopathy of prematurity, and age-related macular degeneration.[66] The binding of prorenin to its receptor, the PRR, has been implicated in the pathogenesis of DR. PRR, also known as ATP6AP2, is shown to interact and colocalize with the β subunit of the pyruvate dehydrogenase (PDH) complex. Previous study showed that PDH activity is downregulated after knockdown of PRR, leading to suppression of glucose-induced ROS generation in RPE. Thus, PRR is considered pathogenic due to its role in RAAS activation and mitochondrial ROS generation. PRR can bind to both renin and prorenin. Therefore, blockade of PRR and other players of the RAAS system might inhibit a series of events vital for neurovascular abnormalities in DR. In DR, increased levels of PRR and Ang II have been detected in vitreous and fibrovascular tissues of patients with PDR, strengthening the evidence for the involvement of PRR in DR. Satofuka et al. investigated the receptor-associated prorenin system (RAPS), which dually activates tissue RAAS and RAAS-independent intracellular signaling. The results showed a significant contribution of RAPS to the pathogenesis of diabetes-induced retinal inflammation, suggesting the possibility of PRR as a novel molecular target for the treatment of DR.[73] Ang II promotes ROS production through Ang II/AT1R-Nox system leading to endothelial cell dysfunction.[74,75] A recent study using mouse models showed that Ang II induces endothelial dysfunction in ophthalmic arteries via AT1R activation and Nox2-dependent ROS formation.[76]

RAAS induces the production of VEGF through ERK1/2, leading to dysfunction of the BRB. Ang II is a potent vasoactive and angiogenic agent. Along with VEGF, Ang II has been reported to be upregulated in the vitreous of patients with PDR. The increase in VEGF and VEGFR-2 expression and an elevation of renin are indicative of the interaction of tissue RAAS and VEGF. Targeting RAAS with angiotensin-converting enzyme inhibitors (ACEIs) and angiotensin II receptor blocker (ARB) has demonstrated a therapeutic effect on DR. For example, ACEIs have been shown to have a beneficial effect on retinopathy development in patients with type 1 DM independent of their reduction in blood pressure. The Daily-Dose Consensus Interferon and Ribavirin: Efficacy of Combined Therapy trial provided evidence that RAAS inhibition is beneficial in DR.[77] EURODIAB Controlled Trial of Lisinopril in Insulin-Dependent Diabetes Mellitus study group reported that ACE inhibition results in a 50% reduction in risk of a one-step retinopathy progression in patients treated with lisinopril, suggesting a potential clinical role for the suppression of RAAS in preventing and treating retinal neovascularization.[78] In the Renin–Angiotensin System Study, the risk of progression was reduced about 65% and 70% for normotensive patients with type 1 DM treated with enalapril and losartan, respectively.[79]

Blockade of the components of RAAS, such as renin, AT1R, ACE, and aldosterone/MR, can reduce retinal edema, retinal vasculopathy, and inflammation, thus significantly slowing or stopping DR. In a rat model of oxygen-induced retinopathy (OIR), spironolactone (MR antagonist) was reported to be antiangiogenic; this might involve the suppression of aldosterone-induced inflammatory pathways and the modulation of glucose-6-phosphate dehydrogenase and NAD(P)H oxidase subunit

4 (Nox 4).[80] Moreover, the aldosterone synthase inhibitor FAD286 reduced neovascularization and neovascular tufts by 89% and 67%, respectively, in OIR rats and decreased VEGF, TNF-α, intercellular adhesion molecule 1 (ICAM-1), vascular cell adhesion molecule 1 (VCAM-1), and MCP-1.[81]

Oxidative stress

The role of oxidative stress in the onset and development of diabetes and its complications is pivotal (Fig. 2.1). Oxidative stress is a cytopathic outcome caused by the imbalance between ROS production and clearance. In normal biological conditions, ROS production and clearance are maintained in an equilibrium state.[82] The increased oxidative stress is involved in the pathogenesis of DR, which is due to both excessive generation of ROS and the downregulation of antioxidant defense system for ROS elimination.[1] The retina is susceptible to oxidative stress not only because of continuous attack by ROS produced by visible light or ultraviolet but also because its large content of easily oxidized polyunsaturated fatty acids (PUFAs). PUFAs are abundant in the outer segment membranes of photoreceptors, making the retina especially sensitive to oxygen and/or nitrogen activated species and lipid peroxidation. The products of lipid peroxidation, such as hydroxyhexenal and hydroxynonenal (HNE), in turn react with cellular macromolecules (DNA and proteins), consequently leading to photoreceptor cell impairments and RPE abnormality. Besides the abundance of PUFAs, high oxygen consumption is essential to the visual imaging function and active metabolism in retina. Notably, the retinal is always under high oxygen tension, which favors the formation of ROS and promotes lipid peroxidation.

Although low concentrations of ROS serve as intracellular signaling molecules to induce repair mechanisms against tissue injury, large amounts of ROS are toxic and can cause cell death. During diabetes, multiple biochemical pathways increase the production of ROS (Fig. 2.1). Meanwhile, the antioxidant defense system is repressed by hyperglycemia-induced epigenetic modification. Increased superoxide in the retinas of diabetics might be from the impairment of antioxidant defense system. Therefore, inhibiting ROS generation and scavenging excessive ROS have each been employed as therapeutic strategies for the treatment of DR. Under normal conditions, the complex antioxidant defense system, including superoxide dismutase, catalase, glutathione peroxidase, glutathione reductase, and glucose-6-phosphate dehydrogenase, helps maintain the intracellular concentration of glutathione and NADPH necessary for maintaining an optimal level of cellular ROS. However, under hyperglycemic condition, downregulation of the defense system may compromise the redox balance and cause oxidative stress, resulting in the overproduction of ROS. Excessive accumulation of ROS induces mitochondrial damage, cellular apoptosis, inflammation, lipid peroxidation, and structural and functional alterations in retina.[1]

The major endogenous ROS are generated from mitochondria. In mitochondria, the proton gradient across the mitochondrial inner membrane is formed by the ETC, which employs NADH and FADH2 as the electron donors and consumes cellular oxygen. The proton gradient drives ATP synthesis via ATP synthase. Under normal condition, only few oxygen molecules accept a donated electron to transform into ROS, such as O_2^-. However, under diabetic condition, excessive glucose is metabolized by the tricarboxylic acid cycle producing large amounts of NADH or FADH2. The increased levels of electron donors (NADH and FADH2) strengthen the proton gradient across the mitochondrial inner membrane, stimulating the production of ROS. It is currently accepted that ROS is induced by hyperglycemia in diabetic patients through mitochondrial respiratory chain enzymes, xanthine oxidases, lipoxygenases, cyclooxygenases, NO synthases, and peroxidases.[83]

The Nox system, as a key enzymatic source of oxidative stress, employs NADPH as an electron donor, and transports electron to oxygen, driving oxygen conversion into superoxide and/or hydrogen peroxide via a single electron reduction.[1,84] The Nox system contains membrane-associated proteins (Nox protein and p22phox) and cytosolic proteins (p47phox, p67phox, and Rac). Nox family includes several isoforms, in which Nox 1, Nox 2, and Nox 4 are highly expressed in the vascular cells.[84] In diabetic mice or rats, Nox 2 is highly activated in retinal cells, augmenting ROS production and enhancing the expression of ICAM-1 and VEGF.[84,85] Nox 1, Nox 4, and Nox 5 aggravate retinal vascular permeability and promote the expression of inflammatory and angiogenic factors that stimulate neovascularization in DR.[84] Nox 4 is upregulated in the retinas of db/db mice, correlating with increased ROS generation, VEGF-A expression, and vascular permeability.[86] Nox-derived ROS seem to particularly contribute to retinal damage by inducing the expression of proangiogenic and proinflammatory factors, such as VEGF-A, erythropoietin, Ang-2, and ICAM-1.[87,88] Thus, the inhibition of Nox is considered to be a potential therapeutic strategy for the treatment of DR.[84] In an OIR mouse model, only genetically modified Nox 1-deficient mice, not Nox 2 or Nox 4 deficiency, were protected from retinal neovascularization.[87] Deletion of the Nox 2 gene in streptozotocin-induced diabetic mice leads to reduced oxidative stress, attenuates vascular permeability, and reduces leucocyte–endothelial interaction and leukostasis.[84] Nox 4 knockdown with small interfering RNA significantly decreased retinal vascular permeability, indicating that Nox 4 contributes to the BRB breakdown in DR.[86] The management of antioxidative stress in DR is further discussed in Chapter 10.

Nitrosative stress

Diabetes is associated with nitrosative stress in multiple tissues including retina.[89] The key intermediate molecule for nitrosative stress is nitric oxide (NO). NO is synthesized from L-arginine via three nitric oxide synthase (NOS) isoforms that are expressed to variable degrees in the retina, that is, endothelial (eNOS), neuronal (nNOS), and inducible (iNOS).[90] Normally, eNOS is expressed in vascular endothelial cells, iNOS is mainly associated with inflammation or pathological states, and nNOS is expressed in the neurons of the peripheral and central nervous system as well as in human skeletal muscles.[90–92] nNOS and eNOS are constitutive, and nNOS is responsible for the largest proportion of constitutive NOS in humans;

iNOS requires induction by immunological factors such as lipopolysaccharide, interferon, and tumor necrosis factor.[93,94]

In diabetic human postmortem retinas, immunoreactivity for iNOS has been detected in RGCs and Müller glial cells, and nitrotyrosine immunoreactivity has been detected in vascular endothelial cells, all indicating the contribution of increased iNOS to neurotoxicity and angiogenesis in DR.[95,96] Oxidative stress has been shown to convert eNOS from an NO-producing enzyme to an enzyme that generates $O2^{\bullet-}$, known as NOS uncoupling[97] that is implicated in vascular diseases, such as DR.[93] For example, a prospective study reported significantly increased NO levels in aqueous humor of diabetic patients when comparing 35 patients with type 2 diabetes with age- and sex-matched healthy subjects for cataract surgery.[98] The NO interacting with the hyperglycemia-induced superoxide anions results in the production of reactive nitrogen species, for example, peroxynitrite (ONOO), causing nitrosative stress.[90,93] Nitrosative stress induces DNA single strand breaks and PARP activation, causing endothelial cell dysfunction. Peroxynitrite formation induces cytochrome C release, impairing the respiratory chain and inducing cell death.[99] Peroxynitrous acid (ONOOH), also called peroxynitrite conjugate acid, can form hydroxyl radical ($^{\bullet}OH$) and nitrogen dioxide ($^{\bullet}NO_2$), which can initiate fatty acid oxidation and amino acid nitration.[93]

Increased NO level is correlated with the severity of DR. Sharma et al. showed that increased plasma NO plasma concentrations are associated with an increased DR severity.[100] Increased NO can directly react with proteins. S-nitrosation is a reaction of NO moiety with low-molecular thiols or cysteine amino acid residues of proteins to form S-nitrosothiols. An important intermediate reaction product in nitrosation is S-nitrosoglutathione.[101] Nitration is a chemical reaction resulting in the formation of products such as 3-nitrotyrosine (3-NT).[101] Both the products of S-nitrosation and nitration may damage the cells. The dysregulation of nitrosation and nitration has been linked to human neurodegenerative disorders and is mostly related to the excessive production of NO that takes place through the excessive nNOS or iNOS activity via neuroinflammatory stimuli or various toxins.[93,102,103] Using vitreous samples, one study found that malondialdehyde, nitrite, and nitrotyrosine are elevated in PDR patients in comparison with type 2 diabetes patients without retinopathy or healthy controls, suggesting a contributing role of nitrosative stress to the pathogenesis of DR.[104]

Nitrosative stress was reported to contribute to aberrant activation of Wnt signaling in experimental DR.[89] Nitrosative stress, induced by peroxynitrite, 4-HNE, or high glucose in retinal cells, activates the canonical Wnt pathway, increasing the expression of phosphorylated low-density lipoprotein receptor-related protein 6 (pLRP6), total and nuclear β-catenin and Wnt target genes such as ICAM-1 and VEGF. Uric acid, a peroxynitrite scavenger, suppresses Wnt signaling and its downstream targets. In streptozotocin-induced diabetic rats, retinal levels of 3-NT, β-catenin, pLRP6, VEGF, and ICAM-1 are increased significantly. Meanwhile, uric acid treatment for 6 weeks ameliorated diabetes-induced Wnt signaling in the diabetic rat retina.[89]

Since nitrosative stress plays an important role in the pathogenesis of DR, targeting NO and its enzymes has been attempted by using antioxidants, NOS inhibitors, and NO scavengers.[105] Nω-Nitro-L-arginine methyl ester (L-NAME), an NOS inhibitor, was shown to decrease the level of oxidized proteins observed in diabetic rat retinas.[106] Aminoguanidine, a pharmacological inhibitor of iNOS and AGEs, was demonstrated to prevent the histological changes induced in diabetic rats, for example, reduction of endothelial proliferation, acellular capillaries, microaneurysms, and pericyte dropout.[107,108] Evidence exists that an iNOS inhibitor (1400 W) can prevent strong H_2O_2-induced degeneration in porcine retinas, implying a promising treatment option for retinal diseases.[109] Recently, the safety and efficacy of intravitreal iNOS inhibitors, such as aminogunidine and 1400 W were tested in preclinical studies.[110] These studies have laid the foundation for further clinical trials of iNOS inhibitors for DR.

Poly(ADP-ribose) polymerase activation

Poly(ADP-ribosyl)ation is an immediate cellular repair response to DNA damage. This response is catalyzed primarily by poly(ADP-ribose) polymerase-1 (PARP-1; EC 2.4.2.30), which is also known as poly(ADP-ribose) synthetase (PARS) or poly(ADP-ribose) transferase (ADPRT). The PARP family consists of 18 isoforms, of which PARP-1 is the major isoform and is one of the most abundant proteins in the nucleus, accounting for more than 90% of the PARP catalytic activity in the nucleus.

PARP-1, a 116 kDa protein, consists of three main domains, that is, the N-terminal DNA-binding domain containing two zinc fingers, the automodification domain, and the C-terminal catalytic domain. The primary structure of the enzyme is highly conserved in eukaryotes with the catalytic domain showing the highest degree of homology among species. PARP is involved in the cellular response to DNA injury, such as that from oxidative stress or nitrosative stress. The oxidative and nitrosative stress are significantly increased in retinas of diabetic animals, causing DNA breaks then leading to PARP activation.[111] PARP activation depletes its substrate, NAD^+, slowing the rate of glycolysis, electron transport, and ATP formation; it also results in the inhibition of GAPDH by poly-ADP-ribosylation. For instance, poly(ADP-ribose)ylated proteins were found abundant in the ganglion cell layer, inner nuclear layer, and outer nuclear layer of the retina as well as endothelial cells and pericytes of retinas from diabetic rats as compared to the controls. PARP activation is a key event causing retinal vascular disfunction in diabetes. The hyperglycemia-induced PARP activation is susceptible to pharmacological PARP inhibition.[112] Inhibition of PARP activity by a specific PARP inhibitor, PJ-34, suppresses the diabetes-induced apoptosis of capillary endothelial cells, pericyte loss, and inhibits the formation of acellular capillaries.[113] PJ-34 inhibits hyperglycemia-induced NF-kappa B activation in cultured bovine retinal endothelial cells and inhibits the diabetes-induced inflammatory proteins such as ICAM-1, and subsequent leukostasis in diabetic rat retinas.[113] Thus, the inhibition of PARP activity may be a therapeutic strategy for diabetic microangiopathy.

Other metabolic alterations in DR

Diabetes mellitus is a group of metabolic diseases. DR is a complication of diabetes. In the diabetic retina, besides altered glucose metabolism, there are also alterations in amino acid, lipid, and nucleotide metabolism. For example (Fig. 2.4), HBP integrates the above four metabolic processes, including carbohydrate (glucose), amino acid (glutamine), lipid (Acetyl-CoA) and nucleotide (UTP). The changes in numerous metabolites are found in plasma, aqueous humor, vitreous, and retina from diabetic patients, which could potentially serve as diagnostic biomarkers or therapeutic targets in DR.[114]

By using high-resolution mass spectrometry coupled with liquid chromatography on plasma of 83 DR patients and 90 diabetic controls without DR, significant alterations were found in the metabolite profiles including amino acids, leukotrienes, niacin, pyrimidines, and purines. In this study, plasma levels of arginine, citrulline, glutamic γ-semialdehyde, and dehydroxycarnitine were significantly altered in DR patients compared with diabetic controls.[114] Between NPDR and PDR, pathway analysis revealed alterations in the β-oxidation of saturated fatty acids, fatty acid metabolism, and vitamin D3 metabolism, in which carnitine was identified to be significantly elevated in PDR patients relative to those with NPDR.[114] Further, in a cross-sectional study using isotope dilution liquid chromatography-tandem mass spectrometry, plasma metabolite levels were quantified in 159 diabetic controls and 156 DR patients, including 92 NPDR and 64 PDR.[115] In this study, plasma arginine and citrulline were significantly elevated in type 2 diabetic patients with DR compared to diabetic controls, showing the dysregulation of amino acid metabolism in DR.[115] Using the aqueous humor of the diabetic patients, the metabolites most altered in DR were lactate, succinate, 2-hydroxybutyrate, asparagine, dimethylamine, histidine, threonine, and glutamine.[116] The metabolomic analyses also indicated an alteration in the metabolic pathways of energy metabolism and amino acid metabolism.[116]

By analyzing the metabolites in vitreous samples from 43 PDR patients and 21 nondiabetic control subjects with epiretinal membrane, 158 metabolites in vitreous samples were found to be altered. Increases in pyruvate, lactate, proline, and allantoin and a decrease in creatine were demonstrated in PDR patients compared with the control subjects.[117] Amino acid metabolism is altered in the posterior segment in DR. For instance, D-serine was increased in the vitreous humor of PDR patients compared with control subjects (patients with idiopathic macular hole and idiopathic epiretinal membrane).[118] The increased D-serine caused neurovascular abnormalities in retinas from diabetic rats.[119,120] D-Serine is degraded by D-amino acid oxidase and synthesized by serine racemase. In diabetic rat, serine racemase was increased, while D-amino acid oxidase was decreased, resulting in the overproduction of D-Serine. Loss-of-function or deletion of serine racemase[121,122] and overexpression of D-amino acid oxidase[119] could provide therapeutic approaches for treating DR (see Chapter 10).

In summary, diabetes drives multiple metabolic disorders. The dysregulation of metabolic pathways has been proven to include amino acid and energy metabolism in DR.[123] Most significantly, the resultant alteration of metabolites in plasma, aqueous humor, vitreous, and retina may serve as potential biomarkers and therapeutic targets for DR. A recent multicenter study demonstrated how the alteration of circulating metabolites can be applied to detect sight-threatening diabetic retinopathy (STDR). This study revealed that the level of plasma cystatin C, a protein conventionally attributed to diabetic kidney, could statistically identify STDR from no DR in clinical practice. This approach may be used to triage who requires prioritization for retinal screening for STDR.[124]

Metabolic memory effect on the progression of DR

Metabolic memory has been observed in both diabetic patients and in diabetic animal models (Fig. 2.7). It refers to the persistent beneficial effect of intensive glycemic control or the persistent deleterious effect of poor glycemic control during the early course of diabetes. This concept arose from the results of multiple large-scale

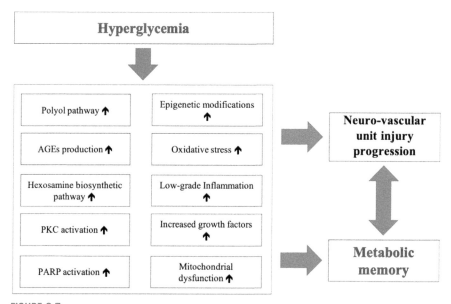

FIGURE 2.7

Metabolic memory effect on the progression of DR. In clinic trials and animal studies, hyperglycemia induces perturbations of various metabolic pathways, include polyol pathway, AGEs production, HBP, PARP activation, epigenetic modifications, oxidative stress, low-grade inflammation, increased growth factor production, mitochondrial dysfunctions, etc. Besides, other mechanisms, such as the epigenetic modification, have also been implicated in the phenomenon of metabolic memory that is due to prior episodes of poor glycemic control, despite subsequent glucose normalization.[125]

clinical trials, which showed that after diabetes onset, diabetic complications persist and progress even when glycemic control is restored through pharmaceutical intervention. Several large-scale clinical trials showed that early intensive glycemic control can reduce the incidence and progression of diabetic complications. However, the epidemiological and prospective data have revealed that after a period of poor glucose control, insulin or diabetes drug treatment fails to prevent the development and progression of DR even when glycemic level has been intensively controlled. The persistent deleterious effects of prior hyperglycemic insult are a metabolic memory phenomenon.[126]

The phenomenon of metabolic memory was reported in diabetic dogs in 1987. In this study, the retinopathy continued to progress even after hyperglycemia was strictly controlled, leading to the concept of "metabolic memory."[127] This phenomenon was also observed in later clinical trials. Two major studies, the Diabetic Complications and Control Trial (DCCT) and Epidemiology of Diabetes Interventions and Complications (EDIC) trial clearly demonstrated the role of metabolic memory in the increased risk of diabetes-related complications. The EDIC trial which extended the work of DCCT showed that individuals under intensive glycemic control during DCCT had a drastic decrease in the risk of developing diabetes-related complications, whereas the individuals who were under conventional treatment during DCCT and intensive glycemic control during EDIC did not have reduced risk of developing complications. These observations clearly indicate the role of metabolic memory in the development of diabetic complications including DR.[128]

As shown in Fig. 2.7, hyperglycemia can induce a variety of epigenetic changes that persist even after the normalization of blood glucose level. Recent studies underline the role of epigenetic modifications as mediators of the metabolic memory. Accumulating evidence suggests a key role for epigenetic mechanisms such as DNA methylation, histone posttranslational modifications in chromatin, and noncoding RNAs such as microRNAs (miRNAs) and long noncoding RNAs (lncRNAs) in the complex interplay between genes and the environment. Several studies have shown that deregulation of the miRNA profile may persist even after normoglycemic restoration. miRNAs participate in metabolic memory by targeting the mRNA of genes encoding enzymes involved in DNA methylation. Meanwhile, miRNAs are extensively regulated at the levels of miRNA promoter transcription, methylation, and miRNA processing.[129] It has been shown that hyperglycemia can alter posttranslational histone modifications and the activity of DNA methyltransferases, thus generate irreversible changes leading to the long-term harmful effects of metabolic memory.[130] Moreover, posttranscriptional epigenetic modification of RNA, mainly N6-methyladenosine (^{m6}A), has a definite effect in various diseases, including DR. The alterations in ^{m6}A modification of RNA have been observed to be associated with inflammation, oxidative stress, angiogenesis, etc., as occur in DR. In fact, various noncoding RNAs such as microRNA, lncRNA, and circular RNA are affected and associated with ^{m6}A modification in DR. Overall, metabolic and epigenetic effects continue to damage the neurovascular unit in retina, enforcing the effects of metabolic memory.

It is proposed that the metabolic memory effect might be better termed "cumulative glycemic effects," instead of "metabolic memory."[131] Targeting epigenetic factors using small molecules or locus-specific epigenetic editing via the clustered regularly interspaced short palindromic repeats (CRISPR)-CRISPR associated protein 9 (Cas9) (CRISPR-Cas9) system or targeting noncoding RNAs using chemically modified antisense oligonucleotides are all potential approaches to manipulate metabolic memory. Therefore, personalized treatment for DR is possible by changing epigenetic profiling through epigenome-wide association studies and RNA profiling (transcriptome) obtained from samples of diabetic patients.

References

1. Kang Q, Yang C. Oxidative stress and diabetic retinopathy: molecular mechanisms, pathogenetic role and therapeutic implications. *Redox Biol*. 2020;37:101799. https://doi.org/10.1016/j.redox.2020.101799.
2. Singh M, Kapoor A, Bhatnagar A. Physiological and pathological roles of aldose reductase. *Metabolites*. 2021;11(10):655. https://doi.org/10.3390/metabo11100655.
3. Lorenzi M. The polyol pathway as a mechanism for diabetic retinopathy: attractive, elusive, and resilient. *Exp Diabetes Res*. 2007;2007:61038. https://doi.org/10.1155/2007/61038.
4. Asnaghi V, Gerhardinger C, Hoehn T, Adeboje A, Lorenzi M. A role for the polyol pathway in the early neuroretinal apoptosis and glial changes induced by diabetes in the rat. *Diabetes*. 2003;52(2):506−511. https://doi.org/10.2337/diabetes.52.2.506.
5. Amano S, Yamagishi S ichi, Kato N, et al. Sorbitol dehydrogenase overexpression potentiates glucose toxicity to cultured retinal pericytes. *Biochem Biophys Res Commun*. 2002;299(2):183−188. https://doi.org/10.1016/s0006-291x(02)02584-6.
6. Song J, Yang X, Yan LJ. Role of pseudohypoxia in the pathogenesis of type 2 diabetes. *Hypoxia Auckl NZ*. 2019;7:33−40. https://doi.org/10.2147/HP.S202775.
7. Williamson JR, Chang K, Frangos M, et al. Hyperglycemic pseudohypoxia and diabetic complications. *Diabetes*. 1993;42(6):801−813. https://doi.org/10.2337/diab.42.6.801.
8. Thamotharampillai K, Chan AKF, Bennetts B, et al. Decline in neurophysiological function after 7 years in an adolescent diabetic cohort and the role of aldose reductase gene polymorphisms. *Diabetes Care*. 2006;29(9):2053−2057. https://doi.org/10.2337/dc06-0678.
9. Zhou M, Zhang P, Xu X, Sun X. The relationship between aldose reductase C106T polymorphism and diabetic retinopathy: an updated meta-analysis. *Invest Ophthalmol Vis Sci*. 2015;56(4):2279−2289. https://doi.org/10.1167/iovs.14-16279.
10. Dagher Z, Park YS, Asnaghi V, Hoehn T, Gerhardinger C, Lorenzi M. Studies of rat and human retinas predict a role for the polyol pathway in human diabetic retinopathy. *Diabetes*. 2004;53(9):2404−2411. https://doi.org/10.2337/diabetes.53.9.2404.
11. Kumar M, Choudhary S, Singh PK, Silakari O. Addressing selectivity issues of aldose reductase 2 inhibitors for the management of diabetic complications. *Future Med Chem*. 2020;12(14):1327−1358. https://doi.org/10.4155/fmc-2020-0032.
12. Lee CA, Li G, Patel MD, et al. Diabetes-induced impairment in visual function in mice: contributions of p38 MAPK, rage, leukocytes, and aldose reductase. *Invest Ophthalmol Vis Sci*. 2014;55(5):2904−2910. https://doi.org/10.1167/iovs.13-11659.

13. Sorbinil Retinopathy Trial Research Group. A randomized trial of sorbinil, an aldose reductase inhibitor, in diabetic retinopathy. *Arch Ophthalmol Chic Ill 1960.* 1990; 108(9):1234−1244. https://doi.org/10.1001/archopht.1990.01070110050024.

14. Hotta N, Kawamori R, Fukuda M, Shigeta Y. Aldose Reductase Inhibitor-Diabetes Complications Trial Study Group. Long-term clinical effects of epalrestat, an aldose reductase inhibitor, on progression of diabetic neuropathy and other microvascular complications: multivariate epidemiological analysis based on patient background factors and severity of diabetic neuropathy. *Diabet Med J Br Diabet Assoc.* 2012;29(12): 1529−1533. https://doi.org/10.1111/j.1464-5491.2012.03684.x.

15. Quattrini L, La Motta C. Aldose reductase inhibitors: 2013-present. *Expert Opin Ther Pat.* 2019;29(3):199−213. https://doi.org/10.1080/13543776.2019.1582646.

16. Kovacikova L, Prnova MS, Majekova M, Bohac A, Karasu C, Stefek M. Development of novel indole-based bifunctional aldose reductase inhibitors/antioxidants as promising drugs for the treatment of diabetic complications. *Mol Basel Switz.* 2021;26(10):2867. https://doi.org/10.3390/molecules26102867.

17. Zeng C, Li Y, Ma J, Niu L, Tay FR. Clinical/translational aspects of advanced glycation end-products. *Trends Endocrinol Metab TEM.* 2019;30(12):959−973. https://doi.org/ 10.1016/j.tem.2019.08.005.

18. Li W, Khatami M, Robertson GA, Shen S, Rockey JH. Nonenzymatic glycosylation of bovine retinal microvessel basement membranes in vitro. Kinetic analysis and inhibition by aspirin. *Invest Ophthalmol Vis Sci.* 1984;25(8):884−892.

19. Ruiz HH, Ramasamy R, Schmidt AM. Advanced glycation end products: building on the concept of the "common soil" in metabolic disease. *Endocrinology.* 2020;161(1): bqz006. https://doi.org/10.1210/endocr/bqz006.

20. Sourris KC, Watson A, Jandeleit-Dahm K. Inhibitors of advanced glycation end product (AGE) formation and accumulation. *Handb Exp Pharmacol.* 2021;264:395−423. https://doi.org/10.1007/164_2020_391.

21. Stitt AW. Advanced glycation: an important pathological event in diabetic and age related ocular disease. *Br J Ophthalmol.* 2001;85(6):746−753. https://doi.org/ 10.1136/bjo.85.6.746.

22. Sharma Y, Saxena S, Mishra A, Saxena A, Natu SM. Advanced glycation end products and diabetic retinopathy. *J Ocul Biol Dis Infor.* 2012;5(3−4):63−69. https://doi.org/ 10.1007/s12177-013-9104-7.

23. Stitt AW. The role of advanced glycation in the pathogenesis of diabetic retinopathy. *Exp Mol Pathol.* 2003;75(1):95−108. https://doi.org/10.1016/s0014-4800(03)00035-2.

24. Fournet M, Bonté F, Desmoulière A. Glycation damage: a possible hub for major pathophysiological disorders and aging. *Aging Dis.* 2018;9(5):880. https://doi.org/10.14336/ AD.2017.1121.

25. Bahmani F, Bathaie SZ, Aldavood SJ, Ghahghaei A. Inhibitory effect of crocin(s) on lens α-crystallin glycation and aggregation, results in the decrease of the risk of diabetic cataract. *Mol Basel Switz.* 2016;21(2):143. https://doi.org/10.3390/molecules21020143.

26. Chaudhuri J, Bains Y, Guha S, et al. The role of advanced glycation end products in aging and metabolic diseases: bridging association and causality. *Cell Metabol.* 2018; 28(3):337−352. https://doi.org/10.1016/j.cmet.2018.08.014.

27. Xie J, Reverdatto S, Frolov A, Hoffmann R, Burz DS, Shekhtman A. Structural basis for pattern recognition by the receptor for advanced glycation end products (RAGE). *J Biol Chem.* 2008;283(40):27255−27269. https://doi.org/10.1074/jbc.M801622200.

28. Xue J, Ray R, Singer D, et al. The receptor for advanced glycation end products (RAGE) specifically recognizes methylglyoxal-derived AGEs. *Biochemistry*. 2014;53(20): 3327−3335. https://doi.org/10.1021/bi500046t.

29. Buetler TM, Leclerc E, Baumeyer A, et al. N(epsilon)-carboxymethyllysine-modified proteins are unable to bind to RAGE and activate an inflammatory response. *Mol Nutr Food Res*. 2008;52(3):370−378. https://doi.org/10.1002/mnfr.200700101.

30. Rowan S, Bejarano E, Taylor A. Mechanistic targeting of advanced glycation end-products in age-related diseases. *Biochim Biophys Acta, Mol Basis Dis*. 2018; 1864(12):3631−3643. https://doi.org/10.1016/j.bbadis.2018.08.036.

31. Giardino I, Edelstein D, Brownlee M. Nonenzymatic glycosylation in vitro and in bovine endothelial cells alters basic fibroblast growth factor activity. A model for intracellular glycosylation in diabetes. *J Clin Invest*. 1994;94(1):110−117. https://doi.org/10.1172/JCI117296.

32. Loho T, Venna V, Setiabudy RD, et al. Correlation between vitreous advanced glycation end products, and D-dimer with blood HbA1c levels in proliferative diabetic retinopathy. *Acta Med Indones*. 2018;50(2):132−137.

33. Ferrington DA, Sinha D, Kaarniranta K. Defects in retinal pigment epithelial cell proteolysis and the pathology associated with age-related macular degeneration. *Prog Retin Eye Res*. 2016;51:69−89. https://doi.org/10.1016/j.preteyeres.2015.09.002.

34. Dyer DG, Dunn JA, Thorpe SR, et al. Accumulation of Maillard reaction products in skin collagen in diabetes and aging. *J Clin Invest*. 1993;91(6):2463−2469. https://doi.org/10.1172/JCI116481.

35. Kalfa TA, Gerritsen ME, Carlson EC, Binstock AJ, Tsilibary EC. Altered proliferation of retinal microvascular cells on glycated matrix. *Invest Ophthalmol Vis Sci*. 1995; 36(12):2358−2367.

36. Tsilibary EC. Microvascular basement membranes in diabetes mellitus. *J Pathol*. 2003; 200(4):537−546. https://doi.org/10.1002/path.1439.

37. Sell DR, Monnier VM. Molecular basis of arterial stiffening: role of glycation—a minireview. *Gerontology*. 2012;58(3):227−237. https://doi.org/10.1159/000334668.

38. Stitt A, Gardiner TA, Alderson NL, et al. The AGE inhibitor pyridoxamine inhibits development of retinopathy in experimental diabetes. *Diabetes*. 2002;51(9): 2826−2832. https://doi.org/10.2337/diabetes.51.9.2826.

39. Jud P, Sourij H. Therapeutic options to reduce advanced glycation end products in patients with diabetes mellitus: a review. *Diabetes Res Clin Pract*. 2019;148:54−63. https://doi.org/10.1016/j.diabres.2018.11.016.

40. Aldini G, Vistoli G, Stefek M, et al. Molecular strategies to prevent, inhibit, and degrade advanced glycoxidation and advanced lipoxidation end products. *Free Radic Res*. 2013; 47(Suppl 1):93−137. https://doi.org/10.3109/10715762.2013.792926.

41. Xue M, Weickert MO, Qureshi S, et al. Improved glycemic control and vascular function in overweight and obese subjects by glyoxalase 1 inducer formulation. *Diabetes*. 2016;65(8):2282−2294. https://doi.org/10.2337/db16-0153.

42. Kanazawa I, Yamamoto M, Yamaguchi T, Sugimoto T. Effects of metformin and pioglitazone on serum pentosidine levels in type 2 diabetes mellitus. *Exp Clin Endocrinol Diabetes Off J Ger Soc Endocrinol Ger Diabetes Assoc*. 2011;119(6):362−365. https://doi.org/10.1055/s-0030-1267953.

43. Gurel Z, Sheibani N. O-Linked β-N-acetylglucosamine (O-GlcNAc) modification: a new pathway to decode pathogenesis of diabetic retinopathy. *Clin Sci Lond Engl 1979*. 2018;132(2):185−198. https://doi.org/10.1042/CS20171454.

44. Campbell S, Mesaros C, Izzo L, et al. Glutamine deprivation triggers NAGK-dependent hexosamine salvage. *eLife*. 2021;10:e62644. https://doi.org/10.7554/eLife.62644.

45. Peterson SB, Hart GW. New insights: a role for O-GlcNAcylation in diabetic complications. *Crit Rev Biochem Mol Biol*. 2016;51(3):150–161. https://doi.org/10.3109/10409238.2015.1135102.

46. Furo K, Nozaki M, Murashige H, Sato Y. Identification of an N-acetylglucosamine kinase essential for UDP-N-acetylglucosamine salvage synthesis in Arabidopsis. *FEBS Lett*. 2015;589(21):3258–3262. https://doi.org/10.1016/j.febslet.2015.09.011.

47. Nakamura M, Barber AJ, Antonetti DA, et al. Excessive hexosamines block the neuroprotective effect of insulin and induce apoptosis in retinal neurons. *J Biol Chem*. 2001;276(47):43748–43755. https://doi.org/10.1074/jbc.M108594200.

48. Gurel Z, Zaro BW, Pratt MR, Sheibani N. Identification of O-GlcNAc modification targets in mouse retinal pericytes: implication of p53 in pathogenesis of diabetic retinopathy. *PLoS One*. 2014;9(5):e95561. https://doi.org/10.1371/journal.pone.0095561.

49. Donovan K, Alekseev O, Qi X, Cho W, Azizkhan-Clifford J. O-GlcNAc modification of transcription factor Sp1 mediates hyperglycemia-induced VEGF-A upregulation in retinal cells. *Invest Ophthalmol Vis Sci*. 2014;55(12):7862–7873. https://doi.org/10.1167/iovs.14-14048.

50. Gurel Z, Sieg KM, Shallow KD, Sorenson CM, Sheibani N. Retinal O-linked N-acetylglucosamine protein modifications: implications for postnatal retinal vascularization and the pathogenesis of diabetic retinopathy. *Mol Vis*. 2013;19:1047–1059.

51. Dierschke SK, Miller WP, Favate JS, et al. O-GlcNAcylation alters the selection of mRNAs for translation and promotes 4E-BP1-dependent mitochondrial dysfunction in the retina. *J Biol Chem*. 2019;294(14):5508–5520. https://doi.org/10.1074/jbc.RA119.007494.

52. Dierschke SK, Toro AL, Barber AJ, Arnold AC, Dennis MD. Angiotensin-(1-7) attenuates protein O-GlcNAcylation in the retina by EPAC/Rap1-dependent inhibition of O-GlcNAc transferase. *Invest Ophthalmol Vis Sci*. 2020;61(2):24. https://doi.org/10.1167/iovs.61.2.24.

53. Dorfmueller HC, Borodkin VS, Blair DE, Pathak S, Navratilova I, van Aalten DMF. Substrate and product analogues as human O-GlcNAc transferase inhibitors. *Amino Acids*. 2011;40(3):781–792. https://doi.org/10.1007/s00726-010-0688-y.

54. Lenzen S, Panten U. Alloxan: history and mechanism of action. *Diabetologia*. 1988;31(6):337–342. https://doi.org/10.1007/BF02341500.

55. Sinha K, Das J, Pal PB, Sil PC. Oxidative stress: the mitochondria-dependent and mitochondria-independent pathways of apoptosis. *Arch Toxicol*. 2013;87(7):1157–1180. https://doi.org/10.1007/s00204-013-1034-4.

56. Geraldes P, King GL. Activation of protein kinase C isoforms and its impact on diabetic complications. *Circ Res*. 2010;106(8):1319–1331. https://doi.org/10.1161/CIRCRESAHA.110.217117.

57. Yuan T, Yang T, Chen H, et al. New insights into oxidative stress and inflammation during diabetes mellitus-accelerated atherosclerosis. *Redox Biol*. 2019;20:247–260. https://doi.org/10.1016/j.redox.2018.09.025.

58. Nogueira-Machado JA, Chaves MM. From hyperglycemia to AGE-RAGE interaction on the cell surface: a dangerous metabolic route for diabetic patients. *Expert Opin Ther Targets*. 2008;12(7):871–882. https://doi.org/10.1517/14728222.12.7.871.

59. George A, Pushkaran S, Konstantinidis DG, et al. Erythrocyte NADPH oxidase activity modulated by Rac GTPases, PKC, and plasma cytokines contributes to oxidative stress in sickle cell disease. *Blood*. 2013;121(11):2099−2107. https://doi.org/10.1182/blood-2012-07-441188.

60. Geraldes P, Hiraoka-Yamamoto J, Matsumoto M, et al. Activation of PKC-delta and SHP-1 by hyperglycemia causes vascular cell apoptosis and diabetic retinopathy. *Nat Med*. 2009;15(11):1298−1306. https://doi.org/10.1038/nm.2052.

61. Sarikaya M, Yazihan N, Daş Evcimen N. Relationship between aldose reductase enzyme and the signaling pathway of protein kinase C in an in vitro diabetic retinopathy model. *Can J Physiol Pharmacol*. 2020;98(4):243−251. https://doi.org/10.1139/cjpp-2019-0211.

62. Lin CM, Titchenell PM, Keil JM, et al. Inhibition of atypical protein kinase C reduces inflammation-induced retinal vascular permeability. *Am J Pathol*. 2018;188(10):2392−2405. https://doi.org/10.1016/j.ajpath.2018.06.020.

63. Singh RK, Kumar S, Tomar MS, et al. Putative role of natural products as Protein Kinase C modulator in different disease conditions. *Daru J Fac Pharm Tehran Univ Med Sci*. July 3, 2021. https://doi.org/10.1007/s40199-021-00401-z.

64. Gálvez MIL. Protein kinase C inhibitors in the treatment of diabetic retinopathy. Review. *Curr Pharmaceut Biotechnol*. 2011;12(3):386−391. https://doi.org/10.2174/138920111794480606.

65. Deissler HL, Lang GE. The protein kinase C inhibitor: ruboxistaurin. *Dev Ophthalmol*. 2016;55:295−301. https://doi.org/10.1159/000431204.

66. Wilkinson-Berka JL, Suphapimol V, Jerome JR, Deliyanti D, Allingham MJ. Angiotensin II and aldosterone in retinal vasculopathy and inflammation. *Exp Eye Res*. 2019;187:107766. https://doi.org/10.1016/j.exer.2019.107766.

67. Patel S, Rauf A, Khan H, Abu-Izneid T. Renin-angiotensin-aldosterone (RAAS): the ubiquitous system for homeostasis and pathologies. *Biomed Pharmacother Biomedecine Pharmacother*. 2017;94:317−325. https://doi.org/10.1016/j.biopha.2017.07.091.

68. Wagner J, Jan Danser AH, Derkx FH, et al. Demonstration of renin mRNA, angiotensinogen mRNA, and angiotensin converting enzyme mRNA expression in the human eye: evidence for an intraocular renin-angiotensin system. *Br J Ophthalmol*. 1996;80(2):159−163. https://doi.org/10.1136/bjo.80.2.159.

69. Patel VB, Zhong JC, Grant MB, Oudit GY. Role of the ACE2/angiotensin 1-7 axis of the renin-angiotensin system in heart failure. *Circ Res*. 2016;118(8):1313−1326. https://doi.org/10.1161/CIRCRESAHA.116.307708.

70. Rodrigues Prestes TR, Rocha NP, Miranda AS, Teixeira AL, Simoes-E-Silva AC. The anti-inflammatory potential of ACE2/angiotensin-(1-7)/mas receptor axis: evidence from basic and clinical research. *Curr Drug Targets*. 2017;18(11):1301−1313. https://doi.org/10.2174/1389450117666160727142401.

71. Mirabito Colafella KM, Bovée DM, Danser AHJ. The renin-angiotensin-aldosterone system and its therapeutic targets. *Exp Eye Res*. 2019;186:107680. https://doi.org/10.1016/j.exer.2019.05.020.

72. Fletcher EL, Phipps JA, Ward MM, Vessey KA, Wilkinson-Berka JL. The renin-angiotensin system in retinal health and disease: its influence on neurons, glia and the vasculature. *Prog Retin Eye Res*. 2010;29(4):284−311. https://doi.org/10.1016/j.preteyeres.2010.03.003.

73. Satofuka S, Ichihara A, Nagai N, et al. (Pro)renin receptor-mediated signal transduction and tissue renin-angiotensin system contribute to diabetes-induced retinal inflammation. *Diabetes*. 2009;58(7):1625−1633. https://doi.org/10.2337/db08-0254.

74. Nguyen Dinh Cat A, Montezano AC, Burger D, Touyz RM. Angiotensin II, NADPH oxidase, and redox signaling in the vasculature. *Antioxid Redox Signal*. 2013;19(10):1110−1120. https://doi.org/10.1089/ars.2012.4641.

75. Ding J, Yu M, Jiang J, et al. Angiotensin II decreases endothelial nitric oxide synthase phosphorylation via AT1R Nox/ROS/PP2A pathway. *Front Physiol*. 2020;11:566410. https://doi.org/10.3389/fphys.2020.566410.

76. Birk M, Baum E, Zadeh JK, et al. Angiotensin II induces oxidative stress and endothelial dysfunction in mouse ophthalmic arteries via involvement of AT1 receptors and NOX2. *Antioxid Basel Switz*. 2021;10(8):1238. https://doi.org/10.3390/antiox10081238.

77. Wright AD, Dodson PM. Diabetic retinopathy and blockade of the renin-angiotensin system: new data from the DIRECT study programme. *Eye Lond Engl*. 2010;24(1):1−6. https://doi.org/10.1038/eye.2009.189.

78. Chaturvedi N, Sjolie AK, Stephenson JM, et al. Effect of lisinopril on progression of retinopathy in normotensive people with type 1 diabetes. The EUCLID study group. EURODIAB controlled trial of lisinopril in insulin-dependent diabetes mellitus. *Lancet Lond Engl*. 1998;351(9095):28−31. https://doi.org/10.1016/s0140-6736(97)06209-0.

79. Mauer M, Zinman B, Gardiner R, et al. Renal and retinal effects of enalapril and losartan in type 1 diabetes. *N Engl J Med*. 2009;361(1):40−51. https://doi.org/10.1056/NEJMoa0808400.

80. Wilkinson-Berka JL, Tan G, Jaworski K, Harbig J, Miller AG. Identification of a retinal aldosterone system and the protective effects of mineralocorticoid receptor antagonism on retinal vascular pathology. *Circ Res*. 2009;104(1):124−133. https://doi.org/10.1161/CIRCRESAHA.108.176008.

81. Deliyanti D, Miller AG, Tan G, Binger KJ, Samson AL, Wilkinson-Berka JL. Neovascularization is attenuated with aldosterone synthase inhibition in rats with retinopathy. *Hypertens Dallas Tex 1979*. 2012;59(3):607−613. https://doi.org/10.1161/HYPERTENSIONAHA.111.188136.

82. Kowluru RA, Kowluru A, Mishra M, Kumar B. Oxidative stress and epigenetic modifications in the pathogenesis of diabetic retinopathy. *Prog Retin Eye Res*. 2015;48:40−61. https://doi.org/10.1016/j.preteyeres.2015.05.001.

83. Balaban RS, Nemoto S, Finkel T. Mitochondria, oxidants, and aging. *Cell*. 2005;120(4):483−495. https://doi.org/10.1016/j.cell.2005.02.001.

84. Urner S, Ho F, Jha JC, Ziegler D, Jandeleit-Dahm K. NADPH oxidase inhibition: preclinical and clinical studies in diabetic complications. *Antioxid Redox Signal*. 2020;33(6):415−434. https://doi.org/10.1089/ars.2020.8047.

85. Al-Shabrawey M, Bartoli M, El-Remessy AB, et al. Role of NADPH oxidase and Stat3 in statin-mediated protection against diabetic retinopathy. *Invest Ophthalmol Vis Sci*. 2008;49(7):3231−3238. https://doi.org/10.1167/iovs.08-1754.

86. Li J, Wang JJ, Yu Q, Chen K, Mahadev K, Zhang SX. Inhibition of reactive oxygen species by lovastatin downregulates vascular endothelial growth factor expression and ameliorates blood-retinal barrier breakdown in db/db mice: role of NADPH oxidase 4. *Diabetes*. 2010;59(6):1528−1538. https://doi.org/10.2337/db09-1057.

87. Wilkinson-Berka JL, Deliyanti D, Rana I, et al. NADPH oxidase, NOX1, mediates vascular injury in ischemic retinopathy. *Antioxid Redox Signal*. 2014;20(17):2726−2740. https://doi.org/10.1089/ars.2013.5357.

88. Al-Shabrawey M, Rojas M, Sanders T, et al. Role of NADPH oxidase in retinal vascular inflammation. *Invest Ophthalmol Vis Sci.* 2008;49(7):3239−3244. https://doi.org/10.1167/iovs.08-1755.

89. Liu Q, Li J, Cheng R, et al. Nitrosative stress plays an important role in Wnt pathway activation in diabetic retinopathy. *Antioxid Redox Signal.* 2013;18(10):1141−1153. https://doi.org/10.1089/ars.2012.4583.

90. Opatrilova R, Kubatka P, Caprnda M, et al. Nitric oxide in the pathophysiology of retinopathy: evidences from preclinical and clinical researches. *Acta Ophthalmol.* 2018; 96(3):222−231. https://doi.org/10.1111/aos.13384.

91. Vielma AH, Retamal MA, Schmachtenberg O. Nitric oxide signaling in the retina: what have we learned in two decades? *Brain Res.* 2012;1430:112−125. https://doi.org/10.1016/j.brainres.2011.10.045.

92. Knowles RG, Moncada S. Nitric oxide synthases in mammals. *Biochem J.* 1994;298(Pt 2):249−258. https://doi.org/10.1042/bj2980249.

93. Cantó A, Olivar T, Romero FJ, Miranda M. Nitrosative stress in retinal pathologies: review. *Antioxid Basel Switz.* 2019;8(11):E543. https://doi.org/10.3390/antiox8110543.

94. Goldstein IM, Ostwald P, Roth S. Nitric oxide: a review of its role in retinal function and disease. *Vision Res.* 1996;36(18):2979−2994. https://doi.org/10.1016/0042-6989(96)00017-x.

95. Abu El-Asrar AM, Desmet S, Meersschaert A, Dralands L, Missotten L, Geboes K. Expression of the inducible isoform of nitric oxide synthase in the retinas of human subjects with diabetes mellitus. *Am J Ophthalmol.* 2001;132(4):551−556. https://doi.org/10.1016/s0002-9394(01)01127-8.

96. Abu El-Asrar AM, Meersschaert A, Dralands L, Missotten L, Geboes K. Inducible nitric oxide synthase and vascular endothelial growth factor are colocalized in the retinas of human subjects with diabetes. *Eye Lond Engl.* 2004;18(3):306−313. https://doi.org/10.1038/sj.eye.6700642.

97. Förstermann U, Sessa WC. Nitric oxide synthases: regulation and function. *Eur Heart J.* 2012;33(7):829−837, 837a-837d. https://doi.org/10.1093/eurheartj/ehr304.

98. Kulaksızoglu S, Karalezli A. Aqueous humour and serum levels of nitric oxide, malondialdehyde and total antioxidant status in patients with type 2 diabetes with proliferative diabetic retinopathy and nondiabetic senile cataracts. *Can J Diabetes.* 2016;40(2):115−119. https://doi.org/10.1016/j.jcjd.2015.07.002.

99. Martínez-Ruiz A, Cadenas S, Lamas S. Nitric oxide signaling: classical, less classical, and nonclassical mechanisms. *Free Radic Biol Med.* 2011;51(1):17−29. https://doi.org/10.1016/j.freeradbiomed.2011.04.010.

100. Sharma S, Saxena S, Srivastav K, et al. Nitric oxide and oxidative stress is associated with severity of diabetic retinopathy and retinal structural alterations. *Clin Exp Ophthalmol.* 2015;43(5):429−436. https://doi.org/10.1111/ceo.12506.

101. Knott AB, Bossy-Wetzel E. Nitric oxide in health and disease of the nervous system. *Antioxid Redox Signal.* 2009;11(3):541−554. https://doi.org/10.1089/ars.2008.2234.

102. McBean GJ, López MG, Wallner FK. Redox-based therapeutics in neurodegenerative disease. *Br J Pharmacol.* 2017;174(12):1750−1770. https://doi.org/10.1111/bph.13551.

103. Bradley SA, Steinert JR. Nitric oxide-mediated posttranslational modifications: impacts at the synapse. *Oxid Med Cell Longev.* 2016;2016:5681036. https://doi.org/10.1155/2016/5681036.

104. Mandal LK, Choudhuri S, Dutta D, et al. Oxidative stress-associated neuroretinal dysfunction and nitrosative stress in diabetic retinopathy. *Can J Diabetes*. 2013;37(6):401−407. https://doi.org/10.1016/j.jcjd.2013.05.004.

105. Zheng L, Kern TS. Role of nitric oxide, superoxide, peroxynitrite and PARP in diabetic retinopathy. *Front Biosci Landmark Ed*. 2009;14(10):3974−3987. https://doi.org/10.2741/3505.

106. Hernández-Ramírez E, Sánchez-Chávez G, Estrella-Salazar LA, Salceda R. Nitrosative stress in the rat retina at the onset of streptozotocin-induced diabetes. *Cell Physiol Biochem Int J Exp Cell Physiol Biochem Pharmacol*. 2017;42(6):2353−2363. https://doi.org/10.1159/000480007.

107. Hammes HP, Martin S, Federlin K, Geisen K, Brownlee M. Aminoguanidine treatment inhibits the development of experimental diabetic retinopathy. *Proc Natl Acad Sci U S A*. 1991;88(24):11555−11558. https://doi.org/10.1073/pnas.88.24.11555.

108. Hammes HP, Strödter D, Weiss A, Bretzel RG, Federlin K, Brownlee M. Secondary intervention with aminoguanidine retards the progression of diabetic retinopathy in the rat model. *Diabetologia*. 1995;38(6):656−660. https://doi.org/10.1007/BF00401835.

109. Mueller-Buehl AM, Tsai T, Hurst J, et al. Reduced retinal degeneration in an oxidative stress organ culture model through an iNOS-inhibitor. *Biology*. 2021;10(5):383. https://doi.org/10.3390/biology10050383.

110. Carr BC, Emigh CE, Bennett LD, Pansick AD, Birch DG, Nguyen C. Towards a treatment for diabetic retinopathy: intravitreal toxicity and preclinical safety evaluation of inducible nitric oxide synthase inhibitors. *Retina Phila Pa*. 2017;37(1):22−31. https://doi.org/10.1097/IAE.0000000000001133.

111. Kiss L, Szabó C. The pathogenesis of diabetic complications: the role of DNA injury and poly(ADP-ribose) polymerase activation in peroxynitrite-mediated cytotoxicity. *Mem Inst Oswaldo Cruz*. 2005;100(Suppl 1):29−37. https://doi.org/10.1590/s0074-02762005000900007.

112. Pacher P, Szabó C. Role of poly(ADP-ribose) polymerase-1 activation in the pathogenesis of diabetic complications: endothelial dysfunction, as a common underlying theme. *Antioxid Redox Signal*. 2005;7(11−12):1568−1580. https://doi.org/10.1089/ars.2005.7.1568.

113. Zheng L, Szabó C, Kern TS. Poly(ADP-ribose) polymerase is involved in the development of diabetic retinopathy via regulation of nuclear factor-kappaB. *Diabetes*. 2004;53(11):2960−2967. https://doi.org/10.2337/diabetes.53.11.2960.

114. Sumarriva K, Uppal K, Ma C, et al. Arginine and carnitine metabolites are altered in diabetic retinopathy. *Invest Ophthalmol Vis Sci*. 2019;60(8):3119−3126. https://doi.org/10.1167/iovs.19-27321.

115. Peters KS, Rivera E, Warden C, et al. Plasma arginine and citrulline are elevated in diabetic retinopathy. *Am J Ophthalmol*. 2022;235:154−162. https://doi.org/10.1016/j.ajo.2021.09.021.

116. Jin H, Zhu B, Liu X, Jin J, Zou H. Metabolic characterization of diabetic retinopathy: an 1H-NMR-based metabolomic approach using human aqueous humor. *J Pharm Biomed Anal*. 2019;174:414−421. https://doi.org/10.1016/j.jpba.2019.06.013.

117. Tomita Y, Cagnone G, Fu Z, et al. Vitreous metabolomics profiling of proliferative diabetic retinopathy. *Diabetologia*. 2021;64(1):70−82. https://doi.org/10.1007/s00125-020-05309-y.

118. Jiang H, Du J, He T, Qu J, Song Z, Wu S. Increased D-serine in the aqueous and vitreous humour in patients with proliferative diabetic retinopathy: role of D-serine in retinal ganglion cell death. *Clin Exp Ophthalmol*. 2014;42(9):841−845. https://doi.org/10.1111/ceo.12329.

119. Jiang H, Zhang H, Jiang X, Wu S. Overexpression of D-amino acid oxidase prevents retinal neurovascular pathologies in diabetic rats. *Diabetologia*. 2021;64(3): 693−706. https://doi.org/10.1007/s00125-020-05333-y.

120. Jiang H, Fang J, Wu B, et al. Overexpression of serine racemase in retina and overproduction of D-serine in eyes of streptozotocin-induced diabetic retinopathy. *J Neuroinflammation*. 2011;8(1):119. https://doi.org/10.1186/1742-2094-8-119.

121. Jiang H, Du J, Song J, et al. Loss-of-function mutation of serine racemase attenuates retinal ganglion cell loss in diabetic mice. *Exp Eye Res*. 2018;175:90−97. https://doi.org/10.1016/j.exer.2018.06.017.

122. Ozaki H, Inoue R, Matsushima T, Sasahara M, Hayashi A, Mori H. Serine racemase deletion attenuates neurodegeneration and microvascular damage in diabetic retinopathy. *PLoS One*. 2018;13(1):e0190864. https://doi.org/10.1371/journal.pone.0190864.

123. Hou XW, Wang Y, Pan CW. Metabolomics in diabetic retinopathy: a systematic review. *Invest Ophthalmol Vis Sci*. 2021;62(10):4. https://doi.org/10.1167/iovs.62.10.4.

124. Gurudas S, Frudd K, Maheshwari JJ, et al. Multicenter evaluation of diagnostic circulating biomarkers to detect sight-threatening diabetic retinopathy. *JAMA Ophthalmol*. May 5, 2022. https://doi.org/10.1001/jamaophthalmol.2022.1175.

125. Natarajan R. Epigenetic mechanisms in diabetic vascular complications and metabolic memory: the 2020 Edwin Bierman award lecture. *Diabetes*. 2021;70(2):328−337. https://doi.org/10.2337/dbi20-0030.

126. Reddy MA, Zhang E, Natarajan R. Epigenetic mechanisms in diabetic complications and metabolic memory. *Diabetologia*. 2015;58(3):443−455. https://doi.org/10.1007/s00125-014-3462-y.

127. Engerman RL, Kern TS. Progression of incipient diabetic retinopathy during good glycemic control. *Diabetes*. 1987;36(7):808−812. https://doi.org/10.2337/diab.36.7.808.

128. Nathan DM, Cleary PA, Backlund JYC, et al. Intensive diabetes treatment and cardiovascular disease in patients with type 1 diabetes. *N Engl J Med*. 2005;353(25): 2643−2653. https://doi.org/10.1056/NEJMoa052187.

129. Breving K, Esquela-Kerscher A. The complexities of microRNA regulation: miranderring around the rules. *Int J Biochem Cell Biol*. 2010;42(8):1316−1329. https://doi.org/10.1016/j.biocel.2009.09.016.

130. Brasacchio D, Okabe J, Tikellis C, et al. Hyperglycemia induces a dynamic cooperativity of histone methylase and demethylase enzymes associated with gene-activating epigenetic marks that coexist on the lysine tail. *Diabetes*. 2009;58(5):1229−1236. https://doi.org/10.2337/db08-1666.

131. Miller RG, Orchard TJ. Understanding metabolic memory: a tale of two studies. *Diabetes*. 2020;69(3):291−299. https://doi.org/10.2337/db19-0514.

Diabetic retinopathy, a neurovascular unit disease

3

Impairment of diverse cell types, rather than just vascular cells, in the diabetic retina has led to a new paradigm that diabetic retinopathy (DR) should be defined as a disease of the neurovascular unit (NVU). The concept of NVU, which was originally applied to the central nervous system (CNS), has now been utilized to understand retinal circuits and the blood–retinal barrier (BRB).[1–3] The distinct molecular characteristics of NVU depend on the segmentally specific vasculature of CNS. Because of the heterogeneity of cellular components of CNS, no single prototype of NVU is replicated at all levels of the vascular network. However, the concept of any specific NVU module has to be understood that neuronal signals regulate nearby microvessels to support the metabolic needs of the cells of CNS.[4] In this regard, the inner retinal NVU (iNVU) comprises vascular cells, neurons, Müller glia, astrocytes, and extracellular matrix (ECM), while the outer retina/choroid neurovascular unit (oNVU), which was previously called neurovascular complex,[5] consists of photoreceptors, Müller glia, retinal pigment epithelium (RPE) with its ECM, and choriocapillaris. These cellular and extracellular components of iNVU and oNVU interact each other and integrate to form inner and outer BRB (oBRB) to maintain normal retinal functions (Fig. 3.1).

Diabetes impacts the iNVU and oNVU, causing disturbance of neurovascular coupling, resulting in dysfunction of BRB. The inner and outer BRB (iBRB and oBRB) are not merely selective diffusion barriers but also a coupling between neurosensory retina and peripheral circulations. The dysfunction of iBRB and oBRB results in dysregulation of retinal blood flow (RBF) and choroidal blood flow (ChBF), respectively. In diabetic retina, the altered iBRB function and RBF are characterized as an increase in vessel permeability and vascular abnormalities, representing hemorrhage, hard exudates, retinal edema, microaneurysms, cotton wool spots, venous beading, intraretinal microvascular abnormalities, and ultimately neovascularization. The altered oBRB and abnormal ChBF in diabetic animal models lead to disturbance of electrochemical impulses in response to light stimulation and to interruption of diffusion of nutrients and oxygen from choroidal vessels through RPE, resulting in decreased visual functions.[7,8] Therefore, disruption of iNVU and oNVU may contribute to the pathogenesis of microangiopathy and neurodegeneration of diabetic retina and may be considered as therapeutic targets.

Therapeutic Targets for Diabetic Retinopathy. https://doi.org/10.1016/B978-0-323-93064-2.00005-6

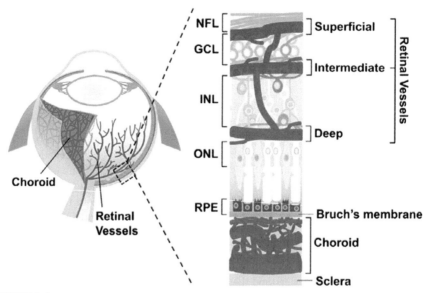

FIGURE 3.1

Schematic drawing of retinal and choroidal circulations. These two are completely separated vascular systems comprising inner and outer blood–retinal barrier (BRB). GCL, ganglion cell layer; INL, inner nuclear layer; NFL, nerve fiber layer; ONL, outer nuclear layer.

Modified from Xia and Rizzolo.[6]

Embryonic origins of neurosensory retina and RPE

Based on the definition of NVU, there must be an interface between the CNS and the peripheral circulatory system. The physical and functional barrier of the neurosensory retina is located at the level of retinal capillary endothelial cells (ECs) with tight junctions as iBRB and RPE cells with tight junctions as oBRB. The neurosensory retina and RPE are part of the CNS due to its embryological origins.[9,10] The intimate anatomic relationship between retinal neurons and RPE starts from early embryonic development through the process of organogenesis of the eye, which begins at embryonic day 25. As the neural tube closes, the optic vesicles remain attached to the neural tube by optic stalks composed of neuroectodermal cells. As the optic vesicle approaches the outer wall of the embryo, cell populations in the optic vesicle differentiate and extend, resulting in the invagination of its temporal and lower walls and the formation of the two-layered optic cup. Neuroectodermal cells of the inner layer of the optic cup evolve as the neurosensory retina. Differentiation of the neurosensory retina begins at the center of the optic cup and gradually expands peripherally. Photoreceptors are neurons located at the outermost layer of the neurosensory retina. Differentiation of the photoreceptors and glial cells in the fovea occurs simultaneously. Among different cell types, synapses as well as intercellular junctions are established by 15 weeks of gestation. The fovea becomes the focal point of the retina. The highest concentration of photoreceptors is in the central retina, which facilitates central vision and permits high-resolution visual acuity. On the other hand, RPE is derived from the outer layer of the optic cup. By eight weeks of gestation, RPE is organized as a single layer of hexagonal columnar cells adjacent to the developing neurosensory retina. RPE cells are polarized epithelial cells. They have long, microvillous processes on their apical surfaces interdigitating with the outer segments of photoreceptors. The basement membrane of the RPE becomes the inner portion of Bruch's membrane. The outer layer of Bruch's membrane is also a basement membrane, which is laid down by the choriocapillaris. Thus, the development of RPE cells has a profound impact on the development of both the choroid and neurosensory retina.

Inner and outer blood—retinal barrier

The inner retina circulation has superficial, intermediate, and deep capillary plexus in the ganglion cell layer and inner nuclear layer. The glial components in iNVU, including astrocytes, Müller cells, and microglia, reside in close proximity to microvascular segments and retinal neurons. The iBRB provides tight control of the neuronal environment regulating the flux of blood borne materials into the neural parenchyma.

We know that the outer retina relies on choroidal circulation, but studies on oBRB are limited. The outer retina comprises photoreceptors, RPE cells, Müller cells, and microglia. The functions of oBRB, specifically the tight junctions of the RPE, include protection of the retina from oxidative stress, facilitation of nutrient delivery and waste disposal, ionic homeostasis, phagocytosis of shed photoreceptor outer segments, synthesis and reisomerization of all-trans-retinal during the visual cycle, and establishment of ocular immune privilege. The RPE is the major component of the oBRB and lies between the choroid and retinal photoreceptors. It is also the key player in the maintenance of retinal tissue integrity because this barrier maintains proper neural homeostasis and protects the neural tissue from potentially harmful factors. The external limiting membrane (ELM) is also part of the oBRB, formed by heterotypic tight-like and adherens junctions, located at the interface between Müller cells and photoreceptor inner segment.[11] And the ELM serves as an important barrier to free protein diffusion across the retina from the inner retina to the subretinal space and *vice versa*. In addition, RPE cells interact with Müller cells. Although these two types of cells do not directly contact each other, they are the major contributors to the pool of secreted molecules, that is, secretome, in the retinal milieu.[12] Secreted trophic factors are key to maintaining the structural and functional integrity of the retina, as they regulate cellular pathways responsible for survival, functionality, and response to injury.

The iBRB and oBRB share important common features as highly selective barriers (Fig. 3.1). They regulate flux of solutes, known as the net quantity over time across a barrier, and permeability, known as the property of the barrier. Changes in permeability across the vessels may occur through changes in transport across the cells, that is, transcytosis, or through changes in the junctional complex connecting cells, leading to flux around the cells or paracellular permeability. Both transcellular and paracellular routes contribute to altered flux.[13] In both iBRB and oBRB, the tight control of solute and fluid flux across the endothelium or RPE layer is conferred by well-developed tight junctions. Tight junctions serve two main functions: gate function that restricts the passage of molecules through the paracellular space and fence function that confers cell polarity by preventing movement of lipids and proteins between the apical and basolateral plasma membrane.[14,15]

Meanwhile, the retinal and choroidal vasculatures differ in several anatomic and physiologic features. Retinal circulation is characterized by a low blood flow, while blood flow in the choroid is high.[16,17] Retinal vessels lack autonomic innervation,[18] whereas the choroidal circulation is innervated by both sympathetic and parasympathetic nerves. In addition, autoregulation is present in the retinal circulation but is lacking in choroidal vessels.[19] Responses to light stimulation also differ. As described below, functional hyperemia (FH) is the coupling mechanism between neural activity and blood flow. The test of retinal FH is the response of the retinal vasculature to light stimulation. Although the choroidal blood flow does not respond well to flickering light stimuli, choroidal vessels do respond to the adaptation state of the eye. A higher choroidal blood flow is observed in the light than in the dark.[20,21] The retinal and choroidal vasculatures are two separate vascular systems with different hierarchies, hemodynamic properties, and regulatory mechanisms. For example, retinal and choroidal vessels have different embryological development. After maturation of these two vascular systems, the ratio of pericytes to ECs (P/E) is about 1:1 in retina, which is the highest in the body, whereas that ratio in choriocapillaris is only a fraction of the P/E ratio in retina.[22–24] Whether and how the high density of retinal capillary pericytes contributes to neurovascular coupling require further exploration, but the contractile dynamics of pericytes suggest that they have a greater impact on resting microvascular perfusion than on fast hemodynamic responses.[4,25] These data suggest that retinal and choroidal, that is, inner and outer neurovascular systems, are distinct but codependent to maintain their homeostasis.

Neurovascular coupling in inner and outer retina

The retina is a specialized neural tissue that senses light and initiates image transmission to the brain. Light-stimulated neuronal activity within the retina evokes local increase of blood flow known as FH. FH in the retina is typically studied by stimulating the eye with a flickering light. The resultant increase in blood flow ensures that active neurons receive sufficient oxygen and nutrients to maintain retinal function. FH maximally activates amacrine cells and retinal ganglion cells (RGCs) in the inner retina.[26] A flickering stimulus dilates the arterioles in both the superficial and deep capillary plexus. Flickering light also increases blood flow in the capillaries of the optic disc.[19]

FH is mediated, either directly or indirectly, by signaling from neurons to blood vessels. Early studies favored a metabolic negative feedback mechanism.[27] It was proposed that the increased neuronal activity leads to a deficit in energy reserves in active neurons. The activated neurons generate metabolic signals that dilate local controlled blood vessels. The resultant increase in blood flow augments glucose and oxygen supplies and restores the energy reserves of the active neurons.[28] Several metabolism-related molecules whose alterations serve as neurovascular coupling signals have been identified, such as a lack of O_2 or glucose, or increases in CO_2 or lactate levels. However, the effects of these direct metabolism-related molecules on vessel dilation may be transitory, probably because the increase in blood flow elicited by neural activity washes them away rapidly, as shown by the rapid washout of elevated CO_2 levels.[27] More recent work has shown that control of the vascular energy supply by neural activity is largely mediated by feedforward mechanisms. The signaling pathways that mediate neurovascular coupling in the neurosensory retina are summarized in Fig. 3.2. In these processes, neurons either signal directly to blood vessels or activate astrocytes to release vasoactive agents onto the vessels. For both of these signaling routes, the coupling mechanisms involve neurotransmitter, particularly glutamate signaling pathway (Fig. 3.2). An alternative to the metabolic negative feedback mechanism of neurovascular coupling is a feedforward mechanism. Evidence exists that multiple signaling pathways contribute to feedforward neurovascular coupling in the CNS. Active neurons release nitric oxide (NO) and prostaglandin E2 (PGE2), both of which relax vascular pericytes or smooth muscle cells and result in vasodilation (Fig. 3.2). Active neurons also release a number of transmitters that act on glial metabotropic receptors, evoking Ca^{2+} increases in glial cells. These Ca^{2+} increases lead to the release of vasodilatory agents from glial cells, including K^+ and the arachidonic acid metabolites PGE2 and epoxyeicosatrienoic acids. The process of FH requires highly complex communication among different cell types in NVU involving neurons and blood vessels, with glial cells playing a central role in the signaling pathway. Fig. 3.2 depicts an example of the feedforward mechanisms mediating neurovascular coupling in the inner retina.[19]

On the other hand, the mechanism that mediates neurovascular coupling between photoreceptors and choroidal circulation is complicated and goes beyond the FH theory.[30] An interaction between ChBF and light-induced photoreceptor activity, a physiological coupling, also exists. Choroidal vessels can respond to the adaptation state of the eye, with higher ChBF observed in the light than in the dark; the choroidal blood supply does not respond well to flickering light stimuli.[31] Lovasik et al. observed that when increasing the blue flicker luminance from low to high in a cohort of healthy individuals, subfoveal ChBF, in terms of volume and velocity, was attenuated.[31] This finding indicates that at the subfoveal region with dense cone population, the outer retina neurovascular coupling might still follow the mechanism of FH. Meanwhile, this finding argues against a dark-induced or flicker-induced FH in the choroid as a result of the demands of the whole outer retina because the ChBF

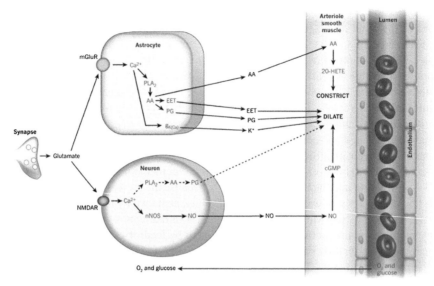

FIGURE 3.2

Summary of signaling pathways that mediate neurovascular coupling by feedforward mechanism in the central nervous system including neurosensory retina. Synaptically released glutamate acts on NMDA receptors in neurons (NMDARs) to raise $[Ca^{2+}]i$, causing neuronal nitric oxide synthase (nNOS) to release NO, which activates smooth muscle guanylate cyclase. Raised $[Ca^{2+}]i$ may also (*dashed line*) generate arachidonic acid (AA) from phospholipase A2 (PLA2), which is converted to prostaglandins (PGss) that dilate vessels. Glutamate also raises $[Ca^{2+}]i$ in astrocytes by activating metabotropic glutamate receptors (mGluRs), generating arachidonic acid and three types of AA metabolites: prostaglandins and EETs in astrocytes, which dilate vessels, and 20-HETE in smooth muscle, which constricts vessels. A rise of $[Ca^{2+}]i$ in astrocyte endfeet may also activate Ca^{2+}-gated K^+ channels (gK(Ca); alternative abbreviation, BK), releasing K^+, which also dilates vessels. In the retina, Müller glial cells are activated by ATP rather than glutamate released from neurons. Calcium increases in Müller cells result in the release of PG and EETs onto smooth muscle cells, which dilate vessels, and 20-HETE production, which constricts vessels; from Attwell *et al.*[27]

Modified from Kur et al.[29]

is not statistically different with flicker stimulation or dark adaptation.[30] Another explanation of this phenomenon is that the blue light-induced photoreceptor response is associated with a differential distribution of the ChBF across the ocular fundus from subfoveal region to the periphery.[31] Indeed, the mechanism of blood distribution is important to regulate ChBF. By using indocyanine green fluorescence angiography, it has been shown that choriocapillaris lobules fill and dissipate the blood entering the choroid during each cardiac cycle. Depending upon the distribution of pressure gradients across a group of lobules, choroidal blood may be regulated to flow from one lobule into others.[32]

Taken together, the available evidence suggests that outer retinal oxygen/glucose consumption is increased when the retina is fully dark adapted, but that ChBF is unchanged. The neurovascular coupling between the photoreceptors and choriocapillaris does not show a clear response to the outer retinal metabolism because signaling pathways from the photoreceptors would have to cross the RPE/Bruch's membrane to affect the regulatory system in the choroid. The signal may become insignificant due to enzymatic degradation, impaired uptake systems, and choriocapillaris washout over the long diffusion distance. It has been proposed that the high basal ChBF is sufficient to maintain adequate oxygen supplies irrespective of light or dark adaptation.[30]

Altered neurovascular coupling of inner retina in DR

The diabetic disturbance of neurovascular coupling in inner retina mainly consists of altered basal blood flow and loss of FH. Studies on the basal blood flow in diabetic retina have generated controversial results, with both increases and decreases being reported. The cause of this discrepancy is complex, probably related to different diabetes type, stage, and severity, and the various measuring techniques utilized.[33] However, a consensus was reached based on a cohort study of diabetic patients. In the early stages of diabetes, RBF decreases by ∼33% compared to the healthy controls, then increases in the advanced stages.[34] Importantly, the increases in the basal blood flow correlate with the severity of retinopathy. Interestingly, the magnitude of decrease in RBF in diabetic animals with experimental non-proliferative diabetic retinopathy (NPDR) shows a similar decrement (∼33%) of retinal flow.[35] The FH response is altered dramatically in diabetic retinas. In nondiabetic subjects, light stimulation produces pronounced vasodilation, while in diabetic patients, light-evoked vasodilation is significantly reduced.[36–38] The light-evoked vasodilation is reduced by ∼60% in arteries and ∼30% in veins of patients with both type 1 and type 2 diabetes.[37,38] Importantly, these reductions in FH occur before the appearance of overt clinical retinopathy in patients.[39] The early loss of FH may be a useful indicator for the onset and progression of DR.[28,29]

The loss of FH in diabetic retina is due to an upregulation of inducible nitric oxide synthase (iNOS) in retinal neurons and glial cells, resulting in an increase in NO levels in the retina (Fig. 3.2).[29,40] The increased NO reduces neurovascular coupling, leading to diminished light-evoked arteriole dilation.[41] The mechanism for the NO-induced reduction in neurovascular coupling is complex and in part modulated by glial cells that regulate vasomotor responses.[41] Using experimental diabetic animal models, inhibition of iNOS, which leads to a reduction in retinal NO levels, results in a restoration of neurovascular coupling in diabetic retinas. For instance, an iNOS inhibitor, aminoguanidine (AMG), restores light-evoked vasodilation to the baseline in isolated diabetic rat retina.[42] In diabetic animals, AMG is able to restore light-evoked vasodilation to control levels.[42,43]

Overall, targeting dysregulation of neurovascular coupling of inner retina is a conceptual approach for treatment of early DR, specifically through control of basal blood flow and/or FH. The loss of light-evoked increases in blood flow in diabetic retina may reduce the supply of oxygen and nutrients to the retina and lead to retinal hypoxia. It has been suggested that hypoxia could exacerbate or even be a root cause of DR. As described above, inhibiting iNOS with AMG, which restores FH in animal models of diabetes, was also used in a clinical trial.[44] The study did not demonstrate statistically significant beneficial effects on the slowing of retinopathy, and some patients receiving high-dose AMG experienced glomerulonephritis.[43] More works need to be done with different agents that can regulate inner RBF in diabetic patients.

Altered neurovascular coupling of outer retina in DR

In contrast to the inner retina, the choroidal circulation, the only blood supply of outer retina, is controlled by extrinsic autonomic innervation. As the choroid is behind the retina and cannot respond readily to retinal metabolic signals, its innervation is important for adjustments of flow required by either retinal activity or by fluctuations in the systemic blood pressure that drive choroidal perfusion. The parasympathetic innervation has been shown to vasodilate and increase ChBF; the sympathetic input has been shown to vasoconstrict and decrease ChBF.[16] The metabolic demand of neurosensory retina and systemic blood pressure triggers neurogenic control that ensures the blood supply to the retina and the stability of ChBF despite fluctuations in ocular perfusion pressure. These key factors have characterized the neurovascular coupling between outer retina neuronal/glial cells and ChBF.[29] Basal neurogenic choroidal tone and/or adaptive ChBF neural control may be impaired by aging or diseases. For example, reductions in basal ChBF occur in the aging macula and in diabetic retina.[33] The diminished ChBF and/or its neural control plays an important role in the progression of DR because the resultant increase in blood viscosity is a possible contributing factor to hypoperfusion to the retina.[45] Although it is uncertain whether ChBF declines in DR stem from disturbed neural control, vascular pathology, or both, improving ChBF and its adaptive regulation may be a viable therapeutic strategy.[29]

There are two specific cellular and molecular features of choroidal vasculature that differ from the retinal vasculature. First, it is the absence of choroidal pericyte desmin expression, which is an intermediate filament responsible for the control of vascular tone.[46] Second, the pericyte ensheathment of choroidal vessels is scarce in comparison with that of retinal pericytes.[47] What is the functional significance of the lack of desmin in choroidal pericytes and the infrequency of pericyte ensheathment? What is the pathologic significance of these special features of choroidal vessels in control of choroidal blood flow in diabetes? In addition to these questions, further study on diabetic oNVU in regards to the understanding of pericyte—EC interaction in choriocapillaris, neural control of ChBF, and choroidal blood viscosity and perfusion is required.

Compromised intercellular communication and BRB breakdown in DR

The NVU refers to interdependency among the vascular cells including ECs and pericytes, neurons, glia, RPE cells, and retina-resident immune cells. The interdependent vascular cells of NVU construct BRB. The BRB structurally consists of inner and outer components, the iBRB being formed by pericytes and EC with tight junctions and the oBRB of tight junctions between RPE cells. The function of BRB, that is, iBRB connecting the inner retina and retinal vasculature, and oBRB linking outer retina and choroidal circulation, is to maintain the integrity of the entire retina. This section focuses on compromised intercellular communication within the NVU in DR.[48−50]

Pericyte−EC interaction in DR

Accelerated apoptosis of retinal vascular cells is a key feature of DR.[51] Metabolic abnormalities in diabetic retina, including apoptotic signaling pathways in both pericytes and ECs, lead to inadequate accessibility of cell survival molecules due to compromised BRB.[51−53] Critical functions of pericyte−EC interaction depend on gap junction intercellular communication (GJIC). GJIC is mediated by docking of connexin hemichannels on two adjacent cells. Through the gap junctions, membrane channels directly connect the cytoplasms of the two cell types. This kind of conduit allows communication of electrical signals between cells and the exchange of selected molecules (Fig. 3.3).[50,54]

The association of pericytes and ECs facilitates their communication through direct contact and GJIC such as connexin 43. High glucose concentrations can induce downregulation of connexin 43 expression and inhibition of GJIC in human cultured retinal pericytes.[55] The decreased connexin 43 levels lead to a significant increase in apoptosis of microvascular cells because the disturbed interaction of GJIC with tight junction proteins causes breakdown of BRB.[56] It has also been shown that high glucose induced oxidative stress hyperphosphorylates connexin 43, leading to the disassembly of gap junctions and degradation of connexin 43 through the proteasome pathway.[50,54,57] Growing evidence shows that the application of a connexin 43 mimetic peptide, peptide 5 that blocks hemichannels, reduces vascular leakage induced by ischemia-reperfusion injury and increases astrocyte cell survival. Another gap junction blocker, carbenoxolone, is able to block intrauterine hypoxia-ischemia induced neuronal apoptosis.[58] These studies point to connexin 43 hemichannels as a potential pharmacological target for the treatment of ischemic retinal damage and DR.[50]

Early pericyte loss, a hallmark of DR pathology, is the consequence of failed pericyte−EC interaction. High glucose levels, *in vitro* as well as *in vivo*, induce pericyte apoptosis,[51] leading to pathological alterations of retinal microvasculature. Regarding the underlying mechanisms, one could surmise that the association of pericyte−EC determines pericyte survival and ECs proliferation through the

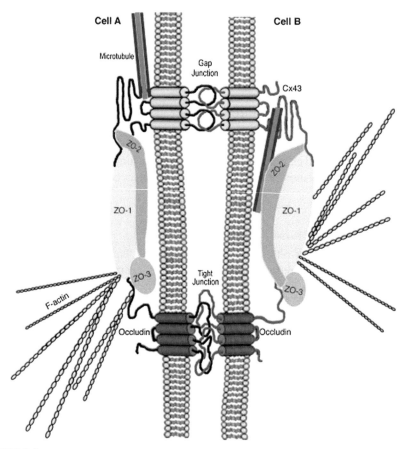

FIGURE 3.3

Schematic representation of gap junction and tight junction organization. Gap junction proteins, such as connexin 43 (Cx43), can directly interact with tight junction proteins and thereby impact barrier characteristics.

Modified from Roy et al.[50]

transforming growth factor β (TGF-β)—mediated signaling pathway.[59] Evidence exists that in the process of angiogenesis, high numbers of pericytes participate in sprouting and remodeling blood vessels. Pericyte coverage is required for the survival of ECs and the stabilization of immature endothelial tubes.[60] Numerous factors including vascular endothelial growth factor (VEGF), angiopoietin-2, TGF-β, platelet-derived growth factor B (PDGF-B), and metalloproteinases are required for the survival and differentiation of both pericytes and ECs. Particularly, PDGF-B, secreted by ECs, and its receptor PDGFR expressed by pericytes are essential to the proliferation, migration, and recruitment of pericytes to the vasculature.[61] On the other hand, pericyte-produced VEGF stimulates ECs proliferation, while TGF-β inhibits ECs proliferation. When pericytes drop out in early diabetic retina, the pericyte—EC interaction is disturbed and BRB maintenance becomes unbalanced, leading to abnormal retinal vasculature.[52,59] Retinal vascular cell apoptosis and angiogenesis in DR are discussed in Chapters 4 and 7, respectively.

Interdependent vascular, neuronal, and glial cells in diabetic inner retina

As described above, DR is considered to be a disorder of both iNVU and oNVU, involving both neurodegeneration and microangiopathy. Clinically, prior to abnormalities in retinal vasculature, changes of visual function have been observed in diabetic patients. Electrophysiologic function testing such as pattern electroretinogram, microperimetric and perimetric testing specifically points to deficits of RGCs.[62] Other cellular testing specific for the inner retina also reveals alterations in diabetic retina such as increased implicit times and reduction in oscillatory potentials in the multifocal ERG.[63] Other less cellular-specific testing such as abnormal dark adaptation, contrast sensitivity, and color vision is also used to detect early DR.[64,65] Optical coherence tomography (OCT) has become the most widely utilized method for imaging studies of individual retinal layers. Currently, several OCT-detected alterations are used to characterize neurons, neuronal synapses, and glial cells in the diabetic retina. These OCT characteristics of diabetic retina include ganglion cell/ nerve fiber layer thinning, disorganization of the retinal inner layers (DRILs), photoreceptor disruption, and hyperreflective foci (HRF) in the inner and/or outer retinal layers, an indicator of microglia activation and migration.[66-69] With improving OCT/OCT angiography (OCTA) techniques, more rapid and precise biomarkers of DR may be utilized to discover early diabetic retinal neurodegeneration.

In the process of neurodegeneration, Müller glia activation is an important event. Müller cells are the primary macroglial cells in the retina, representing 90% of the retinal glia. Since Müller cells have contacts with virtually every cell type in the retina including neurons and vascular cells, they are uniquely positioned to perform a wide variety of functions necessary to maintaining retinal homeostasis. One of the early signs of retinal metabolic stress is the upregulation of glial fibrillary acidic protein (GFAP) by Müller cells. GFAP, a common marker of reactive gliosis and Müller cell activation, was reported to be upregulated in diabetic animal models as well as in tissues from diabetic patients with no to mild NPDR.[70-73] Furthermore, a progressive increase in the expression of GFAP is correlated with diabetes progression in animal models.[74] Müller cells are a primary site of energy metabolism for the inner retina. Müller cells depend primarily on glycolysis rather than oxidative phosphorylation (OxPhos). This is essential as it spares oxygen for retinal neurons and other cell types that use OxPhos for ATP production.[75] Müller cells are also the primary site of glycogen storage in the retina.[75] When nutrient supplies are low, Müller cells can utilize this glycogen storage to provide metabolites for other cell types. Furthermore, the large amounts of lactate that Müller cells produce via glycolysis and irreversible conversion of pyruvate to lactate by a specific lactate dehydrogenase isoform can be transported to photoreceptors to be used as a potential alternative source of energy in case of need.[75,76] Therefore, Müller cells are the center of glucose, nutrient, and energy ecosystems of the retinal NVU (Fig. 3.4).[77]

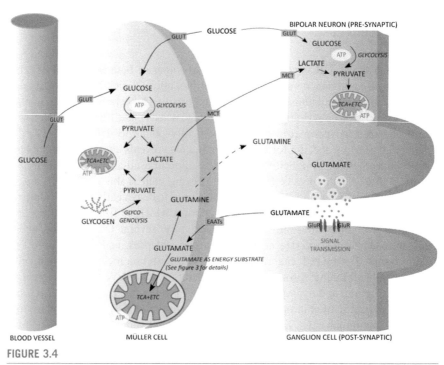

FIGURE 3.4

An illustration of the metabolic coupling between Müller cells and retinal neurons in an intimate partnership with the retinal blood vessel. Glucose is transferred from the circulation to the Müller cells and metabolized via glycolysis. Subsequently, lactate can be transported to retinal neurons as well as glucose from the extracellular environment. The transportation of lactate from Müller cells to neurons is referred to as the lactate shuttle. In contrast to retinal neurons, the Müller cells hold an intracellular glycogen reservoir as an additional energy source. Nevertheless, Müller cells rely mainly on glycolytic derived energy, whereas the viability of retinal neurons depends primarily on oxidative metabolism. Müller cells play a key role in the maintenance of the glutamine–glutamate cycling, since glutamate is eliminated from the extracellular space and taken up by the Müller cells. Glutamate is converted to glutamine and transferred back to retinal neurons, deamidated to glutamate, and thereby the neurotransmitter pool is replenished. Preliminary experiments demonstrate that glutamate is metabolized in a truncated TCA cycle in Müller cells and thus functions as an alternative energy substrate during glucose deprivation.

ATP, adenosine triphosphate; EAATs, excitatory amino acid transporters; ETC, electron transport chain; GluR, glutamate receptor; GLUT, glucose transporter; MCT, monocarboxylate transporter; TCA cycle, tricarboxylic acid cycle.

Modified from Toft-Kehler et al.[77]

Müller cells recycle neurotransmitters, prevent glutamate toxicity, and redistribute ions by spatial buffering. Müller cells also participate in the retinoid cycle and regulate nutrient supplies through multiple mechanisms. In diabetes and diabetic macular edema (DME), Müller cells have been shown to downregulate the inwardly rectifying potassium channel 4.1 (Kir4.1), leading to continued potassium uptake with no release into the microvasculature.[78] This leads to swelling of Müller cells and dysfunction of fluid drainage, contributing to DME. After onset of experimental diabetes, the function of the glutamate transporter in Müller cells is decreased by a mechanism that is likely to involve oxidation (Fig. 3.4).[77,79] When stimulated with stress conditions, such as high glucose levels, Müller cells are a significant source for many growth factors and cytokines.[80] Under diabetic conditions, the gene expression profile of Müller cells from streptozotocin-induced diabetic rats revealed 78 altered genes, of which one-third of their gene products are associated with inflammation, for example, VEGF, intercellular adhesion molecule 1, and interleukin (IL)-1β. Of note, the detrimental effects of some of these cytokines, such as IL-6, have been associated with vascular dysfunction and promotion of angiogenesis.[81−83] On the other hand, some cytokines, including IL-6, could also be responsible for maintaining proper neuronal function as well as stimulating neuroprotective effects.[84] These data indicate that Müller cells are critical in maintaining retinal homeostasis and that their cytokine-specific regulatory events could be targeted as novel therapeutic approaches for diabetic NVU. The fate of Müller cells in diabetes has long been a debate. In general, it has been accepted that Müller cells become activated in diabetic retina. However, recent studies show that over a longer course of DR, Müller cells actually undergo cell death pathway. Notably, death of Müller cells in diabetic retina rapidly accelerates when protective endocrine and paracrine growth factors are blunted.[73,85] Recent studies demonstrated that Müller cells undergo a special cell death pathway other than apoptosis, which is known as pyroptosis. There are two molecular signaling pathways of pyroptosis, the caspase-1-dependent canonical and caspase-4/5/11-dependent noncanonical inflammasome pathways.[86−88] Müller cells show increased caspase-1 activity and IL-1β production under hyperglycemic conditions, and the cells die as a consequence.[89] The consequences of Müller cell death are mixed. On the one hand, it may lead to loss of BRB integrity, increased vascular permeability, and loss of neuroprotective functions for both neurons and vascular cells. On the other hand, diminishing activated Müller cells might decrease the pool of proinflammatory molecules. There are questions worthy of further discussion: how to identify the pyroptosis pathway of Müller cells, how to disclose whether or not all subsets of Müller cells are equally affected by hyperglycemia, and how to control the fate of Müller cells in diabetic retina?

Like Müller cells, astrocytes are connected to both retinal blood vessels and neurons and play a critical role in the maintenance of the integrity of BRB.[90] Astrocytes also play an early and key role in the maintenance of retinal vascular integrity in diabetes. For instance, four weeks after diabetes onset, astrocyte connexin-26 and connexin-43 gene and protein expressions are decreased, an indicator of disruption of vascular integrity before significant astrocyte loss.[91] Two months after diabetes onset, reduced GFAP immunoreactivity correlates with the loss of astrocytes.[92] Cumulative studies showed that high glucose conditions alter the function of retinal astrocytes through increased production of inflammatory cytokines and oxidative stress, thus exerting significant impact on their proliferation, adhesion, migration, and regression. In the retina, individual astrocytes maintain simultaneous contact with axons and blood vessels.[93] When astrocytes are activated under diabetic condition, they produce a variety of proinflammatory factors such as cytokines and chemokines. Cytokines are a class of small proteins that act as signaling molecules at picomolar or nanomolar concentrations, including IL-6, IL-1β, IL-8, cyclooxygenase-2, tumor necrosis factor α, epidermal growth factor, macrophage inflammatory protein 2α, and VEGF.[92,94,95] Apart from inflammatory cytokines, reactive astrocytes can secrete chemokines whose generic function is to induce cell migration.[95] These chemokines are involved in the migration of microglia, monocytes/macrophages, T cells, and dendritic cells, amplifying the inflammatory response. During a long course of diabetes, the number of astrocytes seems to decrease in the retina. The decrease in astrocytes disrupts the iBRB, contributing to vascular leakage and retinal dysfunction.[74]

The third type of glial cells in the retina, microglia, are the resident immune cells. They also become activated and start to produce proinflammatory mediators, exacerbating neuroglial and vascular dysfunction in diabetic retina.[96] The elevated activities of microglia in diabetic retina can now be monitored by the presence of HRF on OCT (see Chapter 5).

Overall, interdependent inner retinal neurons, vessels, and glial cells work together as a unit. Diabetes disturbs this interdependency mainly through glial cell—mediated inflammation and Müller cell—mediated metabolic dysfunction. Müller cells are responsible for the removal of neurotransmitters, buffering of potassium, and providing neurons with adequate energy and essential metabolites as described in Fig. 3.4. Müller cells also provide survival signals to protect retinal neurons. For instance, under nondiabetic conditions, there was no significant increase in apoptotic neurons in the retina of conditional *Vegfr2* KO mice relative to controls. However, loss of VEGFR2-mediated signaling in Müller cells significantly increased neuronal apoptosis four months after the onset of diabetes induced by streptozotocin. These findings indicate that VEGFR2 in Müller cells is a survival factor for retinal neurons against diabetic insult. Additionally, another cellular survival factor, pAKT (phosphorylated protein kinase B), was found to be significantly lower in Müller cells of *Vegfr2* KO mice. Although the neuroprotective mechanism(s) of Müller cells through the VEGFR2-AKT pathway in DR is not completely understood, these findings suggest that Müller cell—mediated neuroprotective strategy could potentially be translated into therapeutic options for protecting inner retinal neurons.[85]

Interdependent photoreceptor, glia, and RPE in diabetic outer retina

Traditionally, DR is considered to be a disorder of the inner retina. However, the OCT era has raised the new concept that DR is both an inner and outer retinal disease because the outer retinal changes in DR are readily visualized by OCT. For instance, DME is characterized by both OCT measurable inner and outer retina morphology. These characteristic features of DME include increased central subfield thickness, presence of septae within the intraretinal cystoid abnormalities, presence of HRF, presence and extent of DRIL, and loss of integrity of the ELM and ellipsoid zone (EZ). The ELM is defined as the first hyperreflective band, representative of the junctional complex between the Müller glia and photoreceptor cells. The EZ is defined as the hyperreflective band below the ELM and clinically represents the integrity of photoreceptor layer.[97,98] It is particularly important that the alterations seen on OCT of ELM and EZ are direct evidence of disrupted integrity of the outer retina in diabetic retina.

Although the study on how the outer retinal pathology contributes to the development of DR is limited, increasing evidence shows that the normal RPE, which is the major component of the oBRB between the choroid and neurosensory retina, is key to maintaining the integrity of the retinal tissues.[6] Still, photoreceptors, RPE, and Müller cells, which are working together as oNVU, are codependent. In DR, as the disease progresses, tight junction complexes between RPE cells are disassembling and paracellular leakage can be detected.[83,6] The first example of the loss of cellular codependency is altered glucose utilization in the diabetic outer retina.[99] Glucose from the blood is largely transported across the RPE to photoreceptors. Glucose metabolites such as pyruvate and lactate are transported by Müller cells to neurons, including photoreceptors (Fig. 3.4). Photoreceptors also use glucose through glycolysis to produce energy and the byproduct lactate. The latter is transported back to the RPE for OxPhos. As OxPhos alters in diabetic RPE mitochondria, ATP production is reduced, forcing RPE to rely on glycolysis to maintain the cell's energy requirement. Thus, the flow of glucose to the photoreceptors is reduced. Consequently, the decreased photoreceptor glycolysis could reduce the production of lactate as an energy source for RPE. In other words, suppression of photoreceptor glycolysis associated with decreased lactate promotes glucose overutilization by the RPE, theoretically inducing neuronal dysfunction.[100] However, studies on whether or not photoreceptor cells die in diabetes have generated conflicting results.[98] The discrepancy is probably due to relatively subtle photoreceptor alterations in diabetic retina, rather than overt cell loss. Furthermore, the biomarkers for photoreceptor changes in diabetic retina, specifically disruption of the ELM and loss of integrity of EZ on spectral-domain OCT imaging, might not be sensitive enough.[101] Cumulative evidence reveals that the photoreceptor damage measured by OCTA appears to directly correlate with hypoperfusion of the choriocapillaris.[102] It is worth to mention that in multiple regression analysis, EZ "normalized" reflectivity, which is calculated by a special software, displayed a significant direct association with choriocapillaris perfusion density in patients with NPDR.[102] To date, the exact cause(s) of neuronal damage in outer retina remain unclear. In addition to counter-actions against hyperglycemia-induced abnormal major metabolic pathways as described in Chapter 2, strategies targeting diabetic choroidopathy and improving choriocapillaris perfusion may be a novel therapeutic approach for the protection of photoreceptors.[102]

The second example of the cellular codependency is the altered profile of secre-tory factors in diabetic inner and outer retina. As described above, both Müller cells and RPE cells secrete a number of growth factors, cytokines, and chemokines, contributing to the pool of secreted molecules in retina.[12] (see Chapter 6). Prote-omics studies of RPE cells in a diabetic condition have implicated these proteins in protecting against/inducing stress, structural modifications, mitochondrial traf-ficking, and apoptosis.[103] Proteomics of cadaver RPE from donors with preclinical DR has also revealed alterations in the proteins involved in membrane dynamics, metabolic events, and cytoskeletal structure.[104] The altered profile of secreted fac-tors in retina is dynamic, varying with the different stages of DR (Fig. 3.5). The imbalanced pairs of "agonist versus antagonist" are exemplified by VEGF:PEDF (pigment epithelium-derived factor) and VEGF:CTGF (connective tissue growth factor) (Fig. 3.5). This altered "secretome" in diabetic retina perturbs the structural and functional integrity of the retina, as these factors regulate cellular pathways responsible for survival, functionality, and responses to metabolic insults.

A third example of the cellular codependency is the interaction between RPE and microglial cells, which participates in maintenance of oBRB integrity. Under dia-betic condition, the tight junction complex by ZO-1 and occludin of RPE is disrup-ted.[105] Recent studies on a diabetic animal model showed that upregulation of VEGF-A in RPE cells leads to increase in microglial cell recruitment. The activated microglia produce various inflammatory cytokines and chemokines such as IL-6, which further attract and activate microglial cells.[83] The evidence exists that after intravitreal injection of IL-6 to diabetic animals, microglial cells were attracted to RPE cells, leading to reduced ZO-1 in RPE cells and disrupted oBRB. Since signal transducer and activator of transcription 3 (STAT3) inhibition can block the activity of IL-6-treated microglial cells on the RPE monolayer in vitro, when a STAT3 inhib-itor was applied for diabetic mice, it effectively reversed ZO-1 disruption of RPE cells.[83] This proof-of-concept approach could be translated to the protection of oBRB in diabetes.

Translational study on keeping integrity of inner and outer NVU in diabetic retina

The concept of NVU of the CNS was applied to retina about two decades ago.[2] Within an NVU, neuronal activity evokes local blood flow alteration. This response is called neurovascular coupling or FH. Since single-cell transcriptomic studies have provided molecular insight into the diversity of CNS vasculature, it has been realized that there is no single NVU model replicated at all levels of the neurovascular activ-ity of CNS.[4] Based on the distinct cellular and molecular characteristics of inner and

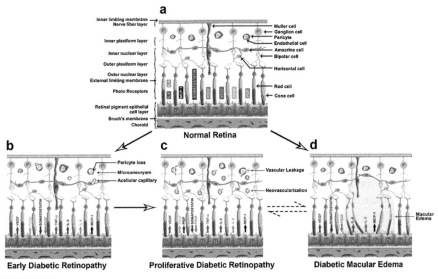

FIGURE 3.5

Schematic representation shows the dynamic profile of retinal secretory factors contributed mainly by Müller and RPE cells in normal retina and DR (A). Schematic representation of the normal retina with the balanced secretion pattern of factors from the RPE toward the neural retina. (B) Illustration of early diabetic retina with loss of pericytes, microaneurysm, acellular capillary formation, and altered secreted factors. (C) Schematic representation of proliferative diabetic retinopathy (PDR) showing clinical manifestations (neovascularization and vitreous hemorrhage) with modulated regulation of antiangiogenic/angiogenic factors, cytokines, and chemokines. VEGF, vascular endothelial growth factor. (D) Schematic representation of diabetic macular edema with an imbalance of secreted factors showing the accumulation of fluid and altered retinal layers.

FGF, fibroblast growth factor; IL, interleukin; MCP-1, monocyte chemoattractant protein-1; PEDF, pigment epithelium-derived factor; PDGF, platelet-derived growth factor; PlGF, placental growth factor; TNF-α, tumor necrosis factor alpha; VEGF, vascular endothelial growth factor. *Solid arrow* represents the sequence of the disease development stages. *Dashed arrow* represents the plausible sequence in advanced DR.

Modified from Ponnalagu et al.[103]

outer retina, the ocular neurovascular coupling may be proposed as inner and outer NVU, respectively. This neurovascular response requires special anatomic relation between CNS and peripheral circulation, such as blood—brain barrier in brain or BRB in retina. The neuron—glia—vascular interaction determines both inner and outer retinal neurovascular coupling, which is protected by inner and oBRB, respectively. The inner retinal vasculature and outer choroidal vasculature are two separate vascular systems with different hierarchies, hemodynamic properties, and regulatory mechanisms. It is well known that diabetes is a systemic metabolic disease. Major hyperglycemia-induced biochemical pathways are activated in the whole retina, affecting all retinal layers, locations, and all types of retinal cells via neuron—glia—vascular interactions. Thus, DR can be defined as a disease of both iNVU and oNVU. With diabetes progression, both inner and outer neurovascular coupling are compromised, leading to retinal neurodegeneration and retina/choroid microangiopathy. Thus, the therapeutic targets for clinical DR are broad, focusing not only on individual cell types or individual pathways but also on the interaction of multiple types of cells and interdependent signaling pathways. Although treatment strategies focusing on NVU disorder are still largely hypothetical, future research may provide insights into neurovascular communication in diabetic retina and choroid, which may have therapeutic value.

First, the future therapies should target both retinal neurodegeneration and retinal vascular abnormalities, particularly targeting signaling pathways that regulate the neuron—glia—vascular axis.[106] For instance, targeting neuroglial cells and regulating amino acid metabolism, it has been evidenced that the decreased D-amino acid oxidase (DAAO) plays a pathogenic role in animal models of DR. D-Serine is degraded by DAAO and synthesized by serine racemase in retinal cells including RGCs, Müller cells, astrocytes, and RPE cells. Intravitreal adenovirus-associated virus 8-mediated DAAO expression (AAV8-DAAO-IRES-ZsGreen) was used to overexpress DAAO, which targets inner and outer NVU and prevents retinal neurovascular abnormalities in diabetic animals.[107]

Second, FH, a regional increase of blood flow, is triggered by local neural activation. This canonical response of neurovascular coupling is clearly shown in the iNVU. Notably, early decrease in FH may be a useful biomarker for the onset and the progression of DR. For instance, in a diabetic animal model and in an isolated retinal tissue, an upregulation of iNOS was detected. Inhibition of iNOS restored both light and glial-evoked vasodilation to control levels, restoring the response of neurovascular coupling in diabetic retinas.[40] In fact, the iNOS selective inhibitor AMG restores light-evoked vasodilation to baseline in isolated diabetic rat retina.[42] In vivo, when AMG was administered chronically through drinking water or by intravenous injection, it also restored light-evoked vasodilation to control levels.[42,108] It should be noted that AMG is also an inhibitor of advanced glycation end products (AGEs). The impact on the normalization of neurovascular coupling in diabetic retina by AMG has been proved to be independent of significant effects on AGEs deposition.[109] Overall, selective iNOS inhibitors, not limited to AMG, require further study.

Third, Müller cells are responsible for the homeostatic and metabolic functions of retinal neurons and vascular cells. In this regard, they act as a linker between neurons and vessels playing an indispensable role in the formation of NVUs. Overall, when retinal neurons such as RGCs are under diabetic stress, Müller cells cannot provide RGCs with sufficient energy sources nor clear excess glutamate from the extracellular space (Fig. 3.4). As the consequences, RGCs may undergo cell death.[110,111] Therefore, improvement of Müller cell functions will have a critical impact on future strategies to treat and prevent RGC death. Recent research has generated more evidence showing the crucial role of Müller cells in repairing neuro-degeneration. A subset of Müller cells can differentiate into neural progenitor/stem cells that regenerate photoreceptors and inner retinal neurons. Because of this potential, Müller cells could be used as cell-based therapy in retinal degenerative diseases including DR. For instance, transdifferentiated Müller cells can be obtained surgically from epiretinal membranes and then identified by neural stem cell marker(s) expressed by Müller cells.[112] Subretinal or intravitreal transplantation may result in migration of this subset of cells into the retinal parenchyma and action of normal neuronal cells.[110]

Fourth, as described above, the impairment of GJIC and the expression of the BRB-specific component connexin 43 have been found in diabetic retina (Fig. 3.3).[113,114] This is a primary mechanism contributing to BRB breakdown and subsequent damage to the NVU in DR. Recent research is exploring whether restoration of diabetes-mediated changes in connexin expression and GJIC may dampen the subsequent effects. For instance, using RNA sequencing, mRNA and miRNA expression profiles of human postmortem retinal samples with various stages of DR were obtained. The data revealed differentially expressed transcripts to be predominantly associated with late-stage DR and related to gap junction signaling. Thus, miR-329 that suppresses expression of CD146, an adhesion molecule acting as a coreceptor for VEGFR2, was used in a mouse model and found to reduce pathological angiogenesis.[115]

Fifth, Müller cells, astrocytes, and microglial cells are all components of NVU. They join in the construction of the BRB. Glial cells monitor the pathological changes of the NVU. They become activated by neuronal stress and cell death in early DR, which is defined as reactive gliosis. Since glial dysfunction is involved in numerous NVU functions, theoretically inhibition of glial activation should be therapeutic, analogous to antiinflammatory therapy for DR. However, the beneficial or destructive effects of pregliotic events under diabetic stress are clinical context dependent. For example, Müller cell activation can contribute to the neuroprotection rather than neuroapoptosis through extracellular signal-related kinase 1/2 activation under hyperglycemic conditions.[116] In contrast, another study using activated Müller cells with VEGF knockout confirmed that the early response of Müller cell−derived VEGF is responsible for vascular leakage and retinal inflammation in DR.[117] Further studies are needed to determine the role of glial cells in different stages of DR and to discover glial cell−specific targets.[48,118]

Sixth, the diabetic impact on oNVU, that is, photoreceptors, RPE, and choriocapillaris, has been documented by OCTA. In NPDR patients, the reduced choriocapillaris density, a biomarker of hypoperfusion is strongly associated with photoreceptor damage.[102] More data showed that oBRB disruption is clearly presented in patients with DME.[11] However, evidence for a pathogenic contribution of oNVU to DR formation is still fragmentary. As existing data showed, 80% of retinal glucose and oxygen supply is from choroidal circulation, for which RPE serves as the most critical monolayer for the transportation and protection of oNVU and photoreceptor survival. It is postulated that the modulation of impaired RPE functions under diabetic conditions is a therapeutic approach for DR. Indeed, clinical photocoagulation that facilitates oxygen perfusion from choroid to neurosensory retina is a proof-of-concept example, although it is tissue-destructive and only appropriate for late-stage DR. On the other hand, the relationship between DR and diabetic choroidopathy remains unclear. Accumulating data show that hyperglycemia affects both the choroidal micro- and macrovasculature, especially via underlying inflammatory mechanisms in choriocapillaris endothelial cells (CECs).[119] Based on early work in our laboratory and other recent reports, CECs respond to mitogens and vasoactive factors differently as compared with retinal capillary ECs.[120,121] This endothelium-specific discrepancy merits further study. For example, single cell RNA sequencing could be used to discover the molecular link between diabetic choroidopathy and retinal neurodegeneration.[120]

Seventh, the imbalance of autoregulation of inner RBF in early DR is usually accompanied with an altered blood distribution and diminished endothelial surface glycoproteins.[34] A recent study revealed the pivotal role of endothelin in the pathogenesis of diabetic complications, particularly in the regulation of the capillary flow, which is affected in the course of DR. There is a correlation between the level of endothelin-1 and the stages of DR.[122] For instance, in preclinical DR, blood concentration of endothelin-1 is increased with worsening microangiopathy. In clinical DR, endothelin-1 is decreased with increased capillary dilation, microaneurysm formation, and fluid leakage. In severe DR, both endothelin-1 and endothelin-3 are increased, accompanied by capillary occlusion, increased retinal ischemia, and neovascularization. Therefore, preventing the early decrease in blood flow and restoring hypoxia and angiogenesis in late-stage DR by targeting the endothelin system may be a useful therapeutic strategy for DR.

References

1. Hawkins BT, Davis TP. The blood-brain barrier/neurovascular unit in health and disease. *Pharmacol Rev.* 2005;57(2):173–185. https://doi.org/10.1124/pr.57.2.4.
2. Metea MR, Newman EA. Signalling within the neurovascular unit in the mammalian retina. *Exp Physiol.* 2007;92(4):635–640. https://doi.org/10.1113/expphysiol.2006.036376.
3. Antonetti DA, Klein R, Gardner TW. Diabetic retinopathy. *N Engl J Med.* 2012;366(13):1227–1239. https://doi.org/10.1056/NEJMra1005073.
4. Schaeffer S, Iadecola C. Revisiting the neurovascular unit. *Nat Neurosci.* 2021;24(9):1198–1209. https://doi.org/10.1038/s41593-021-00904-7.
5. Li W. Age-related macular degeneration. https://www.clinicalkey.com/dura/browse/bookChapter/3-s2.0-C20190040757; 2022. Accessed January 31, 2022.
6. Xia T, Rizzolo LJ. Effects of diabetic retinopathy on the barrier functions of the retinal pigment epithelium. *Vision Res.* 2017;139:72–81. https://doi.org/10.1016/j.visres.2017.02.006.
7. Yu X, Ji C, Shao A. Neurovascular unit dysfunction and neurodegenerative disorders. *Front Neurosci.* 2020;14:334. https://doi.org/10.3389/fnins.2020.00334.

8. Muir ER, Rentería RC, Duong TQ. Reduced ocular blood flow as an early indicator of diabetic retinopathy in a mouse model of diabetes. *Invest Ophthalmol Vis Sci.* 2012;53(10):6488−6494. https://doi.org/10.1167/iovs.12-9758.

9. Jacobson M, Hirose G. Origin of the retina from both sides of the embryonic brain: a contribution to the problem of crossing at the optic chiasma. *Science.* 1978;202(4368):637−639. https://doi.org/10.1126/science.705349.

10. McGill TJ, Osborne L, Lu B, et al. Subretinal transplantation of human central nervous system stem cells stimulates controlled proliferation of endogenous retinal pigment epithelium. *Trans Vis Sci Tech.* 2019;8(3):43. https://doi.org/10.1167/tvst.8.3.43.

11. Daruich A, Matet A, Moulin A, et al. Mechanisms of macular edema: beyond the surface. *Prog Retin Eye Res.* 2018;63:20−68. https://doi.org/10.1016/j.preteyeres.2017.10.006.

12. Araújo RS, Santos DF, Silva GA. The role of the retinal pigment epithelium and Müller cells secretome in neovascular retinal pathologies. *Biochimie.* 2018;155:104−108. https://doi.org/10.1016/j.biochi.2018.06.019.

13. Díaz-Coránguez M, Ramos C, Antonetti DA. The inner blood-retinal barrier: cellular basis and development. *Vis Res.* 2017;139:123−137. https://doi.org/10.1016/j.visres.2017.05.009.

14. Mandel LJ, Bacallao R, Zampighi G. Uncoupling of the molecular "fence" and paracellular "gate" functions in epithelial tight junctions. *Nature.* 1993;361(6412):552−555. https://doi.org/10.1038/361552a0.

15. Dogné S, Flamion B, Caron N. Endothelial glycocalyx as a shield against diabetic vascular complications: involvement of hyaluronan and hyaluronidases. *Arterioscler Thromb Vasc Biol.* 2018;38(7):1427−1439. https://doi.org/10.1161/ATVBAHA.118.310839.

16. Reiner A, Fitzgerald MEC, Del Mar N, Li C. Neural control of choroidal blood flow. *Prog Retin Eye Res.* 2018;64:96−130. https://doi.org/10.1016/j.preteyeres.2017.12.001.

17. Delaey C, Van De Voorde J. Regulatory mechanisms in the retinal and choroidal circulation. *Ophthalmic Res.* 2000;32(6):249−256. https://doi.org/10.1159/000055622.

18. Ye XD, Laties AM, Stone RA. Peptidergic innervation of the retinal vasculature and optic nerve head. *Invest Ophthalmol Vis Sci.* 1990;31(9):1731−1737.

19. Newman EA. Functional hyperemia and mechanisms of neurovascular coupling in the retinal vasculature. *J Cerebr Blood Flow Metabol.* 2013;33(11):1685−1695. https://doi.org/10.1038/jcbfm.2013.145.

20. Fuchsjäger-Mayrl G, Polska E, Malec M, Schmetterer L. Unilateral light-dark transitions affect choroidal blood flow in both eyes. *Vision Res.* 2001;41(22):2919−2924. https://doi.org/10.1016/s0042-6989(01)00171-7.

21. Longo A, Geiser M, Riva CE. Subfoveal choroidal blood flow in response to light-dark exposure. *Invest Ophthalmol Vis Sci.* 2000;41(9):2678−2683.

22. Nag TC, Gorla S, Kumari C, Roy TS. Aging of the human choriocapillaris: evidence that early pericyte damage can trigger endothelial changes. *Exp Eye Res.* 2021;212:108771. https://doi.org/10.1016/j.exer.2021.108771.

23. Shepro D, Morel NML. Pericyte physiology. *Faseb J.* 1993;7(11):1031−1038. https://doi.org/10.1096/fasebj.7.11.8370472.

24. Lutty GA, McLeod DS. Development of the hyaloid, choroidal and retinal vasculatures in the fetal human eye. *Prog Retin Eye Res.* 2018;62:58−76. https://doi.org/10.1016/j.preteyeres.2017.10.001.

25. Caporarello N, D'Angeli F, Cambria MT, et al. Pericytes in microvessels: from "mural" function to brain and retina regeneration. *Int J Mol Sci.* 2019;20(24):E6351. https://doi.org/10.3390/ijms20246351.

26. Werblin FS, Dowling JE. Organization of the retina of the mudpuppy, *Necturus maculosus.* II. Intracellular recording. *J Neurophysiol.* 1969;32(3):339−355. https://doi.org/10.1152/jn.1969.32.3.339.

27. Attwell D, Buchan AM, Charpak S, Lauritzen M, Macvicar BA, Newman EA. Glial and neuronal control of brain blood flow. *Nature.* 2010;468(7321):232−243. https://doi.org/10.1038/nature09613.

28. Nippert AR, Newman EA. Regulation of blood flow in diabetic retinopathy. *Vis Neurosci.* 2020;37:E004. https://doi.org/10.1017/S0952523820000036.

29. Kur J, Newman EA, Chan-Ling T. Cellular and physiological mechanisms underlying blood flow regulation in the retina and choroid in health and disease. *Prog Retin Eye Res.* 2012;31(5):377−406. https://doi.org/10.1016/j.preteyeres.2012.04.004.

30. Shih YYI, Wang L, De La Garza BH, et al. Quantitative retinal and choroidal blood flow during light, dark adaptation and flicker light stimulation in rats using fluorescent microspheres. *Curr Eye Res.* 2013;38(2):292−298. https://doi.org/10.3109/02713683.2012.756526.

31. Lovasik JV, Kergoat H, Wajszilber MA. Blue flicker modifies the subfoveal choroidal blood flow in the human eye. *Am J Physiol Heart Circ Physiol.* 2005;289(2):H683−H691. https://doi.org/10.1152/ajpheart.01187.2004.

32. Flower RW. Extraction of choriocapillaris hemodynamic data from ICG fluorescence angiograms. *Invest Ophthalmol Vis Sci.* 1993;34(9):2720−2729.

33. Pemp B, Schmetterer L. Ocular blood flow in diabetes and age-related macular degeneration. *Can J Ophthalmol.* 2008;43(3):295−301. https://doi.org/10.3129/i08-049.

34. Harris NR, Leskova W, Kaur G, Eshaq RS, Carter PR. Blood flow distribution and the endothelial surface layer in the diabetic retina. *Biorheology.* 2019;56(2−3):181−189. https://doi.org/10.3233/BIR-180200.

35. Clermont AC, Aiello LP, Mori F, Aiello LM, Bursell SE. Vascular endothelial growth factor and severity of nonproliferative diabetic retinopathy mediate retinal hemodynamics in vivo: a potential role for vascular endothelial growth factor in the progression of nonproliferative diabetic retinopathy. *Am J Ophthalmol.* 1997;124(4):433−446. https://doi.org/10.1016/s0002-9394(14)70860-8.

36. Garhöfer G, Zawinka C, Resch H, Kothy P, Schmetterer L, Dorner GT. Reduced response of retinal vessel diameters to flicker stimulation in patients with diabetes. *Br J Ophthalmol.* 2004;88(7):887−891. https://doi.org/10.1136/bjo.2003.033548.

37. Nguyen TT, Kawasaki R, Wang JJ, et al. Flicker light-induced retinal vasodilation in diabetes and diabetic retinopathy. *Diabetes Care.* 2009;32(11):2075−2080. https://doi.org/10.2337/dc09-0075.

38. Pemp B, Garhofer G, Weigert G, et al. Reduced retinal vessel response to flicker stimulation but not to exogenous nitric oxide in type 1 diabetes. *Invest Ophthalmol Vis Sci.* 2009;50(9):4029−4032. https://doi.org/10.1167/iovs.08-3260.

39. Mandecka A, Dawczynski J, Blum M, et al. Influence of flickering light on the retinal vessels in diabetic patients. *Diabetes Care.* 2007;30(12):3048−3052. https://doi.org/10.2337/dc07-0927.

40. Mishra A, Newman EA. Inhibition of inducible nitric oxide synthase reverses the loss of functional hyperemia in diabetic retinopathy. *Glia*. 2010;58(16):1996−2004. https://doi.org/10.1002/glia.21068.

41. Metea MR, Newman EA. Glial cells dilate and constrict blood vessels: a mechanism of neurovascular coupling. *J Neurosci*. 2006;26(11):2862−2870. https://doi.org/10.1523/JNEUROSCI.4048-05.2006.

42. Mishra A, Newman EA. Aminoguanidine reverses the loss of functional hyperemia in a rat model of diabetic retinopathy. *Front Neuroenergetics*. 2011;3:10. https://doi.org/10.3389/fnene.2011.00010.

43. Kern TS, Engerman RL. Pharmacological inhibition of diabetic retinopathy: aminoguanidine and aspirin. *Diabetes*. 2001;50(7):1636−1642. https://doi.org/10.2337/diabetes.50.7.1636.

44. Bolton WK, Cattran DC, Williams ME, et al. Randomized trial of an inhibitor of formation of advanced glycation end products in diabetic nephropathy. *Am J Nephrol*. 2004;24(1):32−40. https://doi.org/10.1159/000075627.

45. Sebag J, Tang M, Brown S, Sadun AA, Charles MA. Effects of pentoxifylline on choroidal blood flow in nonproliferative diabetic retinopathy. *Angiology*. 1994;45(6):429−433. https://doi.org/10.1177/000331979404500603.

46. Hughes S, Chan-Ling T. Characterization of smooth muscle cell and pericyte differentiation in the rat retina in vivo. *Invest Ophthalmol Vis Sci*. 2004;45(8):2795−2806. https://doi.org/10.1167/iovs.03-1312.

47. Chan-Ling T, Koina ME, McColm JR, et al. Role of CD44+ stem cells in mural cell formation in the human choroid: evidence of vascular instability due to limited pericyte ensheathment. *Invest Ophthalmol Vis Sci*. 2011;52(1):399−410. https://doi.org/10.1167/iovs.10-5403.

48. Antonetti DA, Silva PS, Stitt AW. Current understanding of the molecular and cellular pathology of diabetic retinopathy. *Nat Rev Endocrinol*. 2021;17(4):195−206. https://doi.org/10.1038/s41574-020-00451-4.

49. Cunha-Vaz J, Bernardes R, Lobo C. Blood-retinal barrier. *Eur J Ophthalmol*. 2011;21(Suppl 6):S3−S9. https://doi.org/10.5301/EJO.2010.6049.

50. Roy S, Jiang JX, Li AF, Kim D. Connexin channel and its role in diabetic retinopathy. *Prog Retin Eye Res*. 2017;61:35−59. https://doi.org/10.1016/j.preteyeres.2017.06.001.

51. Li W, Yanoff M, Liu X, Ye X. Retinal capillary pericyte apoptosis in early human diabetic retinopathy. *Chin Med J (Engl)*. 1997;110(9):659−663.

52. Beltramo E, Porta M. Pericyte loss in diabetic retinopathy: mechanisms and consequences. *Curr Med Chem*. 2013;20(26):3218−3225. https://doi.org/10.2174/09298673113209990022.

53. Suarez S, McCollum GW, Jayagopal A, Penn JS. High glucose-induced retinal pericyte apoptosis depends on association of GAPDH and Siah1. *J Biol Chem*. 2015;290(47):28311−28320. https://doi.org/10.1074/jbc.M115.682385.

54. Wright JA, Richards T, Becker DL. Connexins and diabetes. *Cardiol Res Pract*. 2012;2012:496904. https://doi.org/10.1155/2012/496904.

55. Li AF, Sato T, Haimovici R, Okamoto T, Roy S. High glucose alters connexin 43 expression and gap junction intercellular communication activity in retinal pericytes. *Invest Ophthalmol Vis Sci*. 2003;44(12):5376−5382. https://doi.org/10.1167/iovs.03-0360.

56. Roy S, Trudeau K, Roy S, Behl Y, Dhar S, Chronopoulos A. New insights into hyperglycemia-induced molecular changes in microvascular cells. *J Dent Res*. 2010;89(2):116−127. https://doi.org/10.1177/0022034509355765.

57. Kowluru RA, Chan PS. Oxidative stress and diabetic retinopathy. *Exp Diabetes Res.* 2007;2007:43603. https://doi.org/10.1155/2007/43603.

58. Danesh-Meyer HV, Zhang J, Acosta ML, Rupenthal ID, Green CR. Connexin43 in retinal injury and disease. *Prog Retin Eye Res.* 2016;51:41−68. https://doi.org/10.1016/j.preteyeres.2015.09.004.

59. Walshe TE, Saint-Geniez M, Maharaj ASR, Sekiyama E, Maldonado AE, D'Amore PA. TGF-beta is required for vascular barrier function, endothelial survival and homeostasis of the adult microvasculature. *PLoS One.* 2009;4(4):e5149. https://doi.org/10.1371/journal.pone.0005149.

60. Gerhardt H, Betsholtz C. Endothelial-pericyte interactions in angiogenesis. *Cell Tissue Res.* 2003;314(1):15−23. https://doi.org/10.1007/s00441-003-0745-x.

61. Hammes HP, Lin J, Renner O, et al. Pericytes and the pathogenesis of diabetic retinopathy. *Diabetes.* 2002;51(10):3107−3112. https://doi.org/10.2337/diabetes.51.10.3107.

62. Verma A, Rani PK, Raman R, et al. Is neuronal dysfunction an early sign of diabetic retinopathy? Microperimetry and spectral domain optical coherence tomography (SD-OCT) study in individuals with diabetes, but no diabetic retinopathy. *Eye.* 2009;23(9):1824−1830. https://doi.org/10.1038/eye.2009.184.

63. van der Torren K, van Lith G. Oscillatory potentials in early diabetic retinopathy. *Doc Ophthalmol.* 1989;71(4):375−379. https://doi.org/10.1007/BF00152764.

64. Sokol S, Moskowitz A, Skarf B, Evans R, Molitch M, Senior B. Contrast sensitivity in diabetics with and without background retinopathy. *Arch Ophthalmol.* 1985;103(1):51−54. https://doi.org/10.1001/archopht.1985.01050010055018.

65. Roy MS, Gunkel RD, Podgor MJ. Color vision defects in early diabetic retinopathy. *Arch Ophthalmol.* 1986;104(2):225−228. https://doi.org/10.1001/archopht.1986.01050140079024.

66. Sun JK, Lin MM, Lammer J, et al. Disorganization of the retinal inner layers as a predictor of visual acuity in eyes with center-involved diabetic macular edema. *JAMA Ophthalmol.* 2014;132(11):1309−1316. https://doi.org/10.1001/jamaophthalmol.2014.2350.

67. Bonnin S, Tadayoni R, Erginay A, Massin P, Dupas B. Correlation between ganglion cell layer thinning and poor visual function after resolution of diabetic macular edema. *Invest Ophthalmol Vis Sci.* 2015;56(2):978−982. https://doi.org/10.1167/iovs.14-15503.

68. Shin HJ, Lee SH, Chung H, Kim HC. Association between photoreceptor integrity and visual outcome in diabetic macular edema. *Graefes Arch Clin Exp Ophthalmol.* 2012;250(1):61−70. https://doi.org/10.1007/s00417-011-1774-x.

69. Yoshitake T, Murakami T, Suzuma K, Dodo Y, Fujimoto M, Tsujikawa A. Hyperreflective foci in the outer retinal layers as a predictor of the functional efficacy of ranibizumab for diabetic macular edema. *Sci Rep.* 2020;10(1):873. https://doi.org/10.1038/s41598-020-57646-y.

70. Mizutani M, Gerhardinger C, Lorenzi M. Müller cell changes in human diabetic retinopathy. *Diabetes.* 1998;47(3):445−449. https://doi.org/10.2337/diabetes.47.3.445.

71. Abu-El-Asrar AM, Dralands L, Missotten L, Al-Jadaan IA, Geboes K. Expression of apoptosis markers in the retinas of human subjects with diabetes. *Invest Ophthalmol Vis Sci.* 2004;45(8):2760−2766. https://doi.org/10.1167/iovs.03-1392.

72. Picconi F, Parravano M, Sciarretta F, et al. Activation of retinal Müller cells in response to glucose variability. *Endocrine*. 2019;65(3):542−549. https://doi.org/10.1007/s12020-019-02017-5.

73. Coughlin BA, Feenstra DJ, Mohr S. Müller cells and diabetic retinopathy. *Vision Res*. 2017;139:93−100. https://doi.org/10.1016/j.visres.2017.03.013.

74. Rungger-Brändle E, Dosso AA, Leuenberger PM. Glial reactivity, an early feature of diabetic retinopathy. *Invest Ophthalmol Vis Sci*. 2000;41(7):1971−1980.

75. Winkler BS, Arnold MJ, Brassell MA, Puro DG. Energy metabolism in human retinal Müller cells. *Invest Ophthalmol Vis Sci*. 2000;41(10):3183−3190.

76. Poitry-Yamate CL, Poitry S, Tsacopoulos M. Lactate released by Müller glial cells is metabolized by photoreceptors from mammalian retina. *J Neurosci*. 1995;15(7 Pt 2):5179−5191.

77. Toft-Kehler AK, Skytt DM, Svare A, et al. Mitochondrial function in Müller cells - does it matter? *Mitochondrion*. 2017;36:43−51. https://doi.org/10.1016/j.mito.2017.02.002.

78. Pannicke T, Iandiev I, Wurm A, et al. Diabetes alters osmotic swelling characteristics and membrane conductance of glial cells in rat retina. *Diabetes*. 2006;55(3):633−639. https://doi.org/10.2337/diabetes.55.03.06.db05-1349.

79. Puro DG. Diabetes-induced dysfunction of retinal Müller cells. *Trans Am Ophthalmol Soc*. 2002;100:339−352.

80. Zong H, Ward M, Madden A, et al. Hyperglycaemia-induced pro-inflammatory responses by retinal Müller glia are regulated by the receptor for advanced glycation end-products (RAGE). *Diabetologia*. 2010;53(12):2656−2666. https://doi.org/10.1007/s00125-010-1900-z.

81. Gerhardinger C, Costa MB, Coulombe MC, Toth I, Hoehn T, Grosu P. Expression of acute-phase response proteins in retinal Müller cells in diabetes. *Invest Ophthalmol Vis Sci*. 2005;46(1):349−357. https://doi.org/10.1167/iovs.04-0860.

82. Rübsam A, Parikh S, Fort PE. Role of inflammation in diabetic retinopathy. *Int J Mol Sci*. 2018;19(4):E942. https://doi.org/10.3390/ijms19040942.

83. Jo DH, Yun JH, Cho CS, Kim JH, Kim JH, Cho CH. Interaction between microglia and retinal pigment epithelial cells determines the integrity of outer blood-retinal barrier in diabetic retinopathy. *Glia*. 2019;67(2):321−331. https://doi.org/10.1002/glia.23542.

84. Zhao XF, Wan J, Powell C, Ramachandran R, Myers MG, Goldman D. Leptin and IL-6 family cytokines synergize to stimulate müller glia reprogramming and retina regeneration. *Cell Rep*. 2014;9(1):272−284. https://doi.org/10.1016/j.celrep.2014.08.047.

85. Fu S, Dong S, Zhu M, et al. Müller glia are a major cellular source of survival signals for retinal neurons in diabetes. *Diabetes*. 2015;64(10):3554−3563. https://doi.org/10.2337/db15-0180.

86. Bergsbaken T, Fink SL, Cookson BT. Pyroptosis: host cell death and inflammation. *Nat Rev Microbiol*. 2009;7(2):99−109. https://doi.org/10.1038/nrmicro2070.

87. Denes A, Lopez-Castejon G, Brough D. Caspase-1: is IL-1 just the tip of the ICEberg? *Cell Death Dis*. 2012;3(7). https://doi.org/10.1038/cddis.2012.86. e338-e338.

88. Galluzzi L, Vitale I, Abrams JM, et al. Molecular definitions of cell death subroutines: recommendations of the Nomenclature Committee on Cell Death 2012. *Cell Death Differ*. 2012;19(1):107−120. https://doi.org/10.1038/cdd.2011.96.

89. Küser-Abali G, Ozcan F, Ugurlu A, Uysal A, Fuss SH, Bugra-Bilge K. SIK2 is involved in the negative modulation of insulin-dependent müller cell survival and implicated in

hyperglycemia-induced cell death. *Invest Ophthalmol Vis Sci.* 2013;54(5):3526. https://doi.org/10.1167/iovs.12-10729.

90. Ridet JL, Malhotra SK, Privat A, Gage FH. Reactive astrocytes: cellular and molecular cues to biological function. *Trends Neurosci.* 1997;20(12):570−577. https://doi.org/10.1016/s0166-2236(97)01139-9.

91. Ly A, Yee P, Vessey KA, Phipps JA, Jobling AI, Fletcher EL. Early inner retinal astrocyte dysfunction during diabetes and development of hypoxia, retinal stress, and neuronal functional loss. *Invest Ophthalmol Vis Sci.* 2011;52(13):9316−9326. https://doi.org/10.1167/iovs.11-7879.

92. Barber AJ, Antonetti DA, Gardner TW. Altered expression of retinal occludin and glial fibrillary acidic protein in experimental diabetes. The Penn State Retina Research Group. *Invest Ophthalmol Vis Sci.* 2000;41(11):3561−3568.

93. Rungger-Brändle E, Messerli JM, Niemeyer G, Eppenberger HM. Confocal microscopy and computer-assisted image reconstruction of astrocytes in the mammalian retina. *Eur J Neurosci.* 1993;5(8):1093−1106. https://doi.org/10.1111/j.1460-9568.1993.tb00963.x.

94. Pekny M, Wilhelmsson U, Pekna M. The dual role of astrocyte activation and reactive gliosis. *Neurosci Lett.* 2014;565:30−38. https://doi.org/10.1016/j.neulet.2013.12.071.

95. Rothhammer V, Quintana FJ. Control of autoimmune CNS inflammation by astrocytes. *Semin Immunopathol.* 2015;37(6):625−638. https://doi.org/10.1007/s00281-015-0515-3.

96. Langmann T. Microglia activation in retinal degeneration. *J Leukoc Biol.* 2007;81(6):1345−1351. https://doi.org/10.1189/jlb.0207114.

97. Saxena S, Meyer CH, Akduman L. External limiting membrane and ellipsoid zone structural integrity in diabetic macular edema. *Eur J Ophthalmol.* June 16, 2021. https://doi.org/10.1177/11206721211026106.

98. Tonade D, Kern TS. Photoreceptor cells and RPE contribute to the development of diabetic retinopathy. *Prog Retin Eye Res.* November 12, 2020:100919. https://doi.org/10.1016/j.preteyeres.2020.100919.

99. Kanow MA, Giarmarco MM, Jankowski CS, et al. Biochemical adaptations of the retina and retinal pigment epithelium support a metabolic ecosystem in the vertebrate eye. *Elife.* 2017;6:e28899. https://doi.org/10.7554/eLife.28899.

100. Antonetti DA, Barber AJ, Bronson SK, et al. Diabetic retinopathy: seeing beyond glucose-induced microvascular disease. *Diabetes.* 2006;55(9):2401−2411. https://doi.org/10.2337/db05-1635.

101. Jain A, Saxena S, Khanna VK, Shukla RK, Meyer CH. Status of serum VEGF and ICAM-1 and its association with external limiting membrane and inner segment-outer segment junction disruption in type 2 diabetes mellitus. *Mol Vis.* 2013;19:1760−1768.

102. Borrelli E, Palmieri M, Viggiano P, Ferro G, Mastropasqua R. Photoreceptor damage in diabetic choroidopathy. *Retina.* 2020;40(6):1062−1069. https://doi.org/10.1097/IAE.0000000000002538.

103. Ponnalagu M, Subramani M, Jayadev C, Shetty R, Das D. Retinal pigment epithelium-secretome: a diabetic retinopathy perspective. *Cytokine.* 2017;95:126−135. https://doi.org/10.1016/j.cyto.2017.02.013.

104. Decanini A, Karunadharma PR, Nordgaard CL, Feng X, Olsen TW, Ferrington DA. Human retinal pigment epithelium proteome changes in early diabetes. *Diabetologia.* 2008;51(6):1051−1061. https://doi.org/10.1007/s00125-008-0991-2.

105. Zhang C, Xie H, Yang Q, et al. Erythropoietin protects outer blood-retinal barrier in experimental diabetic retinopathy by up-regulating ZO-1 and occludin. *Clin Exp Ophthalmol.* 2019;47(9):1182−1197. https://doi.org/10.1111/ceo.13619.

106. Kimura H. Signaling molecules: hydrogen sulfide and polysulfide. *Antioxidants Redox Signal.* 2015;22(5):362−376. https://doi.org/10.1089/ars.2014.5869.

107. Jiang H, Zhang H, Jiang X, Wu S. Overexpression of D-amino acid oxidase prevents retinal neurovascular pathologies in diabetic rats. *Diabetologia.* 2021;64(3): 693−706. https://doi.org/10.1007/s00125-020-05333-y.

108. Elucidation of pathophysiology and novel treatment for diabetic macular edema derived from the concept of neurovascular unit. *JMA J.* 2020;3(3):201−207. https://doi.org/10.31662/jmaj.2020-0022.

109. Reckelhoff JF, Hennington BS, Kanji V, et al. Chronic aminoguanidine attenuates renal dysfunction and injury in aging rats. *Am J Hypertens.* 1999;12(5):492−498. https://doi.org/10.1016/s0895-7061(98)00264-7.

110. Reichenbach A, Bringmann A. New functions of Müller cells. *Glia.* 2013;61(5): 651−678. https://doi.org/10.1002/glia.22477.

111. Toft-Kehler AK, Skytt DM, Kolko M. A perspective on the müller cell-neuron metabolic partnership in the inner retina. *Mol Neurobiol.* 2018;55(6):5353−5361. https://doi.org/10.1007/s12035-017-0760-7.

112. Johnsen EO, Frøen RC, Albert R, et al. Activation of neural progenitor cells in human eyes with proliferative vitreoretinopathy. *Exp Eye Res.* 2012;98:28−36. https://doi.org/10.1016/j.exer.2012.03.008.

113. Huang CY, Zhou T, Li G, et al. Asymmetric dimethylarginine aggravates blood-retinal barrier breakdown of diabetic retinopathy via inhibition of intercellular communication in retinal pericytes. *Amino Acids.* 2019;51(10−12):1515−1526. https://doi.org/10.1007/s00726-019-02788-1.

114. Rudraraju M, Narayanan SP, Somanath PR. Regulation of blood-retinal barrier cell-junctions in diabetic retinopathy. *Pharmacol Res.* 2020;161:105115. https://doi.org/10.1016/j.phrs.2020.105115.

115. Becker K, Klein H, Simon E, et al. In-depth transcriptomic analysis of human retina reveals molecular mechanisms underlying diabetic retinopathy. *Sci Rep.* 2021;11(1): 10494. https://doi.org/10.1038/s41598-021-88698-3.

116. Matteucci A, Gaddini L, Villa M, et al. Neuroprotection by rat Müller glia against high glucose-induced neurodegeneration through a mechanism involving ERK1/2 activation. *Exp Eye Res.* 2014;125:20−29. https://doi.org/10.1016/j.exer.2014.05.011.

117. Wang J, Xu X, Elliott MH, Zhu M, Le YZ. Müller cell-derived VEGF is essential for diabetes-induced retinal inflammation and vascular leakage. *Diabetes.* 2010;59(9): 2297−2305. https://doi.org/10.2337/db09-1420.

118. Oshitari T. Neurovascular impairment and therapeutic strategies in diabetic retinopathy. *Int J Environ Res Publ Health.* 2021;19(1):439. https://doi.org/10.3390/ijerph19010439.

119. Lutty GA. Diabetic choroidopathy. *Vision Res.* 2017;139:161−167. https://doi.org/10.1016/j.visres.2017.04.011.

120. Brinks J, van Dijk EHC, Klaassen I, et al. Exploring the choroidal vascular labyrinth and its molecular and structural roles in health and disease. *Prog Retin Eye Res.* July 17, 2021:100994. https://doi.org/10.1016/j.preteyeres.2021.100994.

121. Li W, Liu X, Yanoff M. Different responses of choriocapillary endothelial cells and retinal capillary endothelial cells to mitogenic and vasoactive factors. *Chin Med Sci J*. 1994;9(2):96−99.

122. Sorrentino FS, Matteini S, Bonifazzi C, Sebastiani A, Parmeggiani F. Diabetic retinopathy and endothelin system: microangiopathy versus endothelial dysfunction. *Eye*. 2018;32(7):1157−1163. https://doi.org/10.1038/s41433-018-0032-4.

The pathogenic role of apoptosis in the development of diabetic retinopathy

Cell death in the neurovascular unit of the early diabetic retina

Under diabetic stress, the cellular components in the inner neurovascular unit (iNVU) and outer neurovascular unit (oNVU) undergo cell type–specific death. Loss of different types of cells, leading to structural and functional alterations of both iNVU and oNVU, characterizes diabetic retinal microangiopathy and diabetic retinal neuronopathy/neurodegeneration (DRN). Although the underlying mechanisms of cell death in diabetic retina are not completely clear, it has been recognized that the pathophysiological events leading to apoptosis and other modes of cell death begin at the stage of preclinical diabetic retinopathy (DR).

Preclinical DR begins when diabetes is initially diagnosed and lasts until the first vascular abnormalities are detected, which usually takes many years.[1] This is the period stretching from early dysfunction of neurovascular coupling to neuronal and vascular cell death. The evidence of cell death in preclinical DR comes from clinical data and studies of experimental animals. Patients with preclinical DR may experience deficits in visual functions including night vision, color vision, and electrophysiological manifestations.[2,3] These deficits may be correlated with retinal neuronal layer thinning before the development of vascular abnormalities.[3,4] One of the early events is the dysfunction of intercellular communication. The communications between cell types in the integral network of the NVU are neurochemical (synapses) and electrical (gap junctions). This network of cells is affected early after the onset of hyperglycemia, resulting in disturbed neuroglial regulations of blood flow, that is, functional hyperemia based on metabolic demand of the neurosensory retina. In general, the correlative relationship between structural and functional changes is observed at molecular, cellular, and tissue levels in early diabetic retina.[5] However, the progression of DR is not necessarily linear, but may follow a series of steps that evolve over the course of multiple years. For instance, one of the earliest functional changes in diabetic retina is decreased nitric oxide (NO) bioavailability, which correlates with decreased vascular diameter,

Therapeutic Targets for Diabetic Retinopathy. https://doi.org/10.1016/B978-0-323-93064-2.00008-1

resulting in decreased retinal blood flow. NO bioavailability is a biomarker of retinal vascular cells that utilize NO as a vasodilator.[6] Multiple events occur sequentially as follows: downregulation of connexin 43 (see Chapter 3), retinal ganglion cell (RGC) apoptosis, pericyte/endothelial cell dropout, functional changes such as decreased vascular connectivity (see gap junction in Chapter 3), increased gamma-aminobutyric acid (GABA) sensitivity, deficits in rod pathway, and decreased vasomotor response. GABA sensitivity and rod pathway refer to GABA-mediated light-evoked inhibition, which regulates rod bipolar output to amacrine cells. In early diabetes, the reduced GABA inhibition leads to increased rod pathway signaling, resulting in visual disturbance and reduced contrast sensitivity in diabetic patients.[7] At this point, retinal blood vessels exhibit deficits in light-induced dilation suggesting that neurovascular coupling is already compromised.[8] Functional deficits of retinal neurons recorded by increased implicit time Z-scores on multifocal electroretinogram (mfERG) are predictive of clinical microangiopathy, indicating that neuronal deficits contribute to vasculopathy.[9] It is important to note that NVU function can be compromised in early stage before overt changes in neuronal morphology are observed.[7] During diabetes progression and often prior to onset of clinical DR, apoptosis of RGCs, dopaminergic amacrine cells, and pericytes/endothelial cells in the inner retina becomes evident.[5] At the same time, retinal glia cells are activated, followed by astrocyte apoptosis and Müller cell pyroptosis (see Chapter 3). The gradually progressive neurodegeneration, reactive gliosis, and neuroinflammation precede the observable vascular pathologies, that is, mild nonproliferative diabetic retinopathy by Early Treatment Diabetic Retinopathy Study classification (see Chapter 1).

Photoreceptors and retinal pigment epithelial (RPE) cells work together as a unit in the outer retina. Although there is growing evidence that photoreceptors and RPE cells undergo numerous pathologic events in diabetes, studies focusing on the pathogenic role of outer retina in DR development are still fragmentary. It is of note that the modest photoreceptor degeneration detected in early diabetes may not be enough to explain the structural and functional alterations on diabetic retina as compared with other retinal degenerative diseases such as dry age-related macular degeneration.[10] Since optical coherence tomography (OCT) has enabled direct visualization of the RPE, the role of dysfunction of RPE cells in diabetic macular edema (DME) has drawn great attention. Since the tight junctions between RPE cells comprise the outer blood—retinal barrier (BRB), the macular edema is attributed to diabetes-induced increase in permeability or loss of integrity of RPE.[11] For instance, insufficient activity of Na^+/K^+-ATPase in the RPE could contribute to the disruption of the outer BRB in diabetes, resulting in retinal edema.

Thus, DR is a disease of the retinal NVU, in which specific mode of cell death particularly apoptosis is critical. The complex consequences of apoptosis of specific cell types contribute to the development and progression of DR.

Apoptosis of retinal vascular pericytes and endothelial cells

In the normal microvasculature of human retina, the average endothelial—pericyte ratio is approximate one (1:1). Among retinas of patients with diabetes, as compared with those without diabetes, the mean endothelial—pericyte ratio was increased to 4.2.[12] Therefore, in the diabetic retinal vasculature, a phenomenon of selective loss of pericyte has been defined as a pathologic hallmark of early retinopathy.[13] The nature of preferential dropout of pericytes in the early stage of DR is not completely understood. Yanoff in 1966 described the typical pathological changes of retinal microvasculature in diabetes, such as "ghost cell" pericytes and pyknotic endothelial cells.[14] These morphologic findings imply that diabetic retinal pericytes and endothelial cells may undergo a special process of cell death, later called apoptosis.[15]

Apoptosis is a type of cell death in which a series of molecular events in a cell lead to its death. Morphologically, apoptosis is characterized by cellular shrinking, condensation, and margination of the chromatin and ruffling of the plasma membrane. Then the cell becomes divided into apoptotic bodies that consist of cell organelles and/or nuclear material surrounded by a plasma membrane.[16] Biochemically, apoptosis is a type of programmed cell death, which comprises cell-specific pathways leading to death of cells. The final common apoptotic pathway is the activation of caspases, a family of nucleophilic proteases, leading to the characteristic nuclear changes observed during programmed cell death.[16] The purpose of apoptosis is to eliminate unneeded or abnormal cells.

To understand the nature of the increased endothelial cell—pericyte ratio during diabetes, extensive studies using in vitro and in vivo diabetic models and human postmortem retinas were independently conducted in the 1990s.[17–20] Li et al. studied neural retinas of 12 postmortem eyes of 6 patients (3 diabetic and 3 nondiabetic).[19] In our laboratories, the eyes were first fixed in buffered formaldehyde and then digested with trypsin. Flat-mounts of trypsin-digested retinal blood vessels were studied with periodic acid—Schiff (PAS)-hematoxylin staining. A variety of typical diabetic microvascular changes were observed. These changes included thickened capillary walls, microaneurysms, "ghost-cell"-appearance of pericytes, acellular segments of capillaries, and an increased ratio of retinal capillary endothelial cells to pericytes. All of these changes are characteristics of diabetic microvascular abnormalities (Fig. 4.1).

In a separate study, flat-mounts of trypsin-digested retinal vessels of postmortem eyes were stained first with the end labeling (TUNEL) technique of terminal deoxynucleotidyl transferase-mediated dUTP nick, a specific test for cells undergoing apoptosis, then with PAS, and eventually counterstained with hematoxylin to evaluate DNA fragmentation of cell nuclei and diabetic changes in the retinal capillaries. TUNEL-positive apoptotic pericytes were observed in retinal capillaries in all three diabetic patients in this study. The nuclei of TUNEL-positive pericytes were darker than other pericytes stained with PAS-hematoxylin. TUNEL-positive retinal capillary endothelial cells were also discovered in eyes of the three diabetic patients

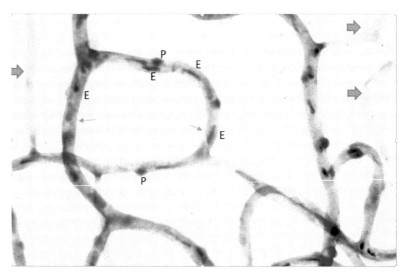

FIGURE 4.1

A representative flat-mount retinal vessels from a postmortem retina of a diabetic patient without history of clinical DR, stained with PAS-hematoxylin-eosin and viewed by light microscopy (200X). Pericytes (p) showing round nuclei, enclosed by basement membrane, perivascular location appearing to protrude from the vessels wall; endothelial cells (e) showing oval nuclei, an intralumen location appearing to be in the vessel wall. In the vessel loop indicated with *small blue arrows*, the number of pericytes is much less than that of endothelial cells, that is, an increased ratio between E and P. The *wide arrows* in the figure indicate acellular capillaries.

Data from Li.

(Fig. 4.2A). No TUNEL-positive pericytes or endothelial cells were found in the three nondiabetic controls. These findings indicate that both pericytes and endothelial cells undergo a specific form of cell death, namely apoptosis, which occurs during the early development of DR (Fig. 4.2A). The significant increase in the ratio of endothelial cells to pericytes and the predominant TUNEL-positive pericytes over endothelial cells give rise to three possibilities (Fig. 4.2).[19] First, a greater impact of apoptosis-related mechanisms may exist in pericytes than in endothelial cells under diabetic condition (vide infra). Second, since only endothelial cells, not pericytes, are located inside of capillary wall, they are directly exposed to blood flow. The blood flow could take dead endothelial cells away, leading to fewer TUNEL-positive endothelial cells than pericytes in microvessel samples. Third, in contrast to pericytes, endothelial cells possess measurable regenerative capacity in vivo, which may contribute to an elevated endothelial—pericyte ratio.[21,22] For these possible reasons, a much decrease in number of pericytes takes place in early diabetic retinal vasculature.[19]

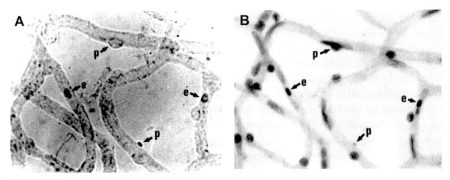

FIGURE 4.2

Comparison of TUNEL and PAS-hematoxylin staining for the same retinal microvessel preparation of a diabetic patient without history of retinopathy. The microvessel preparation was first stained with TUNEL and then PAS-hematoxylin. TUNEL technique was carried out with fluorescein-conjugated dUTP and the enzyme TdT. In (A) positive TUNEL cells of retinal vessels were visualized with an alkaline phosphatase-substrate system showing dark *purple* nuclei. Nonapoptotic pericytes and endothelial cell nuclei do not stain with the TUNEL. Both apoptotic pericytes and endothelial cells are present. In (B) the number of endothelial cells is much higher than that of pericytes with PAS-hematoxylin staining. The microscopic photographs (400X) are used in both (A and B). Apoptotic pericytes (p) and apoptotic endothelial cells (e) are indicated in each photo.

Data from Li.

Based on these studies, apoptosis of retinal vascular cells has been proved to be an important reason of the altered ratio of pericytes over endothelial cells, presenting a phenomenon called selective dropout of pericytes in diabetic retina. Although the underlying mechanisms by which vascular cells undergo apoptosis are still not completely clear, overwhelming evidence points to the contribution of hyperglycemia and related metabolic aberrations (see Chapter 2). A crucial risk factor for vascular complications of diabetes is hyperglycemia-induced oxidative stress.[23] However, despite diabetic oxidative stress, clinically some subsets of patients remain complication-free for a long time. Thus, it seems that the balance between hyperglycemia-induced oxidative stress and antioxidant defense determines the development of vascular complications.[20,24] Li et al. reported a study utilizing human retinal pericytes freshly isolated from postmortem diabetic and nondiabetic eyes.[20] Total mRNA of the purified pericytes was isolated for quantitative reverse transcription polymerase chain reaction assay. mRNA levels of caspase-3, the major enzyme that initiates the proteolytic cascade leading to cell death, were determined in association with the expression of genes encoding antioxidative enzymes, including glutathione peroxidase (GSH-Px), glutathione reductase, CuZn superoxide dismutase (CuZnSOD), manganese superoxide dismutase (MnSOD), and catalase in pericytes. In comparison with pericytes from nondiabetic retinas, pericytes from diabetic retinas highly expressed *caspase-3* genes ($P < .01$, n = 9). In diabetic pericytes, upregulation of glutathione peroxidase (*GSH-Px*, $P < .01$, n = 9) and downregulation of glutathione reductase (*Gr*, $P < .05$, n = 9) and *CuZnSOD* ($P < .05$, n = 9) were observed. mRNA levels of MnSOD and catalase of diabetic pericytes did not differ significantly from those of nondiabetic pericytes. Overexpression of caspase-3 indicated that the pericytes from diabetic retinas are in a preapoptotic state, called proapoptosis. In these cells, upregulation of GSH-Px indicates a compensation mechanism to meet the demand for excessive reduced glutathione. Decreased levels of both glutathione reductase and CuZnSOD, despite the oxidative stress in the diabetic condition, suggest the breakdown of the antioxidant defense in pericytes. Most importantly, the altered gene profile of scavenging enzymes under diabetic conditions, correlating with overexpression of the cell death protease gene, together suggest that increased oxidative stress is an etiological factor in pericyte dropout in DR.[20] Kowluru et al. conducted a therapeutic exploration targeting antioxidative defense systems of diabetic animals in an attempt to rescue caspase-3-mediated apoptosis. Caspase-3 was activated in the rat retina at 14 months of diabetes ($P < .05$ vs. normal control) but not at two months of diabetes, and the administration of antioxidants for the entire duration of the caspase-3 activation. In isolated retinal capillary cells incubated in a high level (25 mM) glucose medium, caspase-3 activity was increased by 50% in comparison with the cells incubated in 5 mM glucose ($P < .02$). Addition of antioxidants or a caspase-3 inhibitor diminished this increase. These findings suggest that increased oxidative stress in diabetes is involved in the activation of retinal caspase-3-mediated apoptosis of endothelial cells and pericytes. Further, these experiments indicate that antioxidants and antiapoptosis agents may be appropriate treatments for the prevention or amelioration of DR.[25,26]

Accumulating evidence shows that both pericytes and endothelial cells undergo apoptosis in diabetic retina. In the early literature, necrotic cell death of pericytes was also implicated in DR.[27] This type of pericyte death was later described as "selective necrosis," referring to a regulated form of cell death under diabetic conditions. Pericyte and endothelial cell death has great consequences for microvascular remodeling. In microvessels, pericytes, specialized contractile mesenchymal cells of mesodermal origin, function similar to smooth muscle cells in larger vessels, regulating vascular tone and perfusion pressure. In retinal microvasculature, their perivascular localization and expression of contractile proteins suggest that pericytes participate in capillary blood flow regulation and neurovascular coupling.[28] Thickening of the basement membrane, together with systemic and local hypertension, hyperglycemia, advanced glycation end products, and hypoxia, may act to disrupt the cell−cell connection between pericytes and endothelial cells. Endothelium that is deprived of proliferative control by pericytes can give rise to microaneurysms in the early stages and, eventually, new vessels in later stages of retinopathy.[26] For the survival and differentiation of pericytes, vascular endothelial growth factor (VEGF), transforming growth factor β (TGF-β) and platelet-derived growth factor subunit B (PDGF-B) are essential. Particularly, PDGF-B, secreted by the endothelium, and its receptor PDGFR-β (expressed in pericytes only) are important in the proliferation, migration, and recruitment of pericytes. Pericyte-produced VEGF stimulates endothelial proliferation, and endothelial cell—pericyte interaction is responsible for the activation of TGF-β, which induces the differentiation of pericytes, while suppressing endothelial proliferation and migration.[23]

In addition to endothelium, pericytes are also in contact with Müller cells, which contribute to the stability of the BRB and the maintenance of retinal homeostasis. Müller cells have been shown to support and protect both neurons and vascular cells from damage caused by diabetic oxidative stress.[29] Taken together, apoptosis of retinal pericytes and endothelial cells, which interact with neurons and glial cells as a unit, contributes to the development of microangiopathy in diabetes.

Apoptosis of retinal neurons and dysfunction of glia cells

The complex pathology and pathogenesis of DR affect both the vascular and neural systems of the retina. Traditionally, DR was considered to be simply a microvascular disease. However, abnormal visual functions detected by electrophysiology/psychophysics tests manifest in the early phase of diabetic retina and progress throughout the disease, demonstrating dysfunction of the retinal neuronal network.[30]

Electroretinography (ERG) is an objective measurement of retinal function which documents the complex electrical responses of retinal neurons such as photoreceptors, bipolar, amacrine, and ganglion cells when stimulated by light.[31] In diabetics, the oscillatory potential is reduced and the b-wave latency is delayed before retinopathy occurs.[32] When measured with a mfERG, local mfERG implicit times are significantly prolonged in the eyes of diabetic patients even without retinopathy, compared to that of normal control subjects (Fig. 4.3).[33]

Functional tests of dark adaptation, contrast sensitivity, color vision, blue-on-yellow perimetry, and standard perimetry also deteriorate in diabetics, supporting a pervasive diabetic impact on retinal neurons. In the era of OCT, these visual disturbances detected by functional tests have been correlated with anatomic OCT/OCT angiography (OCTA) data on diabetic retina.[34] Sohn et al. reported a cohort study on 45 patients with diabetes but with no or minimal retinopathy over 4-year follow-up. Despite stable and minimal retinopathy in these patients, significant, progressive loss of the retinal nerve fiber layer (RNFL) and the ganglion cell layer (GCL)/inner plexiform layer (IPL) were observed from OCT analysis.[34] On the other hand, diabetic animal models with inner retinal thinning on OCT or ganglion cell loss by immunohistochemistry were not associated with retinal vascular abnormalities in the early phase after diabetes onset. Therefore, they proposed that DRN precedes microangiopathy. The recent study by van de Kreeke et al. found retinal layer alterations of type 1 diabetes mellitus patients. The follow-up period was 5 to 7 years. Based on their spectral-domain OCT (SD-OCT) findings, the tomographic features consist of gradual RNFL and GCL thinning and slight IPL thickening over time. It is worth to note that this study was able to measure IPL separately from GCL—IPL complex. These changes were more pronounced for GCL and IPL, specifically corresponding to eyes/quadrants with DR in

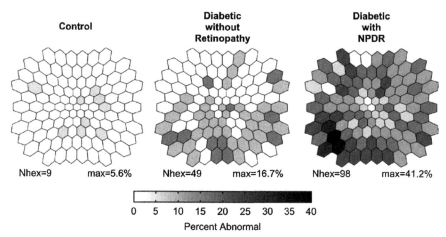

FIGURE 4.3

Frequency of P1 component of the "slow flash" mfERG (sf-mfERG P1) implicit time abnormalities at each of the 103 retinal locations. Results are shown for control subjects (*left*), diabetic subjects without retinopathy (*middle*), and diabetic subjects with mild or moderate nonproliferative diabetic retinopathy (*right*). Each frequency map is plotted as a left eye observed in retinal view. For each retinal map, "Nhex" is the number of locations with at least one abnormality and "max" is the maximum frequency of abnormality. In both groups of diabetic subjects, abnormal P1 implicit times are not uniformly distributed, occurring more frequently within the inferior retina.

Modified from Bearse et al.[33]

a spatial and temporal manner.[35] To establish the correlative relation between ERG-revealed function and OCTA measurable morphology, Kim et al. reported a cohort study of type 2 diabetes mellitus patients and nondiabetic controls, in which the amplitude and implicit time of the rod and cone and combined response ERG b-wave were significantly reduced and prolonged in the eyes of patients with diabetes. There was a positive correlation between the amplitude on ERG and vessel density (VD) of the superficial capillary plexus as acquired from OCTA. A negative correlation between the implicit time and superficial VD in the scotopic and combined response b-wave was also found. However, these correlative relationships between retinal function and vascular morphology were not found in the VD of deep capillary plexus (DCP), although capillary dropout is dominant in DCP in early DR.[36] These findings suggest that functional and structural impairments of retinal neurons do not run parallel with the development of microangiopathy in type 2 diabetes.[37,38] Meanwhile, there are some inconsistent results regarding the temporal and spatial relationship between retinal function and neuronal injury. For instance, the German Diabetes Study reported that visual function does not relate to measurable changes of thickness of retinal layers in early diabetes (within one year of onset).[39] Notably, this study has several limitations that need to be discussed. First, the visual function tests used in this study may not be sensitive nor specific enough for the assessment of diabetic retinal neurodegeneration because only visual acuity and contrast sensitivity are utilized. Second, the OCT measurable retinal layer thickness was restricted to the nasal pericentral segment, which means the research may have overlooked the changes of other quadrant-specific thickness in diabetic retina.[35] Third, in order to improve this study, a longitudinal observation, not cross-sectional study, is needed. Since DRN is the earliest event, responsible for the visual impairment at the early stage of DR, a sensitive and specific clinical assessment of DRN needs to be developed. In this book, diabetic retinal neuropathy and diabetic neurodegeneration are used synonymously (DRN). Recently, a systematic search of the medical literature since 1984 was performed on PUBMED and EMBASE. In the prediabetic retina, color vision changes, flash ERG b-wave latency, multifocal b-wave latency, scotopic b-wave and oscillatory potentials in ERG, and contrast sensitivity changes are confirmed as practical approaches for the assessment of DRN.[40] The correlation of OCT measurable changes in retinal layers with functional abnormalities from multimodal tests may strengthen the capability of recognizing DRN in a timely manner. Since DRN precedes microangiopathy, the gap from neurodegeneration to nascent vasculopathy may be a therapeutic window for early phase of DR.[41]

The direct evidence of retinal neuronal apoptosis largely depends on animal studies.[42] Animal models can also offer the opportunity to examine pathways of cell death in far greater detail than studies in humans.[43] At the same time, identification of apoptosis in vivo for research and clinical practice is essential.[44] For example, the **d**etection of **a**poptotic **r**etinal **c**ells (DARC) technique is a noninvasive method that uses fluorescently conjugated annexin V, which retains a phosphatidylserine binding site for apoptotic cells. The fluorescent apoptotic cells in retina can be visualized by using a wide-angle confocal laser scanning ophthalmoscope (Fig. 4.4).

Besides significant loss of RGCs, photoreceptor disruption in the early phase of diabetes can be visualized on SD-OCT, presenting as loss of integrity of the external limiting membrane, ellipsoid zone, and interdigitation zone. Substantial numbers of apoptotic photoreceptors in diabetic retina have been documented in animal models. For instance, in streptozotocin-induced diabetic rats, photoreceptor apoptosis was documented by histology including immunohistochemical TUNEL technique only 4 weeks after diabetes onset. These findings imply that the visual disturbance in diabetic patients is attributed to substantial photoreceptor apoptosis (TUNEL-positive cells) in early phase because the vascular abnormalities have not developed yet.[45] Changes in the photoreceptors might be directly visualized in diabetic patients prior to clinical retinopathy but require special imaging techniques for detection. The newly developed adaptive optics (AO) scanning laser ophthalmoscope (AOSLO) is one noninvasive method to visualize microcirculation and retinal structures including individual cells of the outer retina. Lammer et al. used high-resolution AOSLO imaging to identify changes in retinal cone density and irregularity of cone spacing in diabetic eyes.[46] These changes as viewed by AO imaging in patients with DR are shown in Fig. 4.5.[47,48]

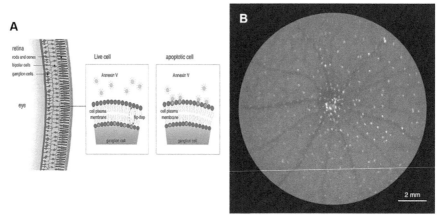

FIGURE 4.4

A schematic diagram of the DARC technology (A). After injection of fluorescent-labeled annexin V, apoptotic cells are identified by the binding of annexin to translocated phosphatidylserine on the outer leaflet of the membrane of retinal ganglion cells. These show up as bright *white* spots in rat retina images from a wide-angle confocal laser scanning ophthalmoscope (B).

Modified from Galvao et al.[44]

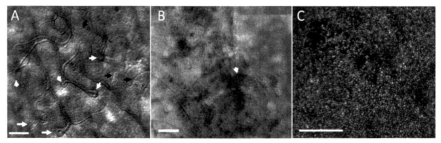

FIGURE 4.5

The microvascular changes and cone density and irregularity changes viewed by AO imaging in patients with DR. (A) An example of a region of multiple vascular anomalies, including looping and doubling of capillaries (*white arrows*) and nonperfused capillaries (*black arrows*) in early DR. (B) A region of microcystic changes (dark regions), not visible at normal magnification but seen with AO retinal imaging. There is a small capillary loop present at the edge of the foveal avascular zone. (C) The localized regions of dark cones are apparent in diabetic patients. The dark cones that fail to guide light are consistent with an early stage of failure of the outer BRB. Scale bars for all panels 100 μm.

Modified from Burns et al.[47]

In the outer retina, the ultrastructure of RPE cells in diabetic retina shows an irregular arrangement of plasma membrane infoldings, degeneration of mitochondria and nuclei, and increased permeability to fluorescein.[11,49] It is suggested that in high glucose conditions, RPE cells downregulate glucose transporter protein 1 (GLUT-1) and reduce the levels of antioxidants, leading to retinal tissue damage.[50,51] Omri et al. utilized a spontaneous type 2 diabetes rat model to document the interaction between microglia/macrophages in the subretinal space and RPE cells. At the early phase of hyperglycemia (5 months after onset of diabetes), a few microglia/macrophages migrated to the subretinal space and numerous pores formed in RPE cells, allowing inflammatory cell traffic between the retina and choroid. With increasing duration of hyperglycemia, the number of microglia/macrophages increased, but reduced pore density and increased vacuolization of RPE cells were observed. The dysfunction and structural damage of RPE contribute to photoreceptor damage.[52] Importantly, the resultant outer BRB breakdown and proinflammatory response in DME are attributed to diabetes-induced abnormal RPE permeability.[53]

During the course of DRN development, synaptic degeneration of RGCs is the earliest event, representing changes in the thickness of IPL by SD-OCT. The IPL is formed by the synaptic connections of ganglion cells, bipolar cells, and amacrine cells. The synaptic structures composing the IPL contain many membranes, a high density of vesicles, and numerous mitochondria. All these components may be the origin of the hyperreflectivity seen in OCT (Fig. 4.6).

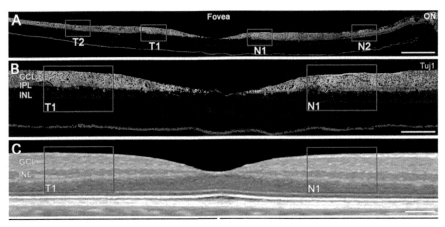

FIGURE 4.6

Changes of the ganglion cell layer (GCL) and RNFL along the retina studied with immunostaining. (A) Panoramic view of a human central retina section stained with Tuj 1 (*green*) and RBPMS (*red*) antibodies, differentiating the nasal (N1, N2) and temporal zones (T1, T2). (B) Ganglion cells in the fovea and (C) the corresponding OCT profile. High magnification images of ganglion cells (*red*) and nerve fibers (*green*). Scale bars: (A) 500 μm; (B, C) 200 μm.

Modified from Cuenca et al.[54]

As seen in Fig. 4.6B, the IPL is very thin at the fovea and gradually becomes thicker. The maximum thickness of the IPL is reached at the point of maximum thickness of the GCL, and the IPL becomes thinner toward more peripheral regions. In clinical practice, the central IPL and GCL together are frequently measured as GCL–IPL complex.[54] Zhu et al. observed that synaptic dysfunction of RGCs is an early sign of neurodegeneration, seen prior to RGC apoptosis in diabetic retina.[55] These findings indicate that targeting synaptic dysfunction and synaptic degeneration of RGCs could be a novel treatment strategy in early DRN.[56]

Müller glial cells and astrocytes are the two types of macroglia cells in retinal NVU. Together with microglia, the resident immune cells in the retina, the macroglia cells provide structural support and functional maintenance of metabolic homeostasis. The different glial cell types react differentially to diabetic stress at different stages of the disease, which may lead to different modes of cell death. Although the soma of Müller cells reside in the inner nuclear layer (INL), the whole Müller glia span all retinal layers and engage processes contacting all types of cells, including neurons, vascular cells, participating in the formation of NVU in the retina.[57,58] Ninety percent of retinal glia cells are Müller cells that react to diabetic stress in the early phase of DR.[59] In addition to glial fibrillary acidic protein (GFAP) upregulation, the activated Müller cells synthesize acute-phase response proteins[60] and many growth factors and cytokines.[61] A gene expression study of Müller cells from diabetic rats showed that one-third of diabetes-induced genes are associated with inflammation, including complement factors, VEGF, intercellular adhesion molecule 1 (ICAM-1), and interleukin (IL)-1β.[62] DR is a special pathological condition, in which the fate of Müller cells is complex.[29] In a diabetic animal model representing progressive diabetes, the number of Müller glia dropped after 7 months of diabetes. In addition to the mode of apoptosis,[63] there is evidence that Müller cells in diabetic retina undergo caspase-1/IL-1β pathway-mediated cell death, a process known as pyroptosis (vide infra). Since pyroptosis is a lytic type of cell death initiated by inflammatory caspases, the Müller cell loss in diabetic retina emphasizes the role of inflammation in DR progression.[64] However, Müller cells may survive in diabetic retina and reenter the proliferation cycle to establish a glial scar. The glial scars are one reason for the failure of the central nervous system (including retina) to regenerate because the machinery of neurotropic production by Müller cells has been damaged in later phase of DR.[29]

Similar to Müller cells, astrocytes contact both retinal blood vessels and neurons and play a critical role in maintenance of BRB.[65] In contrast to Müller cells, they are largely restricted to the RNFL and GCL, while Müller cells are connected with all types of retinal neurons. Retinal astrocytes strikingly associate with blood vessels and are involved in the loss of integrity of the BRB in diabetic retina. In the early phase of diabetes, evidence exists that astrocytes become activated and produce a variety of proinflammatory cytokines, such as IL-6, IL1β, IL-8, cyclooxygenase-2, TGF-β, epidermal growth factor, macrophage inflammatory protein 2α, and VEGF.[66,67] Reactive astrocytes also can secrete chemokines that recruit microglia, monocytes/macrophages, and T cells, amplifying the inflammatory responses.[68]

If astrocyte activation and reactive gliosis are not controlled in early diabetes, astrocyte number seems to progressively decrease in DR patients. Astrocytes may undergo apoptosis, which can be demonstrated by dual immune-labeling of GFAP and TUNEL reaction (Fig. 4.7). This astrocyte loss results in disruption of the inner BRB, contributing to vascular leakage in the retina.[69,70]

After diabetes onset, persistent hyperglycemia activates multiple cellular pathways, leading to increased inflammation, oxidative stress, and vascular dysfunction. Therefore, DR has been delineated as "chronic, low-grade inflammatory disease of the retina" (see Chapter 5). An increasing body of evidence suggests that inflammation and neurodegeneration both occur in human diabetes even before the development of clinical signs of DR. One of the first signs of inflammation in diabetes mellitus is the activation of retinal microglia. Activated microglia release cytotoxic substances responsible for the recruitment of leukocytes, BRB breakdown, glial dysfunction, and neuronal cell death. Among the three types of retinal glial cells, microglia are recruited and activated via a complex interaction among diabetes-induced pathological pathways. Transcriptional changes in the activated microglia result in release of various proinflammatory mediators, including cytokines, chemokines, caspases, and glutamate.[71] The activated microglia in early DR may be tracked by their characteristic hyperreflective foci (HRFs) seen by OCT.[72] In a cohort study, the number of HRF was significantly higher in diabetics with retinopathy versus diabetics without retinopathy ($P < .05$). The number of HRF of both diabetics with and without retinopathy was also significantly higher as compared to controls ($P < .05$). The HRFs are mainly located in the inner retina layers, that is, internal limiting membrane, GCL, and INL, where the resident microglia are present.[72] However, over time or in eyes with DME, HRF became evident in both inner and outer retinal layers,[73] forming multiple inflammatory foci due to the migration

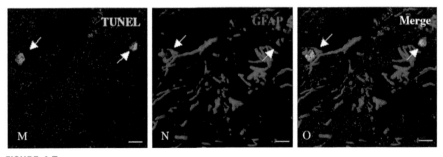

FIGURE 4.7

Representative immunohistochemistry study showing apoptotic astrocytes in central nervous system (CNS) with diabetes. Positive double labeling for TUNEL (*green*) and for GFAP (*red*) in the cerebellum of a rat with diabetes for 8 weeks. *Solid arrows* indicate TUNEL and GFAP double-labeled apoptotic astrocytes. Scale bar = 30 μm in the panel of M, N, and O.

Modified from Lechuga-Sancho et al.[69]

of activated microglia. Importantly, when DME was treated with anti-VEGF agents, disappearance or reduction in HRF is the first obvious change in the retina. Therefore, HRF may represent a clinical biomarker of inflammatory response.[74] Recently, many inflammatory mediators, growth factors, and other molecules have been found in human vitreous and aqueous humor samples. The study of multiple pathways and mechanisms indicates that DME is the result of chronic inflammation of diabetic retina. In fact, the detection of HRF confirms the hypothesis that neuroinflammation and neurodegeneration occur in the early course of human diabetes. These new emerging insights foster a better understanding of the pathogenesis of DR, which can no longer be considered as a pure retinal vascular complication of diabetes.[75]

The complex multicellular dysfunction and death in NVU of diabetic retina are summarized in Fig. 4.8. The outer NVU comprising photoreceptors and RPE cells is

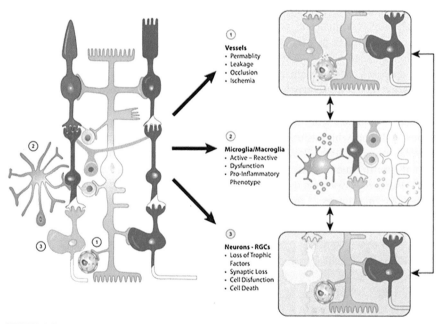

FIGURE 4.8

The complex multicellular dysfunction and death in DR. Diabetes virtually affects all retinal cells in a sequence that remains hard to elucidate as they function as an NVU and influence each other. (1) Vessel dysfunction reflects pericytes and endothelial cells dysfunction and loss, a phenomenon influenced by factors secreted by dying neurons and activated microglia and macroglia. (2) Microglia (*brown*) and macroglia (*green*) become activated in response to the alteration of the retinal environment associated with diabetes, a phenomenon enhanced by neuronal cell death and vascular perturbations. (3) Alteration of the retinal homeostasis by diabetes leads to neuronal dysfunction and ultimately cell death, a phenomenon enhanced by the increasingly proinflammatory environment and vascular perturbations.

Modified from Pan et al.[3]

not included in this figure. The inner NVU has three constituent parts: vessels, glial cells, and neurons. Under the diabetic condition, neuronal degeneration and glial activation precede the microvascular destruction. There are three cellular interplays in the NVU contributing to DR development. The sequence and relative importance of these three factors remain uncertain. First, the dysfunction and apoptotic cell death of pericytes and endothelial cells of vessels are induced by multiple factors that are synthesized by dying neurons and activated microglia and macroglia. The compromised BRB results in increased permeability and leakage of lipoproteins. The accelerated apoptosis of vascular cells leads to vessel occlusion, acellular capillaries, and retinal tissue ischemia. Second, activation of microglia and macroglia in response to acute diabetic stress triggers neuronal and microvascular apoptosis pathways. Over time, the dysfunction of glial cells generates proinflammatory factors and amplifies the inflammatory reactions. Müller cells undergo hyperplasia preceding GFAP expression, and microglial cells are activated, whereas astrocytes regress. This glial behavior may contribute decisively to the onset and development of DRN.[59] Third, the diabetic stress and altered retinal homeostasis induce loss of tropic factors, causing synaptic dysfunction and degeneration, which is prior to RGC apoptosis. Overall, multicellular dysfunction and death are involved in the development and progression of DR. Among multiple modes of cellular death, apoptosis being the main mode for various cells is the anatomic basis of retinal NVU disruption.

Protecting the NVU as therapeutic strategy for DRN

Abundant experimental and clinical data indicate that DRN precedes microangiopathy. In the study on DRN pathogenesis, we have learned that synaptic degeneration of RGCs and activation of glial cells may represent some of the earliest pathophysiological events in diabetic retina. For instance, the synaptic degeneration is prior to RGC apoptosis. Therefore, targeting the pathogenic events in temporal sequence is a therapeutic approach for DRN. The earliest event in the initiation of neurodegeneration may be dysfunction of mitochondria in retinal neuronal and glial cells.[55,76] The mitochondrial dysfunction is caused by altered diabetes-driven metabolic stress. Potential therapeutic interventions targeting mechanisms underlying retinal neurodegeneration in the early stages of DRN are summarized in Fig. 4.9. Diabetes-induced stress can aggravate production and accumulation of reactive oxygen species due to hyperglycemia and/or dyslipidemia.[77] For example, glucolipotoxicity in an animal model induced by high-fat diet (HFD) causes both glial cell activation and abnormal glycogen synthase kinase-3β (GSK-3β) activation in neurons.[55,76] GSK-3β is a proline-directed serine-threonine kinase. In diabetes, GSK-3β is activated and translocated into mitochondria, where it interacts with mitochondrial proteins and components of the respiratory chain.[78] GSK-3β activation induces loss of β-catenin and tau hyperphosphorylation (Fig. 4.9).[55] β-catenin is a dual function protein, involved in regulation and coordination of cell−cell adhesion and gene

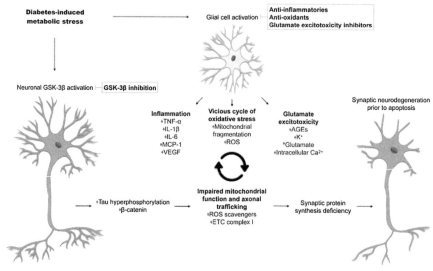

FIGURE 4.9

Potential pharmacological interventions based on mechanisms underlying retinal neurodegeneration in the early stages of DR. Diabetes induced metabolic stress triggers glial cell activation and abnormal GSK-3β activation. Glial cell activation leads to secretion of proinflammatory factors, reactive oxygen species (ROS), and glutamate accumulation, while abnormal GSK-3β activation causes tau hyperphosphorylation and β-catenin loss, followed by impaired mitochondrial function and axonal trafficking, thus resulting in decreased synaptic targeting of mitochondria, reduced localized synaptic protein synthesis, and a vicious cycle of oxidative stress. Therefore, GSK-3β inhibition and other antiglial cell activation agents, such as antiinflammatories, antioxidants, and glutamate excitotoxicity inhibitors might be capable of preventing synaptic neurodegeneration in early DR. Note: ↑ upregulation; ↓ downregulation.

Modified from Rolev et al.[56]

transcription. In humans, β-catenin is encoded by the *CTNNB1* gene. In the HFD-induced diabetic mouse model, Shu et al. discovered that the hyperglycemia- or hyperlipidemia-induced mitochondrial impairment in RGCs is instigated by abnormal loss of β-catenin due to GSK-3β activation (Fig. 4.9).[76] Among GSK-3β activation-dependent events, hyperphosphorylation of tau protein controls mitochondrial function and axonal trafficking. Neurons are rich in tau proteins. Tau proteins regulate microtubule stability through phosphorylation. Hyperphosphorylation of tau proteins can cause the helical and straight filaments to tangle. Tau proteins are mainly active in the distal portions of axons where they stabilize microtubules and also provide flexibility. Therefore, glucolipotoxicity causes hyperphosphorylation of tau, which can destabilize microtubule tracks, impair microtubule-dependent synaptic functions, and disrupt mitochondrial bioenergetics (Fig. 4.9).[78] Under diabetic stress, the mitochondrial impairment of retinal neurons is also instigated by glial cell activation.

Activated glial cells lead to upregulation of VEGF, proinflammatory factors, and the vicious cycle of oxidative stress (Fig. 4.9). The neurons interacting with activated glial cells also alter glial cell glutamate transporter expression, causing further glutamate accumulation and neuronal excitotoxicity (Fig. 4.9).[79,80]

The understanding of underlying mechanisms, which cause retinal neuronal synaptic degeneration, neuronal apoptosis, and eventually neurodegeneration, has become a major focus of DR research. The resultant data are being translated into therapeutic strategies for DRN and microangiopathy. In Fig. 4.9, diabetes-induced GSK-3β activation is shown to be an important limb of pathogenesis of DRN. Thus, GSK-3β inhibition is a prominent target for treating DRN, using siRNA targeting GSK-3β (si-GSK-3β) or specific GSK-3β inhibitors.[76] In targeting pathways downstream of neuronal GSK-3β activation, inhibition of tau hyperphosphorylation is effective in treating neurodegeneration.[81] In order to restore the loss of β-catenin, besides implementing GSK-3β inhibition, various strategies are being explored, including activating β-catenin in early diabetes to protect RGCs.[76] Diabetes-induced glial cell activation, another limb of pathogenesis of DRN, causes accelerated oxidative stress, glutamate excitotoxicity, and proinflammation, resulting in neurodegeneration (Fig. 4.9). Therefore, antioxidants, glutamate excitotoxicity inhibitors, replacement of neuroprotective factors, and antiinflammatory agents are all being studied actively as potential therapies for DRN.[56,82]

Antiapoptotic protein BcL-xL to restore vasoregression and attenuate pathological angiogenesis in diabetic retina

Targeting both vasoregression in early DR and pathological angiogenesis in late stages of DR is an ideal strategy for treating DR. The bottle neck in this approach is the difficulty of distinguishing normal and diseased vascular cells in retinal microvessels, which can often evoke off-target side effects. Crespo-Garcia et al. discovered that diseased blood vessels such as those in DR or retinopathy of prematurity always contain senescent cells expressing p16[INK4A] and simultaneously upregulate the prosurvival protein BcL-xL.[83] Based on these findings, small molecule inhibitors of BcL-xL were administered. A single intravitreal dose of the BcL-xL inhibitor UBX1967 triggered intrinsic pathways of apoptosis through the activation of caspase-3 and caspase-7 within senescent endothelial cells. Ultimately, treatment with BcL-xL inhibitors, which drives selectively induced death of senescent cells, suppresses pathological angiogenesis and facilitates vascular repair, allowing for regrowth of functional blood vessels into the acellular and ischemic retina. These studies indicate that BcL-xL inhibitors may be capable of playing the dual role of treating both early vasoregression and late proliferation in DR. This significant work is illustrated in Fig. 4.10.

Taken together, the retinal NVU in diabetes is characterized by cell-specific and overlapping modes of cell death. Among the multiple modes of cell death, apoptosis

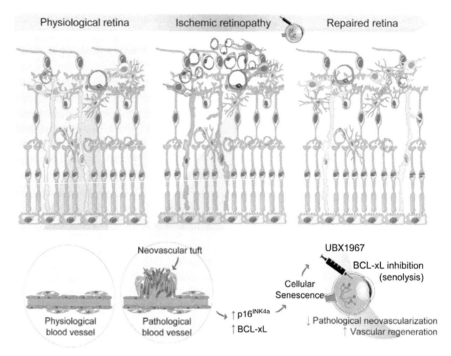

FIGURE 4.10

Antiapoptotic BcL-xL inhibitor (UBX1967) can discriminate diseased blood vessels by their propensity to engage pathways of cellular senescence. It is shown that targeting senescence effector/antiapoptotic protein BCL-xL suppresses pathological angiogenesis and repairs damaged vasculature, providing a therapy for neovascularization-associated retinal diseases, including DR. p16INK4a, activation of p16INK4a expression as one of the most useful in vivo markers of senescence; Senolysis, small-molecules selectively induced death of senescent cells.

Modified from Crespo-Garcia et al.[83]

of vascular pericytes, endothelial cells, RGCs, and photoreceptors is the dominant mode in the early phase of DR. Glial cells, specifically Müller cells undergo reactive gliosis and different modes of cell death. Under diabetic stress, specific types of cells undergo highly controlled apoptosis pathways comprising both extrinsic and intrinsic pathways. Mitochondria function as central regulators of the intrinsic pathway and participate in the extrinsic pathway of apoptosis through their role in energy production, calcium homeostasis, and compartmentalization of cell death activators. Targeting apoptogenic factors from both the intrinsic and extrinsic pathways and controlling the balance of pro- and antiapoptotic gene products are practical approaches for DR management. For further discussion of these approaches, please see Chapters 9 and 10.

References

1. Abcouwer SF, Gardner TW. Diabetic retinopathy: loss of neuroretinal adaptation to the diabetic metabolic environment. *Ann N Y Acad Sci.* 2014;1311:174–190. https://doi.org/10.1111/nyas.12412.
2. Jackson GR, Barber AJ. Visual dysfunction associated with diabetic retinopathy. *Curr Diab Rep.* 2010;10(5):380–384. https://doi.org/10.1007/s11892-010-0132-4.
3. Pan WW, Lin F, Fort PE. The innate immune system in diabetic retinopathy. *Prog Retin Eye Res.* January 8, 2021:100940. https://doi.org/10.1016/j.preteyeres.2021.100940.
4. Adams AJ, Bearse MA. Retinal neuropathy precedes vasculopathy in diabetes: a function-based opportunity for early treatment intervention? *Clin Exp Optom.* 2012;95(3):256–265. https://doi.org/10.1111/j.1444-0938.2012.00733.x.
5. Eleftheriou CG, Ivanova E, Sagdullaev BT. Of neurons and pericytes: the neuro-vascular approach to diabetic retinopathy. *Vis Neurosci.* 2020;37:E005. https://doi.org/10.1017/S0952523820000048.
6. Guthrie MJ, Osswald CR, Kang-Mieler JJ. Inverse relationship between the intraretinal concentration of bioavailable nitric oxide and blood glucose in early experimental diabetic retinopathy. *Invest Ophthalmol Vis Sci.* 2014;56(1):37–44. https://doi.org/10.1167/iovs.14-15777.
7. Moore-Dotson JM, Beckman JJ, Mazade RE, et al. Early retinal neuronal dysfunction in diabetic mice: reduced light-evoked inhibition increases rod pathway signaling. *Invest Ophthalmol Vis Sci.* 2016;57(3):1418–1430. https://doi.org/10.1167/iovs.15-17999.
8. Mishra A, Newman EA. Inhibition of inducible nitric oxide synthase reverses the loss of functional hyperemia in diabetic retinopathy. *Glia.* 2010;58(16):1996–2004. https://doi.org/10.1002/glia.21068.
9. Harrison WW, Bearse MA, Ng JS, et al. Multifocal electroretinograms predict onset of diabetic retinopathy in adult patients with diabetes. *Invest Ophthalmol Vis Sci.* 2011;52(2):772–777. https://doi.org/10.1167/iovs.10-5931.
10. Tonade D, Kern TS. Photoreceptor cells and RPE contribute to the development of diabetic retinopathy. *Prog Retin Eye Res.* 2021;83:100919. https://doi.org/10.1016/j.preteyeres.2020.100919.
11. Zhang J, Wu Y, Jin Y, et al. Intravitreal injection of erythropoietin protects both retinal vascular and neuronal cells in early diabetes. *Invest Ophthalmol Vis Sci.* 2008;49(2):732–742. https://doi.org/10.1167/iovs.07-0721.
12. Speiser P. Studies on diabetic retinopathy: III. Influence of diabetes on intramural pericytes. *Arch Ophthalmol.* 1968;80(3):332. https://doi.org/10.1001/archopht.1968.00980050334007.
13. Cogan DG, Toussaint D, Kuwabara T. Retinal vascular patterns. IV. Diabetic retinopathy. *Arch Ophthalmol.* 1961;66:366–378. https://doi.org/10.1001/archopht.1961.00960010368014.
14. Yanoff M. Diabetic retinopathy. *N Engl J Med.* 1966;274(24):1344–1349. https://doi.org/10.1056/NEJM196606162742403.
15. Wyllie AH, Kerr JF, Currie AR. Cell death: the significance of apoptosis. *Int Rev Cytol.* 1980;68:251–306. https://doi.org/10.1016/s0074-7696(08)62312-8.
16. Van Cruchten S, Van Den Broeck W. Morphological and biochemical aspects of apoptosis, oncosis and necrosis. *Anat Histol Embryol.* 2002;31(4):214–223. https://doi.org/10.1046/j.1439-0264.2002.00398.x.

17. Li W, Liu X, Yanoff M, Cohen S, Ye X. Cultured retinal capillary pericytes die by apoptosis after an abrupt fluctuation from high to low glucose levels: a comparative study with retinal capillary endothelial cells. *Diabetologia*. 1996;39(5):537−547. https://doi.org/10.1007/BF00403300.

18. Mizutani M, Kern TS, Lorenzi M. Accelerated death of retinal microvascular cells in human and experimental diabetic retinopathy. *J Clin Invest*. 1996;97(12):2883−2890. https://doi.org/10.1172/JCI118746.

19. Li W, Yanoff M, Liu X, Ye X. Retinal capillary pericyte apoptosis in early human diabetic retinopathy. *Chin Med J (Engl)*. 1997;110(9):659−663.

20. Li W, Yanoff M, Jian B, He Z. Altered mRNA levels of antioxidant enzymes in pre-apoptotic pericytes from human diabetic retinas. *Cell Mol Biol (Noisy-le-grand)*. 1999;45(1):59−66.

21. Engerman RL, Pfaffenbach D, Davis MD. Cell turnover of capillaries. *Lab Invest*. 1967;17(6):738−743.

22. Gökçinar-Yagci B, Uçkan-Çetinkaya D, Çelebi-Saltik B. Pericytes: properties, functions and applications in tissue engineering. *Stem Cell Rev Rep*. 2015;11(4):549−559. https://doi.org/10.1007/s12015-015-9590-z.

23. Huang H. Pericyte-endothelial interactions in the retinal microvasculature. *Int J Mol Sci*. 2020;21(19):E7413. https://doi.org/10.3390/ijms21197413.

24. Li C, Miao X, Li F, et al. Oxidative stress-related mechanisms and antioxidant therapy in diabetic retinopathy. *Oxid Med Cell Longev*. 2017;2017:9702820. https://doi.org/10.1155/2017/9702820.

25. Kowluru RA, Koppolu P. Diabetes-induced activation of caspase-3 in retina: effect of antioxidant therapy. *Free Radic Res*. 2002;36(9):993−999. https://doi.org/10.1080/1071576021000006572.

26. Beltramo E, Porta M. Pericyte loss in diabetic retinopathy: mechanisms and consequences. *Comput Mater Continua (CMC)*. 2013;20(26):3218−3225. https://doi.org/10.2174/09298673113209990022.

27. Addison DJ, Garner A, Ashton N. Degeneration of intramural pericytes in diabetic retinopathy. *Br Med J*. 1970;1(5691):264−266. https://doi.org/10.1136/bmj.1.5691.264.

28. *Pericyte Biology in Different Organs*Birbrair A, edVol 1122. Springer International Publishing; 2019. https://doi.org/10.1007/978-3-030-11093-2.

29. Bringmann A, Pannicke T, Grosche J, et al. Müller cells in the healthy and diseased retina. *Prog Retin Eye Res*. 2006;25(4):397−424. https://doi.org/10.1016/j.preteyeres.2006.05.003.

30. de Moraes G, Layton CJ. Therapeutic targeting of diabetic retinal neuropathy as a strategy in preventing diabetic retinopathy. *Clin Exp Ophthalmol*. 2016;44(9):838−852. https://doi.org/10.1111/ceo.12795.

31. Birch DG, Anderson JL. Standardized full-field electroretinography. Normal values and their variation with age. *Arch Ophthalmol*. 1992;110(11):1571−1576. https://doi.org/10.1001/archopht.1992.01080230071024.

32. Simonsen SE. The value of the oscillatory potential in selecting juvenile diabetics at risk of developing proliferative retinopathy. *Acta Ophthalmol (Copenh)*. 1980;58(6):865−878. https://doi.org/10.1111/j.1755-3768.1980.tb08312.x.

33. Bearse MA, Adams AJ, Han Y, et al. A multifocal electroretinogram model predicting the development of diabetic retinopathy. *Prog Retin Eye Res*. 2006;25(5):425−448. https://doi.org/10.1016/j.preteyeres.2006.07.001.

34. Sohn EH, van Dijk HW, Jiao C, et al. Retinal neurodegeneration may precede microvascular changes characteristic of diabetic retinopathy in diabetes mellitus. *Proc Natl Acad Sci U S A*. 2016;113(19):E2655–E2664. https://doi.org/10.1073/pnas.1522014113.

35. van de Kreeke JA, Darma S, Chan Pin Yin JMPL, et al. The spatial relation of diabetic retinal neurodegeneration with diabetic retinopathyLewin AS, ed. *PLoS One*. 2020; 15(4):e0231552. https://doi.org/10.1371/journal.pone.0231552.

36. Kaizu Y, Nakao S, Arima M, et al. Capillary dropout is dominant in deep capillary plexus in early diabetic retinopathy in optical coherence tomography angiography. *Acta Ophthalmol*. 2019;97(5):e811–e812. https://doi.org/10.1111/aos.14041.

37. Kim M, Kim RY, Park W, Park YG, Kim IB, Park YH. Electroretinography and retinal microvascular changes in type 2 diabetes. *Acta Ophthalmol*. 2020;98(7):e807–e813. https://doi.org/10.1111/aos.14421.

38. Cordeiro MF, Migdal C, Bloom P, Fitzke FW, Moss SE. Imaging apoptosis in the eye. *Eye*. 2011;25(5):545–553. https://doi.org/10.1038/eye.2011.64.

39. Schröder K, Szendroedi J, Benthin A, et al. German Diabetes Study—baseline data of retinal layer thickness measured by SD-OCT in early diabetes mellitus. *Acta Ophthalmol*. 2019;97(2):e303–e307. https://doi.org/10.1111/aos.13851.

40. Jenkins KS, Steel JC, Layton CJ. Systematic assessment of clinical methods to diagnose and monitor diabetic retinal neuropathy. *J Ophthalmol*. 2018;2018:8479850. https://doi.org/10.1155/2018/8479850.

41. Frydkjaer-Olsen U, Hansen RS, Peto T, Grauslund J. Structural neurodegeneration correlates with early diabetic retinopathy. *Int Ophthalmol*. 2018;38(4):1621–1626. https://doi.org/10.1007/s10792-017-0632-1.

42. Adamiec-Mroczek J, Zając-Pytrus H, Misiuk-Hojło M. Caspase-dependent apoptosis of retinal ganglion cells during the development of diabetic retinopathy. *Adv Clin Exp Med*. 2015;24(3):531–535. https://doi.org/10.17219/acem/31805.

43. Borrie SC, Duggan J, Cordeiro MF. Retinal cell apoptosis. *Expert Rev Ophthalmol*. 2009; 4(1):27–45. https://doi.org/10.1586/17469899.4.1.27.

44. Galvao J, Davis BM, Cordeiro MF. In vivo imaging of retinal ganglion cell apoptosis. *Curr Opin Pharmacol*. 2013;13(1):123–127. https://doi.org/10.1016/j.coph.2012.08.007.

45. Park SH, Park JW, Park SJ, et al. Apoptotic death of photoreceptors in the streptozotocin-induced diabetic rat retina. *Diabetologia*. 2003;46(9):1260–1268. https://doi.org/10.1007/s00125-003-1177-6.

46. Lammer J, Prager SG, Cheney MC, et al. Cone photoreceptor irregularity on adaptive optics scanning laser ophthalmoscopy correlates with severity of diabetic retinopathy and macular edema. *Invest Ophthalmol Vis Sci*. 2016;57(15):6624–6632. https://doi.org/10.1167/iovs.16-19537.

47. Burns SA, Elsner AE, Sapoznik KA, Warner RL, Gast TJ. Adaptive optics imaging of the human retina. *Prog Retin Eye Res*. 2019;68:1–30. https://doi.org/10.1016/j.preteyeres.2018.08.002.

48. Arroba AI, Mazzeo A, Cazzoni D, et al. Somatostatin protects photoreceptor cells against high glucose-induced apoptosis. *Mol Vis*. 2016;22:1522–1531.

49. Vinores SA, Gadegbeku C, Campochiaro PA, Green WR. Immunohistochemical localization of blood-retinal barrier breakdown in human diabetics. *Am J Pathol*. 1989;134(2): 231–235.

50. Kim DI, Lim SK, Park MJ, Han HJ, Kim GY, Park SH. The involvement of phosphatidylinositol 3-kinase/Akt signaling in high glucose-induced downregulation of GLUT-1

expression in ARPE cells. *Life Sci*. 2007;80(7):626−632. https://doi.org/10.1016/j.lfs.2006.10.026.

51. Madsen-Bouterse SA, Kowluru RA. Oxidative stress and diabetic retinopathy: pathophysiological mechanisms and treatment perspectives. *Rev Endocr Metab Disord*. 2008;9(4):315−327. https://doi.org/10.1007/s11154-008-9090-4.

52. Omri S, Behar-Cohen F, de Kozak Y, et al. Microglia/macrophages migrate through retinal epithelium barrier by a transcellular route in diabetic retinopathy: role of PKCζ in the Goto Kakizaki rat model. *Am J Pathol*. 2011;179(2):942−953. https://doi.org/10.1016/j.ajpath.2011.04.018.

53. Ponnalagu M, Subramani M, Jayadev C, Shetty R, Das D. Retinal pigment epithelium-secretome: a diabetic retinopathy perspective. *Cytokine*. 2017;95:126−135. https://doi.org/10.1016/j.cyto.2017.02.013.

54. Cuenca N, Ortuño-Lizarán I, Sánchez-Sáez X, et al. Interpretation of OCT and OCTA images from a histological approach: clinical and experimental implications. *Prog Retin Eye Res*. 2020;77:100828. https://doi.org/10.1016/j.preteyeres.2019.100828.

55. Zhu H, Zhang W, Zhao Y, et al. GSK3β-mediated tau hyperphosphorylation triggers diabetic retinal neurodegeneration by disrupting synaptic and mitochondrial functions. *Mol Neurodegener*. 2018;13(1):62. https://doi.org/10.1186/s13024-018-0295-z.

56. Rolev KD, Shu XS, Ying Y. Targeted pharmacotherapy against neurodegeneration and neuroinflammation in early diabetic retinopathy. *Neuropharmacology*. 2021;187:108498. https://doi.org/10.1016/j.neuropharm.2021.108498.

57. Goldman D. Müller glial cell reprogramming and retina regeneration. *Nat Rev Neurosci*. 2014;15(7):431−442. https://doi.org/10.1038/nrn3723.

58. Le YZ. VEGF production and signaling in Müller glia are critical to modulating vascular function and neuronal integrity in diabetic retinopathy and hypoxic retinal vascular diseases. *Vision Res*. 2017;139:108−114. https://doi.org/10.1016/j.visres.2017.05.005.

59. Rungger-Brändle E, Dosso AA, Leuenberger PM. Glial reactivity, an early feature of diabetic retinopathy. *Invest Ophthalmol Vis Sci*. 2000;41(7):1971−1980.

60. Lorenzi M, Gerhardinger C. Early cellular and molecular changes induced by diabetes in the retina. *Diabetologia*. 2001;44(7):791−804. https://doi.org/10.1007/s001250100544.

61. Zong H, Ward M, Madden A, et al. Hyperglycaemia-induced pro-inflammatory responses by retinal Müller glia are regulated by the receptor for advanced glycation end-products (RAGE). *Diabetologia*. 2010;53(12):2656−2666. https://doi.org/10.1007/s00125-010-1900-z.

62. Gerhardinger C, Costa MB, Coulombe MC, Toth I, Hoehn T, Grosu P. Expression of acute-phase response proteins in retinal Müller cells in diabetes. *Invest Ophthalmol Vis Sci*. 2005;46(1):349. https://doi.org/10.1167/iovs.04-0860.

63. Kusner LL, Sarthy VP, Mohr S. Nuclear translocation of glyceraldehyde-3-phosphate dehydrogenase: a role in high glucose-induced apoptosis in retinal Müller cells. *Invest Ophthalmol Vis Sci*. 2004;45(5):1553−1561.

64. Feenstra DJ, Yego EC, Mohr S. Modes of retinal cell death in diabetic retinopathy. *J Clin Exp Ophthalmol*. 2013;4(5):298. https://doi.org/10.4172/2155-9570.1000298.

65. Ridet JL, Privat A, Malhotra SK, Gage FH. Reactive astrocytes: cellular and molecular cues to biological function. *Trends Neurosci*. 1997;20(12):570−577. https://doi.org/10.1016/S0166-2236(97)01139-9.

66. Pekny M, Wilhelmsson U, Pekna M. The dual role of astrocyte activation and reactive gliosis. *Neurosci Lett*. 2014;565:30−38. https://doi.org/10.1016/j.neulet.2013.12.071.

67. Shin ES, Huang Q, Gurel Z, Sorenson CM, Sheibani N. High glucose alters retinal astrocytes phenotype through increased production of inflammatory cytokines and oxidative stress. *PLoS One*. 2014;9(7):e103148. https://doi.org/10.1371/journal.pone.0103148.

68. Rothhammer V, Quintana FJ. Control of autoimmune CNS inflammation by astrocytes. *Semin Immunopathol*. 2015;37(6):625−638. https://doi.org/10.1007/s00281-015-0515-3.

69. Lechuga-Sancho AM, Arroba AI, Frago LM, et al. Activation of the intrinsic cell death pathway, increased apoptosis and modulation of astrocytes in the cerebellum of diabetic rats. *Neurobiol Dis*. 2006;23(2):290−299. https://doi.org/10.1016/j.nbd.2006.03.001.

70. Yun JH, Park SW, Kim JH, Park YJ, Cho CH, Kim JH. Angiopoietin 2 induces astrocyte apoptosis via αvβ5-integrin signaling in diabetic retinopathy. *Cell Death Dis*. 2016;7:e2101. https://doi.org/10.1038/cddis.2015.347.

71. Altmann C, Schmidt M. The role of microglia in diabetic retinopathy: inflammation, microvasculature Defects and neurodegeneration. *IJMS*. 2018;19(1):110. https://doi.org/10.3390/ijms19010110.

72. Vujosevic S, Bini S, Midena G, Berton M, Pilotto E, Midena E. Hyperreflective intraretinal spots in diabetics without and with nonproliferative diabetic retinopathy: an in vivo study using spectral domain OCT. *J Diabetes Res*. 2013;2013:1−5. https://doi.org/10.1155/2013/491835.

73. Bolz M, Schmidt-Erfurth U, Deak G, et al. Optical coherence tomographic hyperreflective foci: a morphologic sign of lipid extravasation in diabetic macular edema. *Ophthalmology*. 2009;116(5):914−920. https://doi.org/10.1016/j.ophtha.2008.12.039.

74. Framme C, Schweizer P, Imesch M, Wolf S, Wolf-Schnurrbusch U. Behavior of SD-OCT-detected hyperreflective foci in the retina of anti-VEGF-treated patients with diabetic macular edema. *Invest Ophthalmol Vis Sci*. 2012;53(9):5814−5818. https://doi.org/10.1167/iovs.12-9950.

75. Midena E, Pilotto E. Emerging insights into pathogenesis. *Dev Ophthalmol*. 2017;60:16−27. https://doi.org/10.1159/000459687.

76. Shu XS, Zhu H, Huang X, et al. Loss of β-catenin via activated GSK3β causes diabetic retinal neurodegeneration by instigating a vicious cycle of oxidative stress-driven mitochondrial impairment. *Aging (Albany NY)*. 2020;12(13):13437−13462. https://doi.org/10.18632/aging.103446.

77. Kanwar M, Chan PS, Kern TS, Kowluru RA. Oxidative damage in the retinal mitochondria of diabetic mice: possible protection by superoxide dismutase. *Invest Ophthalmol Vis Sci*. 2007;48(8):3805−3811. https://doi.org/10.1167/iovs.06-1280.

78. Yang K, Chen Z, Gao J, et al. The key roles of GSK-3β in regulating mitochondrial activity. *Cell Physiol Biochem*. 2017;44(4):1445−1459. https://doi.org/10.1159/000485580.

79. Lieth E, LaNoue KF, Antonetti DA, Ratz M. Diabetes reduces glutamate oxidation and glutamine synthesis in the retina. The Penn State Retina Research Group. *Exp Eye Res*. 2000;70(6):723−730. https://doi.org/10.1006/exer.2000.0840.

80. Sorrentino FS, Allkabes M, Salsini G, Bonifazzi C, Perri P. The importance of glial cells in the homeostasis of the retinal microenvironment and their pivotal role in the course of diabetic retinopathy. *Life Sci*. 2016;162:54−59. https://doi.org/10.1016/j.lfs.2016.08.001.

81. Ying Y, Zhang YL, Ma CJ, et al. Neuroprotective effects of ginsenoside Rg1 against hyperphosphorylated tau-induced diabetic retinal neurodegeneration via activation of

IRS-1/Akt/GSK3β signaling. *J Agric Food Chem.* 2019;67(30):8348−8360. https://doi.org/10.1021/acs.jafc.9b02954.

82. Simó R, Hernández C. Novel approaches for treating diabetic retinopathy based on recent pathogenic evidence. *Prog Retin Eye Res.* 2015;48:160−180. https://doi.org/10.1016/j.preteyeres.2015.04.003.

83. Crespo-Garcia S, Tsuruda PR, Dejda A, et al. Pathological angiogenesis in retinopathy engages cellular senescence and is amenable to therapeutic elimination via BCL-xL inhibition. *Cell Metabol.* 2021;33(4):818−832.e7. https://doi.org/10.1016/j.cmet.2021.01.011.

Diabetic retinopathy, a disease with low-grade inflammation

5

Diabetic retinopathy (DR) is considered as a disease of chronic microinflammation.[1,2] The microinflammation refers to a low-grade background inflammation. The clinical findings of DR comprise increased systemic inflammatory biomarkers, such as C-reactive protein[3] and neutrophil count,[4] and increased inflammatory biomarkers of the posterior segment.[5,6] In diabetic eyes, increased vitreous levels of inflammatory cytokines, such as interleukin (IL)-1β,[7] IL-6, and tumor necrosis factor-α (TNF-α),[8] along with hyperglycemia-induced activation of retinal microglia and infiltration of immune cells,[9,10] such as macrophages, lymphocytes, and neutrophils, have been reported.[11] In both experimental and clinical DR, upregulation of leukocyte adhesion molecules in the blood vessels,[12] entrapment of neutrophils in the retinal and choroidal microcirculation,[13,14] and activation of the renin—angiotensin—aldosterone system that enhances chronic inflammation,[15] have also been observed. These findings indicate that DR has a chronic inflammatory etiology.[1,2,16,17] The inflammatory etiology of DR is characterized by increased proinflammatory mediators, activated cellular inflammatory processes, and resultant blood—retinal barrier (BRB) breakdown and macular edema.[18—23] Retinal cells participating in the production of proinflammatory mediators, include endothelial cells, Müller cells, microglia, and infiltrating monocytes.[24] The BRB breakdown induced by these inflammatory mediators aggravates leukocyte infiltration, thus producing more cytokines, chemokines, and the worsening of BRB breakdown.

Leukocyte adhesion and leukostasis

Both leukocyte adhesion and leukostasis are inflammatory and pathogenic markers of microvasculature during DR development. The inflammatory nature of DR starts with leukocyte adhesion to the vascular endothelium (leukocyte—endothelium adhesion), which happens in the early stage of the DR (Fig. 5.1). In a postmortem study of human subjects, Lutty et al. demonstrated increased numbers of neutrophils in the choroid and retina of diabetic individuals.[12] Leucocyte—endothelial interaction (leukocyte adhesion) contributes to BRB breakdown and the disruption and downregulation of tight junctions.[25] The adherent leukocytes can occlude retinal capillaries, participating in the development of capillary nonperfusion. Leukocyte adhesion is mediated by the adhesion molecules expressed both on the surface of

Therapeutic Targets for Diabetic Retinopathy. https://doi.org/10.1016/B978-0-323-93064-2.00001-9

113

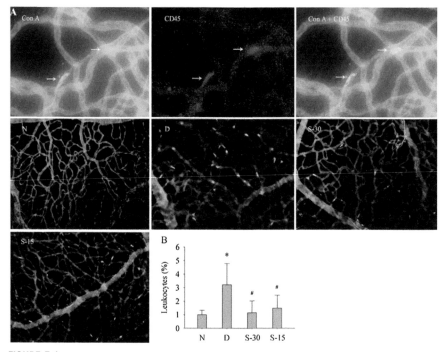

FIGURE 5.1

Leukocyte adhesion in experimental diabetic rat retina. (A) The representative examples of adherent leukocytes with FITC-labeled concanavalin A and anti-CD45 antibody staining in situ in digest retinal preparation (Con A, CD45, and Con A+CD45, X 400; N, D, S-30, and S-15, X 200). (B) Quantitative analysis of the effect of silybin on vascular leukostasis in retinal vasculature.

Con A, FITC-conjugated concanavalin A; Con A+CD45, Con A merged with CD45; CD45, anti-CD45 antibody; D, vehicle-treated diabetic group; N, nondiabetic control group; S-30 (30), S-15 (15) mg/kg/day silybin-treated diabetic group.

Modified from Zhang et al.[27]

leukocytes and endothelial cells.[26] For instance, adhesion molecules, such as inter-cellular adhesion molecule-1 (ICAM-1), are expressed on endothelial cells,[27] which bind to β2 integrins expressed by leukocytes.[26,28] The β2 integrins are heterodimeric receptors, composed of a variable α subunit (CD11a-CD11d) and a constant β2 (CD18) subunit, in which CD18 is critical for the firm attachment of human neutrophils to endothelial cells.[28,29] The β2 integrins consist of lymphocyte function−associated antigen-1 (LFA-1, CD11a/CD18, αLβ2),[26] macrophage-1 antigen (Mac-1, CD11b/CD18), p150/95 (CD11c/CD18), and CD11d/CD18, and mediate leukocyte adhesion, phagocytosis, cytoskeletal organization, and cell signaling.[30] Through binding to β2 integrin of LFA-1, ICAM-1 activates a key adhesion pathway causing upregulation of inflammatory cytokines[31,32] and promotes an inflammatory cascade in retina.[33] Besides ICAM-1/β2 integrin interaction, other molecules also mediate leukocyte adhesion, including vascular cell adhesion molecule-1 (VCAM-1) expressed by endothelial cells and very late antigen-4 (VLA-4) expressed by leukocytes, particularly through their interactions with each other.

The leukocyte adhesion is associated with capillary endothelial cell damage and obstruction of the microvasculature, leading to leukostasis and capillary nonperfusion, vascular leakage, and BRB breakdown.[34] In DR, retinal leukocyte adhesion is implicated in a cascade of retinal vascular events, including leukostasis, vascular endothelial cell injury/death, occlusion, and capillary nonperfusion.[35,36] Retinal leukocyte adhesion was observed less than 3 days after diabetes induction and was temporally and spatially correlated with capillary nonperfusion and BRB breakdown. In fact, the early retinal microvascular alterations in diabetes are induced by low-grade, persistent leukocyte activation, which is resulted from leukocyte—endothelial cell interaction (leukocyte adhesion). Initially, capillary function is maintained due to oxygen demand of retinal tissues. Progressively, this functionality is hindered and intravascular leukocyte arrest (leukostasis) becomes irreversible, followed by vascular leakage and retinal ischemia. It is important to note that increased leukostasis parallels the increase in metabolic abnormalities of diabetes.[37,38] The latter induce loss of endothelial lining such as endothelial hyaluronan-rich glycocalyx (see Chapter 6), leading to reduced capillary density and increased acellular capillaries in the later stages of DR.[11]

Although it is generally assumed that leukocyte adhesion and leukostasis play a critical role in inciting a chronic, low-grade inflammation in DR, van der Wijk et al. offered a different opinion that the increased leukostasis seems to be the result of unspecific endothelial cell dysfunction, rather than a crucial, specific step in the development of DR, and therefore leukostasis is likely an epiphenomenon, or secondary effect, in DR.[39] Thus, further study to elucidate the specific role of leukostasis and low-grade inflammation in the development of DR is needed. On the other hand, the underlying molecular mechanisms, whereby leukocytes are activated and leukocyte—endothelium interaction is enhanced, could be therapeutic targets for early DR. For instance, it has been postulated that inhibition of leukocyte—endothelial cell interaction could reduce retinal leukostasis, lessen BRB breakdown, and decrease macular edema.[33,40] In an experimental diabetic rat model, anti-ICAM-1 antibody prevented the increase in retinal leukostasis and vascular leakage.[33] SAR 1118, a novel small-molecule antagonist of LFA-1, binds to the I-domain of the CD11a subunit of LFA-1. SAR1118 serves as a direct competitive antagonist of LFA-1 binding to ICAM-1.[41] Topical delivery of SAR1118 significantly reduced leukostasis and BRB breakdown in the streptozotocin-induced diabetic rat model.[42] A prospective, randomized, double-masked phase 1b trial showed that topical SAR1118 was safe and well tolerated when applied topically to the human eye, demonstrating favorable pharmacokinetics for the therapeutic use in the anterior segment of the human eye.[43] However, vitreous levels were below the threshold of detection with the concentrations tested. Further investigation to increase its concentration in posterior segment and its efficacy in patients with DR/DME should be explored. Blocking VLA-4 with anti-CD49a significantly attenuated diabetes-induced leukostasis and vascular leakage.[44] Moreover, the anti-CD49a neutralizing antibody reduced the nuclear factor kappa B (NF-κB) activity and protein levels of vascular endothelial growth factor (VEGF) and TNF-α, indicating that leukocyte recruitment has a positive feedback role in the inflammatory pathway in diabetic retina.[45] Risuteganib, an integrin antagonist (formerly ALG-1001, Allegro Ophthalmics, San Juan Capistrano, CA, USA), is a novel, intravitreally administered, synthetic arginine—glycine—aspartic acid (RGD) oligopeptide that effectively binds and inhibits four integrin heterodimers, that is, $\alpha V\beta 3$, $\alpha V\beta 5$, $\alpha 5\beta 1$, and $\alpha M\beta 2$, disrupting cellular interactions involved in the regulation of angiogenesis, inflammation, vascular permeability, and cytotoxicity.[46] The DEL MAR Phase-2b trial using risuteganib as sequential therapy following a single anti-VEGF injection in patients with DME, in comparison with standard anti-VEGF monotherapy, reported sustained and equal visual acuity gains with the combined treatments.[46]

Activation of microglia

Microglia, the primary resident immune cell type, constitute a key population of glia in the retina. Microglia function as the tissue macrophages in retina. Microglia are required for normal retinal growth, the function of the immune system, neurogenesis, and synaptic pruning. Microglia interact with neurons, endothelial cells, and other glial cells, controlling blood vessel formation and participating in aging and retinal functions. Microglia secret growth factors, cytokines, as well as neuroprotective and antiinflammatory mediators.[47] In developing retina, microglia are mainly located in the inner retina, including the nerve fiber layer, the ganglion cell layer, and the inner and outer plexiform layers.[47] In adult retina, microglia gain a highly branched/ramified morphology with small cell bodies and long cellular protrusions that may span both inner and outer nuclear layers. Ramified microglia form an organized territorial network, constantly moving their processes to scan the surface of retinal neurons in a defined area surrounding each single cell.[47] Microglia are sensors of the retinal microenvironment and respond rapidly to various insults with a morphological and functional transformation into reactive phagocytes with ameboid morphology.

Microglia are activated early in streptozotocin-induced diabetic rat retinas.[48] The phenomenon of microglia activation in diabetic retina has been documented by our recent work.[49,50] In the diabetic rat, microglia become activated with increased cell proliferation and enhanced migration from inner to outer retina, even to the subretinal space and retinal pigment epithelial (RPE) layer.[50] In our recent work, it is clearly shown that the activated microglia closely contact the retinal capillaries, especially the deep capillary plexus (Fig. 5.2).[50] This study showed that the activated

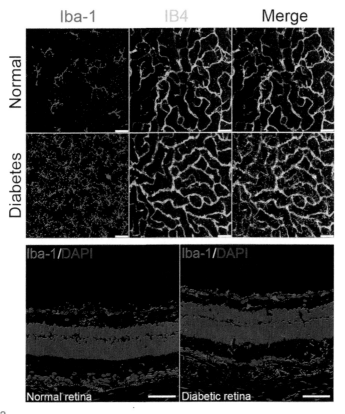

FIGURE 5.2

Activation of microglia in experimental diabetic rat retinas. Compared with normal control, in 8-week diabetic rat retinas, the activated microglia (Iba-1, *red*) proliferated, and migrated from inner retina to out retina even to the subretinal space and retinal pigment epithelium. The morphology was changed from ramified to ameboid. Activated microglia have a close relationship with retinal capillaries (IB4, *green*).

Modified from our recent unpublished data (Zhang and Li et al.).

microglia penetrate the basement membrane of the capillaries and phagocytose endothelial cells, leading to the breakdown of the BRB and the formation of acellular capillaries.[50] This enhanced phagocytosis by microglia is associated with decreased Src/Akt/Cofilin pathway signaling.[50] Besides direct interaction, activated microglia also mediate noncell-autonomous cell death of retinal ganglion cells by releasing TNF-α.[51] Microglia activation, accompanied by increased inflammatory factors and intracellular reactive oxygen species (ROS), was detected in experimental DR. Most importantly, in a proof-of-concept finding, the increased inflammatory factors and intracellular ROS could be prevented in experimental DR by intravitreal injection of fractalkine, an inhibitor of microglia activation.[49]

The Goto Kakizaki rat is a widely used model of spontaneous type 2 diabetes generated by selective breeding of Wistar rats.[47,52] In Goto Kakizaki rats, activated microglia/macrophages gradually accumulate in the subretinal space with diabetes progression. Up to 5 months, sparse microglia/macrophages are detected in the subretinal space, together with numerous pores in RPE cells, allowing inflammatory cell traffic between the retina and choroid. After 12 months of diabetes, numerous microglia are found in the outer retina and in the subretinal space. At this time point, the density of pores is significantly reduced in the RPE cell layer, with microglia/macrophage accumulation in the subretinal space together with vacuolization of RPE cells and disorganization of photoreceptor outer segments.[53] Microglia appear to migrate via "pores" that are present in the RPE layer at earlier time points.[53] These reactive microglia are preferentially located in areas of RPE vacuolization and close to disorganized photoreceptor outer segments. The transcellular migration of microglia is mediated by the PKCζ pathway because intravitreal injection of a PKCζ inhibitor can suppress subretinal trafficking of microglia.[47,53] In DR, the activated microglia that migrate to the subretinal space and accumulate above the RPE cause RPE dysfunction.[53] As DR progresses, the microglia markedly increase in number and become hypertrophic.[54] These cells clustered around the retinal vasculature, especially the dilated veins, microaneurysms, intraretinal hemorrhages, cotton wool spots, and areas of retinal and vitreous neovascularization. In retinas with macular edema, microglia infiltrate the outer retina and subretinal space.[54] Aggregates of activated microglial cells in the diabetic human retina appear as hyperreflective spots or hyperreflective foci (HRFs) by spectral domain optical coherence tomography (SD-OCT) imaging. In patients with DME, there was a strong positive correlation between the level of soluble CD14 (sCD14, a cytokine released by microglia/macrophages) in the aqueous humor and the number of HRFs observed with SD-OCT, indicating that inflammatory cells such as microglia/marcophages are closely involved in the pathogenesis of DME.[6]

Targeting microglia trafficking and activation would be reasonable approaches to control inflammatory events in DR. For example, minocycline, a commonly used second generation semisynthetic tetracycline analog, has potent antiinflammatory and neuroprotective effects. Minocycline has been demonstrated in cell culture and animal models to have antiinflammatory properties that are independent of its antibacterial property. It has high bioavailability and has been used in various animal models, including experimental DR,[48] retinal degeneration,[55,56] endotoxin-induced uveitis,[36] retinal detachment,[57] and glaucoma.[58] For example, a single-centered, prospective, and open-label phase I/II clinical trial (NCT01120899)[59] enrolled five participants with fovea-involving DME who received oral minocycline 100 mg twice daily for 6 months. The result showed that minocycline treatment is associated with improvements in visual function, central macular edema, and vascular leakage. The preliminary result suggested that microglial inhibition with oral minocycline is an applicable strategy, targeting the inflammatory etiology of DME[59] (see Chapter 9).

Inflammatory cytokines and chemokines in diabetic eyes

Activated endothelial cells, microglia, infiltrating monocytes/macrophages, and retinal Müller cells are considered to be the main source of proinflammatory cytokines in the retina.[24] Besides the activation of inflammatory cells, the inflammatory cytokines and chemokines are upregulated and involved in the development of DR.[5] Numerous studies have demonstrated increased levels of inflammation-related factors in the ocular fluid of diabetic patients.[1,60] Hyperglycemia is directly linked to upregulation of various inflammation-related cytokines in retina and ocular fluid.[5,61] Based on previous reports, the list is summarized as follows: hypoxia-induced factor-1α (HIF-1α), VEGF, placental growth factor (PlGF), insulin-like growth factor-1, basic fibroblast growth factor, pigment epithelium-derived factor, IL-1β, IL-2, IL-4, IL-6, IL-8, IL-10, monocyte chemotactic protein 1/2, ICAM-1, VCAM-1, TNF-α, interferon-γ, interferon γ-induced protein 10, regulated upon activation normal T-cell expressed and secreted, complement components 3a and 5a (C3a/5a), CD40, etc.[5] In particular, in DME patients, the levels of inflammatory cytokines, such as VEGF, ICAM-1, IL-1β, IL-6, TNF-α, IL-8, and MCP-1, are elevated in the vitreous.[60−64] Among numerous inflammation-related cytokines that have been discovered in diabetic eyes, the following key factors are further discussed.

Hypoxia-induced factor-1α

In diabetic retina, the hypoxia is aggravated by the increasing expression of HIF-1α.[65] Upregulation of HIF-1α leads to the elevation of several hypoxia-regulated gene products, including VEGF, angiopoietin-2 (Ang-2), IL-6, TNF-α, and vascular endothelial-protein tyrosine phosphatase.[65] During hypoxia, VEGF-A expression is regulated at the transcriptional level via HIF-1α. In contrast, the basal level of VEGF-A is not dependent upon HIF-1α signaling, relying instead on PKCβ/HuR cascade at posttranslational level.[66] A recent study using the Ins2^{Akita} diabetic mouse model revealed the time-dependent regulatory events of HIF-1α in diabetic retina. HIF-1α protein is significantly increased at 9 weeks (early phase of DR), and then gradually decreases to baseline level. On the other hand, protein levels of PKCβ/HuR rose significantly at 46 weeks to maintain VEGF-A level during the late phase of DR. In the context of DR, the early elevated HIF-1α protein level may be protective against neurodegeneration because it appears to favor transcription of VEGF-A isoforms such as VEGF120/121 rather than VEGF164 (equivalent to human VEGF165). As compared to VEGF-A, these isoforms are neuroprotective, antiangiogenic, and antiinflammatory. By using conditional HIF-1α KO mice, it has been proven that Müller cell-derived HIF-1α is a key mediator of retinal angiogenesis and inflammation. Thus, Müller cell-derived HIF-1α is a promising therapeutic target for inflammatory inhibition of diabetic retina.[67]

Versatile functions of VEGF-A

VEGF-A is considered as the central player in the progression of DR.[68,69] VEGF-A possesses versatile functions in ischemia-induced and inflammatory downstream pathways.[70,71] Upon binding VEGF receptors, VEGF-A mainly promotes cell survival via phosphoinositide 3-kinase (PI3K), which is dependent on the activation of the antiapoptotic Akt/protein kinase B (PI3K-Akt) pathway. Akt phosphorylates the proapoptotic Bcl-2-associated death promoter protein, resulting in the inhibition of caspase activity.[72] VEGF/VEGFR also activates phospholipase C (PLC), which stimulates the protein kinase C (PKC) pathway to promote cell proliferation.[73] In addition, VEGF/VEGFR stimulates the mitogen-activated protein kinase (MAPK) signaling pathway, which is involved in endothelial hyperpermeability and angiogenesis.

Thus, VEGF-A has diverse roles. On the one hand, in diabetic retina, excessive VEGF is produced by ischemic Müller cells,[74] ganglion cells,[75] and by activated leukocytes.[76] The activated leukocytes further aggravate Müller cell production of VEGF.[77] Subsequently, VEGF exacerbates leukostasis, a hallmark or inflammation. On the other hand, the aggregated leukocytes that could block the access of VEGF receptors may permit retinal reperfusion.[78]

Overall, VEGF-A is the major therapeutic target for DR. To target VEGF-A, several approaches are being used including the control of upstream HIF-1α and PKCβ/HuR pathways, direct neutralization of VEGF-A, blockade of the VEGF-VEGFR axis, and regulation of VEGF-A downstream pathways. However, a classical study showed that the VEGF concentration in 38% of diabetic patients with quiescent neovascularization of PDR is low, that is, no significant difference from that of the nondiabetic control. This finding indicates that these patients are no longer responsive to anti-VEGF therapy. In other words, the clinical manifestations of these patients may be attributed to non-VEGF pathways.[79] Post hoc analyses of the DRCR.net Protocol T showed that persistent DME existed 24 weeks after regular anti-VEGF treatment in 30%−66% of patients.[80] These findings also suggested that VEGF-independent pathways, specifically inflammatory pathways, significantly contribute to the pathogenesis of DME.[21,81]

Placental growth factor

PlGF, a member of VEGF family, modulates a range of neural, glial, and vascular cell responses that are distinct from VEGF-A. As PlGF expression is selectively associated with pathological angiogenesis and inflammation, its blockade does not affect the healthy vasculature. PlGF actions have been extensively studied in tumor biology. Recently, there has been accumulating preclinical evidence that PlGF could have an important role in retinal diseases.[82] The human PlGF gene is located on chromosome 14q24 and is encoded by seven exons. Due to alternative mRNA splicing, 4 isoforms have been identified, that is, PlGF-1, PlGF-2, PlGF-3, and PlGF-4. PlGF-1 (PlGF131) and PlGF-2 (PlGF152) are the best characterized, whereas the biological relevance of PlGF-3 (PlGF203) and PlGF-4 (PlGF224) remains to be studied.[82] PlGF-1 and PlGF-3 are nonheparin-binding, diffusible proteins, whereas PlGF-2 and PlGF-4 have heparin-binding domains. All PlGF isoforms bind VEGFR-1, while PlGF-2 additionally binds Nrp-1 and Nrp-2 due to an insertion of 21 basic amino acids in its carboxy-terminal region.[83] Upon receptor binding, PlGF can affect the growth, migration, and survival of endothelial cells.[82] The VEGFR-1 pathway has been best described in endothelial cells where it transduces the ligand-induced autophosphorylation on different tyrosine residues in the intracellular domain.[84] This phosphorylation leads to the activation of PLCγ and PI3K, regulating endothelial cell survival and proliferation via the MAPK pathway.[73] VEGFR-1 is mainly expressed in vascular endothelial cells, hematopoietic cells, osteoblasts, monocytes/macrophages, and pericytes.[82]

Under ischemic stress, PlGF can activate monocytes to increase different proinflammatory chemokines (e.g., IL-1β, IL-8, and MCP-1).[85] In the bone marrow, PlGF has been shown to have a role in mobilizing hematopoietic stem cells.[86] After new blood vessel formation, PlGF may also stimulate VEGFR-1 on smooth muscle cells to evoke vessel maturation and stabilization.[87] PlGF was found to be upregulated in ocular samples, such as aqueous humor, vitreous, retina, as well as the retinal cells (e.g., endothelial cells and pericytes), in patients with DR correlating with progressive retinal ischemia.[82,88,89] Despite these data, the exact role of PlGF in pathological angiogenesis in retinal vascular diseases and the benefits of PlGF-specific inhibition in humans with DR remain to be explored (see Fig. 7.4, in Chapter 7).

Intercellular adhesion molecule-1

Hyperglycemia leads to upregulation of ICAM-1 in retina, which is accompanied by markedly increased numbers of leukocytes, causing capillary obstruction, endothelial cell damage, and vascular leakage.[34,36,90] ICAM-1 expression is upregulated in the retinal and choroidal vasculature in diabetic patients and diabetic animal models.[12,33] In patients with DME, vitreous soluble ICAM-1 is significantly increased and correlates with increased retinal thickness at the central fovea.[91] A recent meta-analysis indicated that ICAM-1 generally is increased in the patients with DR, with higher levels associated with more severe DR.[92] In streptozotocin-induced diabetic rats, retinal vascular leakage and nonperfusion are temporally and spatially associated with retinal leukostasis; further, ICAM-1 inhibition prevents diabetic retinal leukostasis and vascular leakage, indicating involvement of ICAM-1 in the inflammatory etiology of DR.[33] Blockade of ICAM-1 function with a monoclonal antibody or knockout reduces leukostasis, vascular leakage, and endothelial cell death, while preserving the integrity of BRB in diabetic animals.[19,33,34]

Monocyte chemotactic protein-1

Monocyte chemotactic protein-1 (MCP-1), also called CCL2, is a member of the C−C chemokine family that plays a vital role in retinal inflammation in DR.

MCP-1 is known to be a potent chemotactic factor that stimulates recruitment and activation of monocytes and macrophages.[60] MCP-1 stimulates monocytes and macrophages to produce superoxide, inflammatory factors, and other mediators.[60] Besides, MCP-1 also promotes fibrosis and angiogenesis.[93] MCP-1 expression is regulated by NF-κB,[94] which upregulates both the activity of the MCP-1 promoter and expression of the MCP-1 protein in glial cells.[95,96] For example, Müller cells in diabetic eyes produce significant levels of MCP-1 in aqueous and vitreous.[97] MCP-1 can increase VEGF expression, contributing to neovascularization.[98]

MCP-1 was detected in the membranes of myofibroblasts and vascular endothelial cells of PDR and proliferative vitreoretinopathy patients.[99] In diabetic retina, retinal neurons are the main source of MCP-1 production, and MCP-1 increases with the progression of disease, subsequently activating retinal microglia.[100]

In diabetic patients, RPE cells, glial cells, and endothelial cells regulate MCP-1 production.[95,96,101,102] Increased MCP-1 exerts its function through its receptor, C−C chemokine receptor type 2 (CCR2). Monocytes and macrophages express CCR2 and are involved in the inflammatory events of DR.[103] The adhesion of macrophages to the capillary endothelium leads to capillary occlusion and consequently to retinal ischemia.[104] Several studies have demonstrated higher MCP-1 levels in the vitreous fluid relative to that in the serum in DR patients, indicating a local vitreous production of MCP-1 expression.[104,105] Furthermore, there is a significant positive association between the vitreous levels of the MCP-1 and the severity of the DR.[106] Overall, MCP-1 plays a pivotal role in vascular inflammation through induction, activation, and recruitment of monocytes and macrophages. In this regard, possible strategies that require further clinical studies include *MCP-1* gene inhibition, inhibition of NF-κB, and inhibition of the MCP-1−CCRs axis.[60]

Tumor necrosis factor-α

TNF-α was found to be upregulated in vitreous and serum of patients with PDR compared with non-PDR (NPDR).[107,108] TNF-α is the inflammatory initiator promoting leukocytes adhesion to retinal blood vessels, which also mediates NF-κB activation in DR. In diabetic rat retinas, TNF-α causes significant pericyte loss and capillary degeneration.[109,110] In contrast, mice genetically deficient in TNF-α showed alleviated leukostasis, reduced vascular leakage, and decreased loss of pericytes and endothelial cells.[111] Intravitreal injection of TNF-α inhibitor also alleviates retinal capillary degeneration and pericyte loss,[109] thus preventing BRB breakdown in experimental diabetic animals. The possible application of TNF-α inhibitors for DR requires further investigation.

Interleukin-1β

IL-1β is mainly produced by macrophages. IL-1β is activated by cleaved caspase-1, prompting NF-κB transcription and increasing expression of IL-6 and IL-8. Thus, increased activity of caspase-1 contributes to the development of inflammation in DR.[112] In a mouse model of oxygen-induced ischemic retinopathy, IL-1β activity is increased while IL-18 activity is decreased, promoting angiogenesis and neovascularization.[113] By using MCC950, an inhibitor of nucleotide-binding domain leucine-rich repeat and pyrin domain containing receptor 3 (NLRP3), the IL-1β/IL-18 activation pattern can be reversed, resulting in the inhibition of retinal neovascularization, decrease in the number of acellular capillaries, and reduced leakage of retinal vessels.[113] In addition, antioxidants or caspase-1 inhibitors can prevent the IL-1β increase in retina and alleviate the degeneration of retinal capillaries in those animals.[114,115] Deletion of the IL-1β receptor also protects against degeneration of capillaries in diabetic retina.[115] Clinically applicable IL-1β inhibitors merit further study.

Interleukin-6

IL-6 is produced by a variety of retinal cells and involved in inflammation, acting as local signal intensifier in the early events of DR. These early events are characterized by increased leukostasis and the presence of inflammatory mediators such as IL-6 and TNF-α, which directly correlate with endothelial cell damage and vascular dysfunction.[19,34,116] Meta-analysis showed that the level of IL-6 in patients with DR is significantly increased relative to that in the control group.[117] Subgroup analysis further showed IL-6 levels in the PDR group are higher than those in the NPDR group, indicating that increased IL-6 is also involved in the progression of DR.[117]

Analysis of the intravitreal concentrations of cytokines in DME with subfoveal neuroretinal detachment (SND) revealed elevated intravitreal concentrations of VEGF, IL-6, and IL-8.[118,119] Among them, the elevated IL-6 has a strong association with the presence of SND, suggesting an inflammatory etiology in the development of this type of DME.[118,119] Disruption of the external limiting membrane in DME with SND is accompanied by outer retina cellular damage. The damaged cells may attract scavenger cells, such as activated microglia and macrophages, which subsequently produce more IL-6.[120]

Angiopoietin-2

The pathway of angiopoietin/tyrosine kinase with immunoglobulin and epidermal growth factor homology domains (Ang/Tie) plays an important role in the maintenance of vascular stability, angiogenesis, and vascular permeability.[121,122] Ang-2 is not just a proangiogenic factor but also an inflammatory factor.[123] Ang-2 is produced mainly by endothelial cells and stored in Weibel–Palade bodies, from which Ang-2 is released rapidly upon stimulus (Fig. 5.3).[124] Ang-2 levels are reported to be upregulated under multiple conditions, including hypoxia,[125] hyperglycemia,[126–128] and oxidative stress.[129] Ang-2 can act either in an autocrine manner on endothelial cells or in a paracrine manner on leukocytes (Fig. 5.3). The autocrine Ang-2

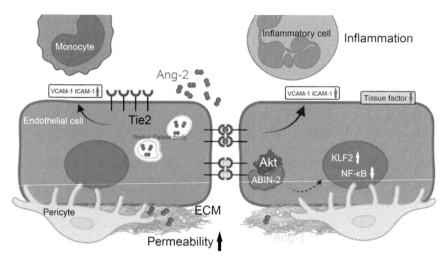

FIGURE 5.3

Diagram for Ang-2 action. Ang-2 is secreted from Weibel—Palade bodies (WPBs) of endothelial cells and sensitizes endothelial cells for interaction with inflammatory cells. Ang-2, as an antagonist of Tie2, can act either in an autocrine manner on endothelial cells (*left*), increasing the expressions of ICAM-1 and VCAM-1, or in a paracrine manner on inflammatory cells (*right*), including monocytes/macrophages and neutrophils. Upon stimulation, inflammatory cells respond with increased adhesion to the endothelium, triggered in a β2 integrin-dependent manner, leading to inflammation and increased permeability of blood vessels. Tie2 inhibition promotes the expression of ICAM-1, VCAM-1, and E-selectin on endothelial cells, enhancing monocyte adhesion to endothelial cells and leading to inflammation.

Ang-1, angiopoietin 1; Ang-2, angiopoietin 2; ECM, extracellular matrix; ICAM-1, intercellular adhesion molecule-1; VCAM-1, vascular adhesion molecule-1.

Modified from Eklund et al.[186]

signaling induces adhesion molecules and vascular leakage. The paracrine signaling is received by monocytes/macrophages and neutrophils. Upon stimulation, innate immune cells can respond with increased adhesion to the vessel wall, triggered in a β2 integrin—dependent manner, leading to inflammation.[123]

Faricimab, previously known as RG7716, is a bispecific antibody that simultaneously binds both VEGF-A and Ang-2. Phase 3 trials for DME (YOSEMITE NCT03622580 and RHINE NCT03622593) showed robust vision gains and anatomical improvements after treatment with faricimab. The personalized treatment interval for faricimab could be extended to 16 weeks for some patients, demonstrating the potential durability of treatment for DME.[130] Faricimab was first approved by FDA for the treatment of patients with neovascular age-related macular degeneration or DME in January 2022.[131] The mechanism of action by Ang/Tie pathway is also discussed in Chapters 7 and 9.

Inflammatory impact on BRB breakdown

One of the pathogenic effects of inflammation in DR is the negative impact on BRB integrity. Chronic low-grade inflammation is present at different stages of DR. Inflammation is responsible for retinal vasculature damage, for example, increased retinal vascular permeability and neovascularization.[18] Increased inflammatory factors induce activation and migration of leukocytes and leukostasis with subsequent capillary occlusion, retinal nonperfusion, and hypoxia. The resultant endothelial cell damage leads to BRB breakdown, retinal edema, microaneurysm, hemorrhages, and exudates.[1,18] Leukocytes contribute to microvascular damage by releasing cytokines and superoxide and by physically blocking the capillary lumen.[1] They interact via integrin with ICAM-1 and VCAM-1 on the surface of endothelial cells, resulting in leukostasis.[1] As mentioned above, leukostasis results in the disruption of tight junctions and BRB breakdown induced by the fenestrations and vesiculovacuolar organelles.[25] The activated leukocytes, especially mononuclear phagocytes/macrophages, release various inflammatory factors, which further damage the endothelial cells, causing the downregulation of tight junctions and BRB breakdown.

Anti-inflammation as a therapeutic strategy

Since inflammation plays a critical role in the pathogenesis of DR and DME, suppression of inflammation seems to be a reasonable approach for treating DR and DME.[1]

Corticosteroids have been proven to be beneficial in treating DR and DME due to their anti-inflammatory and anti-angiogenic properties.[132] Intravitreal injection of sustainable dexamethasone (Ozurdex, Allergen), as an example, was efficacious and safe in the treatment of DME, achieving visual improvement, edema resolution, as well as a decrease in intraocular inflammatory mediators, including VEGF, MCP-1, and IL-6. Intravitreal corticosteroid injections have showed similar effects in human and animal models with DME. In diabetic rats, leukostasis, vascular leakage, and central subfield thickness are decreased after steroid administration.[133–136] In the Ozurdex MEAD Study Group trials, two large double-blind studies evaluated the safety and efficacy of Ozurdex (0.7 and 0.35 mg). In the treatment of patients with DME, both doses of the Ozurdex implant met the primary efficacy endpoint for improvement in visual acuity with acceptable safety profile.[137] FAME study evaluated long-term efficacy and safety of intravitreal inserts of fluocinolone acetonide (Iluvien, Alimera Sciences, Alpharetta, GA, USA). Iluvien inserts releasing 0.2 µg/day (low dose) or 0.5 µg/day (high dose) fluocinolone acetonide were used to treat patients with DME. Iluvien inserts provided substantial visual benefit for up to 3 years, providing a valuable addition to the options available for patients with DME,[138] especially those who do not respond to other therapy, such as anti-VEGF treatment.[139]

In the treatment for DME, anti-VEGF therapy is the first-line therapy due to its great efficacy in blocking VEGF-mediated downstream functions. Despite the high efficacy of the VEGF inhibitors, reported by DRCR.NET Protocol T, about 30% −66% of the DME patients treated with anti-VEGF agents still have persistent macular edema, indicating poor or nonresponse to current anti-VEGF therapy.[80,82] Among those patients with persistent DME, continuous anti-VEGF treatment remains partially beneficial. For instance, when following the treatment protocol used in this trial, the cumulative 3-year probabilities of chronic persistent DME are decreased, and vision is improved.[140] On the other hand, despite timely and appropriate treatment with anti-VEGF drugs, some subsets of patients continue to experience visual loss, indicating the pathogenesis of DME involves more than just VEGF-driven mechanisms. Some studies demonstrated the advantage of combined therapy with corticosteroids and anti-VEGF agents in refractory DME patients.[141−143] Busch et al. demonstrated that DME patients that become refractory to anti-VEGF after three monthly injections might benefit from a switch to a dexamethasone implant early in the treatment.[142] In a pilot study, the combined intravitreal injection of both bevacizumab and triamcinolone could improve vision acuity and decrease central macular thickness in some patients with severe diffuse DME, who were refractory to previous monotherapies.[143] In a nonrandomized retrospective interventional study, Sadhukhan et al. combined monthly intravitreal ranibizumab injection for six doses with a single intravitreal dexamethasone implant at first injection of ranibizumab in patients with refractory DME. The results revealed that 21 patients out of 30 showed encouraging results, demonstrating both visual acuity improvement and central macular thickness reduction.[141]

Thus, preclinical and clinical studies suggest that other factors besides VEGF-A play a pathogenic role in disease progression. Clearly, alternative therapies for DR, especially antiinflammatory therapies are attractive. For example, nonsteroidal antiinflammatory drugs (NSAIDs) are inhibitors of cyclooxygenase (COX) enzymes, which reduce the synthesis of proinflammatory prostaglandins.[2] COX-2 plays a role in the inflammation in DR, thereby NSAIDs may have therapeutic potential in DR.[45] COX-2 expression and its products, such as prostaglandin E2 (PGE2), are increased significantly in diabetic rat retinas and in a retinal Müller cell line (rMC-1) cultured in high glucose.[144,145] COX-2 inhibition reduces the production of PGE2 in diabetic rat retinas[146] and blocks diabetes-induced expression of ICAM-1 and TNF-α.[144,147] Infliximab, a monoclonal antibody directed against TNF-α, was tested in four patients with DME nonresponsive to laser photocoagulation.[148] After 2 months of 5 mg/kg intravenous infliximab, five of the seven symptomatic eyes showed positive responses, including improvement in visual acuity and reduction in macular thickness, with further improvement seen after repeated infusions. Canakinumab (Novartis, Basel, Switzerland), a selective IL-1β antibody, was adjunctively used to treat patients with PDR, showing stabilization of PDR, but without effect on neovascularization, despite demonstrating reduction of macular edema.[149] Other potential therapies targeting proinflammatory factors, such as MCP-1, IL-6 and ICAM-1, merit clinical trials in the future.

Innate and adaptive immunity in DR

As an immune-privileged tissue, the retina is protected from systemic immune attack by a highly complex, sophisticated system.[16] Accumulating evidence shows that immunological mechanisms play a prominent role in the pathogenesis of DR.[21] For instance, BRB breakdown in DR is a prerequisite of inflammation onset in retina. In DR, metabolic disorder in endothelial cells may lead to vascular dysfunction and disruption of tight junctions between endothelial cells and RPE cells. Circulating immune cells, including neutrophils and monocytes are activated, leading to increased leukocyte adhesion, leukostasis, and transmigration of leukocytes into retinal parenchyma.[16] BRB breakdown also results in the leakage of serum proteins, including immunoglobulins and complement proteins into retinal parenchyma.

The immune system consists of innate and adaptive immunity.[16] The role of innate immunity in the development of diabetic complications has been extensively studied.[11] Innate immunity protects the host from both exogenous pathogens, such as the pathogen-associated molecular patterns (PAMPs) and endogenous danger molecules, known as damage-associated molecular patterns (DAMPs). DAMPs that comprise oxidized or glycated proteins, mislocated proteins/antigens, and intracellular contents (e.g., uric acid, DNA, RNA, etc.) are released by necrotic cells and recognized by various pattern recognition receptors (PRRs) expressed by innate immune cells to initiate both rapid defense and more delayed cellular responses.[16,150] The common PRRs responsible for PAMP/DAMP detection include toll-like receptors (TLRs), C-type lectin receptors, receptor for advanced glycation end-products (RAGE), NOD-like receptors (NLRs), RIG-like receptors, etc.[16] The innate immune system provides the first line of defense against DAMPs. NLRP3, a component of the inflammasome, plays a key role in innate immunity.[151] The NLRP3 inflammasome is a multimeric protein complex that initiates an inflammatory form of cell death and triggers the release of proinflammatory cytokines IL-1β and IL-18.[152] The activation of the NLRP3 inflammasome is a two-step process. The initial extracellular priming signal induced by the TLR/NF-κB pathway upregulates cellular transcription of pro-IL-1β and NLRP3 inflammasome component proteins. The secondary activation signal is mediated by numerous PAMP or DAMP stimulation and promotes the assembly of the adapter apoptosis-associated speck-like protein containing a C-terminal caspase recruitment domain (ASC) and procaspase-1, leading to the activation of the NLRP3 inflammasome complex.[153] Common secondary signals include changes in potassium ion flux, ROS, lysosomal destabilization, and certain posttranslational protein modifications.[152]

Dysregulation of innate immunity was reported to be associated with increased inflammatory responses, contributing to DR progression.[16] The activation of the NLRP3 inflammasome may cause the exacerbation of macular edema and angiogenesis in DR.[154,155] During diabetes, metabolic disturbances trigger the release of DAMPs in retina.[16] The released DAMPs could be the ligands for TLRs.[156] The injured cell-released high mobility group box 1 (HMGB1), a DNA-binding protein, is able to bind to its receptors including TLR2, TLR4, TLR9, and RAGE, then activating NLRP3 inflammasome.[156,157] Under inflammatory conditions, extracellular ATP mediates NLRP3 inflammasome activation through the P2X7 receptor.[158] Overall, the activation of NLRP3 inflammasome leads to caspase-1-dependent production of IL-1β and IL-18, resulting in pyroptosis.[159] Several NLRP3 inhibitors have been investigated for the treatment of DR. For example, Zhang et al. demonstrated that MCC950, the inhibitor of NLRP3, has protective effects against high glucose-induced inflammation in human retinal endothelial cells via downregulation of the Nek7-NLRP3 pathway.[160] The activation of hydroxycarboxylic acid receptor 2 by β-hydroxybutyrate inhibits diabetic damage of retina through reduction of the NLRP3 inflammasome activation.[161] The recently discovered Exchange Protein Activated by cAMP (Epac1 and Epac2) are expressed within the retina.[162] Jiang et al. reported that loss of Epac1 in the mouse retinal vasculature significantly increased the inflammatory proteins, including TLR4, HMGB1, NLRP3, cleaved caspase-1, and IL-1β in vascular specific Epac1 knockout mice.[163] Epac1 agonist (8-CPT-2′-O-Me-cAMP) can effectively reduce the expressions of TLR4, HMGB1, cleaved caspase-1, and IL-1β in high glucose-treated retinal endothelial cells. Jiang et al. found that Epac1 requires AMP-activated protein kinase to increase sirtuin 1 (SIRT1) and reduce HMGB1 by using cdh5/Epac1 Cre mice and diabetic mice.[164] Epac1 may serve as a potential antiinflammatory target to inhibit the NLRP3 inflammasome in DR.[163]

The immune suppressive microenvironment of the retina might be compromised in DR. In experimental and clinical DR,[165−167] both neuronal degeneration and loss of synaptic connectivity are observed. Retinal neurons critically control microglial activation through the CD200-CD200R and CX3CL1-CX3CR1 pathways.[16,168] Neuronal degeneration may lead to dysfunction of these pathways, resulting in uncontrolled microglial activation.[166,167] High levels of the soluble form of CD200 have been detected in the vitreous of patients with PDR.[169] Recently discovered 7 histone deacetylases, called SIRTs, are involved in cellular senescence, cell cycle, metabolic pathways, and DNA repair. In DR, SIRT 1, 3, 5, and 6 play regulatory roles in the activation of the inflammatory response, oxidative stress, and both glycolysis and gluconeogenesis. Activators of SIRTs pathways (e.g., antagomiR, resveratrol, or glycyrrhizin) are currently being developed to treat the inflammatory cascade occurring in DR. Therefore, regulation of SIRTs is a novel approach for antiinflammatory therapy[170] (see Chapter 10).

During the course of diabetes, circulating immune cells such as neutrophils and macrophages may infiltrate the retina. Infiltrating immune cells together with activated microglia may contribute to retinal pathologies.[16] It has been reported that M2 macrophages are increased in the vitreous and fibrovascular membranes of patients with PDR.[171] The increased M2 macrophage density is associated with high levels of IL-11, VEGF, and soluble CD163.[172] M2 macrophages promote angiogenesis and fibrosis, which might be exacerbated and prolonged by dysregulated innate immunity.[17] With the breakdown of BRB, serum proteins such as complement, cytokines, and chemokines may leak into the retinal parenchyma causing additional insults. Dysregulated complement activation is known to be involved in DR, and systemic complement activation is positively correlated with the progression of DR.[173] The increased deposition of membrane attack complex and a prominent reduction in CD55 and CD59 are detectable in the retinal vessels of the patients with type 2 diabetes.[174] Increased C5a, C3, and complement factor I have been detected in the vitreous of PDR patients.[175,176]

Autoimmunity as a driver of disease progression in DR has also been proposed. Various autoantibodies, including antialdolase antibody[177] and antipericyte antibody[178] have been detected in the plasma of patients with DR, indicating the association of autoimmunity with DR. Autoantibodies against retinal pericytes may induce vascular damage through classical pathway-mediated complement activation.[178] A previous study reported that increased serum levels of antitype II collagen antibodies were detected in patients with DR.[179] Retinal hypoxia in DR may induce pericytes to express type II collagen, resulting in autoantibody production against type II collagen.[17] As the result of BRB breakdown, anti-type II collagen antibodies in the serum come into contact with type II collagen around the retinal vessels. A continued loss of pericytes and type II collagen around retinal vessels could result in a shift of the immune response site from the retina to the vitreous and vitreoretinal interface, where type II collagen is abundantly present.[180] In addition to autoimmunity, it has been observed that circulating T cells participate in retinal leukostasis. This may create the potential for T cell activation by bone marrow—derived dendritic cells.[11] The T cell participation and activation imply a role of adaptive immunity in DR development.[181]

Since DR has some characteristics implicating both innate and adaptive immunity, it is worthwhile to investigate immunosuppressive or immunomodulating therapies for the treatment of DR.[16,17] Various immunosuppressants including corticosteroids have been shown to be effective in treating DR, especially DME. Intravitreal injection of methotrexate produced anatomical improvement as well as significantly improved vision in 16.6% of eyes in patients with persistent diabetic macular edema nonresponsive to intravitreal bevacizumab.[182] Sirolimus (Rapamune, Wyeth-Ayerst, Madison, NJ) is a potent immunosuppressant that inhibits mammalian target of rapamycin, a multifunctional serine-threonine kinase.[183] Sirolimus has been shown to inhibit the production, signaling, and activity of many growth factors relevant to the development of DR. Subconjunctival or intravitreal injection of a sirolimus formulation appears to be safe for patients with DME.[184] These anti-inflammatory therapies targeting immune regulation are promising and warrant further clinical trials.[185] Overall, it is likely that activation of innate immunity begins the process of DR, whereas any role for adaptive immunity is likely to be in the subsequent progression of the disease.[11]

References

1. Tang J, Kern TS. Inflammation in diabetic retinopathy. *Prog Retin Eye Res*. 2011;30(5): 343−358. https://doi.org/10.1016/j.preteyeres.2011.05.002.
2. Semeraro F, Morescalchi F, Cancarini A, Russo A, Rezzola S, Costagliola C. Diabetic retinopathy, a vascular and inflammatory disease: therapeutic implications. *Diabetes Metab*. 2019;45(6):517−527. https://doi.org/10.1016/j.diabet.2019.04.002.
3. Song J, Chen S, Liu X, Duan H, Kong J, Li Z. Relationship between C-reactive protein level and diabetic retinopathy: a systematic review and meta-analysis. *PLoS One*. 2015; 10(12):e0144406. https://doi.org/10.1371/journal.pone.0144406.
4. Woo SJ, Ahn SJ, Ahn J, Park KH, Lee K. Elevated systemic neutrophil count in diabetic retinopathy and diabetes: a hospital-based cross-sectional study of 30,793 Korean subjects. *Invest Ophthalmol Vis Sci*. 2011;52(10):7697−7703. https://doi.org/10.1167/iovs.11-7784.
5. Rübsam A, Parikh S, Fort PE. Role of inflammation in diabetic retinopathy. *Int J Mol Sci*. 2018;19(4):E942. https://doi.org/10.3390/ijms19040942.
6. Lee H, Jang H, Choi YA, Kim HC, Chung H. Association between soluble CD14 in the aqueous humor and hyperreflective foci on optical coherence tomography in patients with diabetic macular edema. *Invest Ophthalmol Vis Sci*. 2018;59(2):715−721. https://doi.org/10.1167/iovs.17-23042.
7. Mao C, Yan H. Roles of elevated intravitreal IL-1β and IL-10 levels in proliferative diabetic retinopathy. *Indian J Ophthalmol*. 2014;62(6):699−701. https://doi.org/10.4103/0301-4738.136220.
8. Gustavsson C, Agardh CD, Agardh E. Profile of intraocular tumour necrosis factor-α and interleukin-6 in diabetic subjects with different degrees of diabetic retinopathy. *Acta Ophthalmol*. 2013;91(5):445−452. https://doi.org/10.1111/j.1755-3768.2012.02430.x.
9. Esser P, Heimann K, Wiedemann P. Macrophages in proliferative vitreoretinopathy and proliferative diabetic retinopathy: differentiation of subpopulations. *Br J Ophthalmol*. 1993;77(11):731−733. https://doi.org/10.1136/bjo.77.11.731.
10. Tamura K, Yokoyama T, Ebihara N, Murakami A. Histopathologic analysis of the internal limiting membrane surgically peeled from eyes with diffuse diabetic macular edema. *Jpn J Ophthalmol*. 2012;56(3):280−287. https://doi.org/10.1007/s10384-012-0130-y.
11. Forrester JV, Kuffova L, Delibegovic M. The role of inflammation in diabetic retinopathy. *Front Immunol*. 2020;11:583687. https://doi.org/10.3389/fimmu.2020.583687.
12. McLeod DS, Lefer DJ, Merges C, Lutty GA. Enhanced expression of intracellular adhesion molecule-1 and P-selectin in the diabetic human retina and choroid. *Am J Pathol*. 1995;147(3):642−653.
13. Miyamoto K, Hiroshiba N, Tsujikawa A, Ogura Y. In vivo demonstration of increased leukocyte entrapment in retinal microcirculation of diabetic rats. *Invest Ophthalmol Vis Sci*. 1998;39(11):2190−2194.
14. Lutty GA, Cao J, McLeod DS. Relationship of polymorphonuclear leukocytes to capillary dropout in the human diabetic choroid. *Am J Pathol*. 1997;151(3):707−714.

15. Satofuka S, Ichihara A, Nagai N, et al. (Pro)renin receptor-mediated signal transduction and tissue renin-angiotensin system contribute to diabetes-induced retinal inflammation. *Diabetes*. 2009;58(7):1625−1633. https://doi.org/10.2337/db08-0254.

16. Xu H, Chen M. Diabetic retinopathy and dysregulated innate immunity. *Vision Res*. 2017;139:39−46. https://doi.org/10.1016/j.visres.2017.04.013.

17. Ikeda T, Nakamura K, Kida T, Oku H. Possible roles of anti-type II collagen antibody and innate immunity in the development and progression of diabetic retinopathy. *Graefes Arch Clin Exp Ophthalmol Albrecht Von Graefes Arch Klin Exp Ophthalmol*. August 11, 2021. https://doi.org/10.1007/s00417-021-05342-6.

18. Kaštelan S, Orešković I, Bišćan F, Kaštelan H, Gverović Antunica A. Inflammatory and angiogenic biomarkers in diabetic retinopathy. *Biochem Med*. 2020;30(3):030502. https://doi.org/10.11613/BM.2020.030502.

19. Joussen AM, Poulaki V, Le ML, et al. A central role for inflammation in the pathogenesis of diabetic retinopathy. *FASEB J*. 2004;18(12):1450−1452. https://doi.org/10.1096/fj.03-1476fje.

20. Kern TS. Contributions of inflammatory processes to the development of the early stages of diabetic retinopathy. *Exp Diabetes Res*. 2007;2007:95103. https://doi.org/10.1155/2007/95103.

21. Adamis AP, Berman AJ. Immunological mechanisms in the pathogenesis of diabetic retinopathy. *Semin Immunopathol*. 2008;30(2):65−84. https://doi.org/10.1007/s00281-008-0111-x.

22. Spencer BG, Estevez JJ, Liu E, Craig JE, Finnie JW. Pericytes, inflammation, and diabetic retinopathy. *Inflammopharmacology*. 2020;28(3):697−709. https://doi.org/10.1007/s10787-019-00647-9.

23. Altmann C, Schmidt MHH. The role of microglia in diabetic retinopathy: inflammation, microvasculature defects and neurodegeneration. *Int J Mol Sci*. 2018;19(1):E110. https://doi.org/10.3390/ijms19010110.

24. Rivera JC, Dabouz R, Noueihed B, Omri S, Tahiri H, Chemtob S. Ischemic retinopathies: oxidative stress and inflammation. *Oxid Med Cell Longev*. 2017;2017. https://doi.org/10.1155/2017/3940241, 3940241.

25. Ascaso FJ, Huerva V, Grzybowski A. The role of inflammation in the pathogenesis of macular edema secondary to retinal vascular diseases. *Mediat Inflamm*. 2014;2014:432685. https://doi.org/10.1155/2014/432685.

26. Barouch FC, Miyamoto K, Allport JR, et al. Integrin-mediated neutrophil adhesion and retinal leukostasis in diabetes. *Invest Ophthalmol Vis Sci*. 2000;41(5):1153−1158.

27. Zhang HT, Shi K, Baskota A, Zhou FL, Chen YX, Tian HM. Silybin reduces obliterated retinal capillaries in experimental diabetic retinopathy in rats. *Eur J Pharmacol*. 2014;740:233−239. https://doi.org/10.1016/j.ejphar.2014.07.033.

28. Hynes RO. Integrins: a family of cell surface receptors. *Cell*. 1987;48(4):549−554. https://doi.org/10.1016/0092-8674(87)90233-9.

29. Lawrence MB, Smith CW, Eskin SG, McIntire LV. Effect of venous shear stress on CD18-mediated neutrophil adhesion to cultured endothelium. *Blood*. 1990;75(1):227−237.

30. Bednarczyk M, Stege H, Grabbe S, Bros M. β2 integrins-multi-functional leukocyte receptors in health and disease. *Int J Mol Sci*. 2020;21(4):E1402. https://doi.org/10.3390/ijms21041402.

31. Long EO. ICAM-1: getting a grip on leukocyte adhesion. *J Immunol Baltim Md 1950*. 2011;186(9):5021−5023. https://doi.org/10.4049/jimmunol.1100646.

32. Dustin ML, Rothlein R, Bhan AK, Dinarello CA, Springer TA. Induction by IL 1 and interferon-γ: tissue distribution, biochemistry, and function of a natural adherence molecule (ICAM-1). *J Immunol*. 1986;137:245−254. *J Immunol Baltim Md 1950*. 2011;186(9):5024−5033.

33. Miyamoto K, Khosrof S, Bursell SE, et al. Prevention of leukostasis and vascular leakage in streptozotocin-induced diabetic retinopathy via intercellular adhesion molecule-1 inhibition. *Proc Natl Acad Sci U S A*. 1999;96(19):10836−10841. https://doi.org/10.1073/pnas.96.19.10836.

34. Joussen AM, Murata T, Tsujikawa A, Kirchhof B, Bursell SE, Adamis AP. Leukocyte-mediated endothelial cell injury and death in the diabetic retina. *Am J Pathol*. 2001; 158(1):147−152. https://doi.org/10.1016/S0002-9440(10)63952-1.

35. Patel N. Targeting leukostasis for the treatment of early diabetic retinopathy. *Cardiovasc Hematol Disord Drug Targets*. 2009;9(3):222−229. https://doi.org/10.2174/187152909789007052.

36. Schröder S, Palinski W, Schmid-Schönbein GW. Activated monocytes and granulocytes, capillary nonperfusion, and neovascularization in diabetic retinopathy. *Am J Pathol*. 1991;139(1):81−100.

37. Roy S, Kern TS, Song B, Stuebe C. Mechanistic insights into pathological changes in the diabetic retina: implications for targeting diabetic retinopathy. *Am J Pathol*. 2017; 187(1):9−19. https://doi.org/10.1016/j.ajpath.2016.08.022.

38. Kinoshita N, Kakehashi A, Inoda S, et al. Effective and selective prevention of retinal leukostasis in streptozotocin-induced diabetic rats using gliclazide. *Diabetologia*. 2002; 45(5):735−739. https://doi.org/10.1007/s00125-002-0820-y.

39. van der Wijk AE, Hughes JM, Klaassen I, Van Noorden CJF, Schlingemann RO. Is leukostasis a crucial step or epiphenomenon in the pathogenesis of diabetic retinopathy? *J Leukoc Biol*. 2017;102(4):993−1001. https://doi.org/10.1189/jlb.3RU0417-139.

40. Muranaka K, Yanagi Y, Tamaki Y, et al. Effects of peroxisome proliferator-activated receptor gamma and its ligand on blood-retinal barrier in a streptozotocin-induced diabetic model. *Invest Ophthalmol Vis Sci*. 2006;47(10):4547−4552. https://doi.org/10.1167/iovs.05-1432.

41. Gadek TR, Burdick DJ, McDowell RS, et al. Generation of an LFA-1 antagonist by the transfer of the ICAM-1 immunoregulatory epitope to a small molecule. *Science*. 2002; 295(5557):1086−1089. https://doi.org/10.1126/science.295.5557.1086.

42. Rao VR, Prescott E, Shelke NB, et al. Delivery of SAR 1118 to the retina via ophthalmic drops and its effectiveness in a rat streptozotocin (STZ) model of diabetic retinopathy (DR). *Invest Ophthalmol Vis Sci*. 2010;51(10):5198−5204. https://doi.org/10.1167/iovs.09-5144.

43. Paskowitz DM, Nguyen QD, Gehlbach P, et al. Safety, tolerability, and bioavailability of topical SAR 1118, a novel antagonist of lymphocyte function-associated antigen-1: a phase 1b study. *Eye Lond Engl*. 2012;26(7):944−949. https://doi.org/10.1038/eye.2012.68.

44. Iliaki E, Poulaki V, Mitsiades N, Mitsiades CS, Miller JW, Gragoudas ES. Role of alpha 4 integrin (CD49d) in the pathogenesis of diabetic retinopathy. *Invest Ophthalmol Vis Sci*. 2009;50(10):4898−4904. https://doi.org/10.1167/iovs.08-2013.

45. Zhang W, Liu H, Rojas M, Caldwell RW, Caldwell RB. Anti-inflammatory therapy for diabetic retinopathy. *Immunotherapy*. 2011;3(5):609−628. https://doi.org/10.2217/imt.11.24.

46. Shaw LT, Mackin A, Shah R, et al. Risuteganib-a novel integrin inhibitor for the treatment of non-exudative (dry) age-related macular degeneration and diabetic macular edema. *Expert Opin Invest Drugs.* 2020;29(6):547–554. https://doi.org/10.1080/13543784.2020.1763953.

47. Karlstetter M, Scholz R, Rutar M, Wong WT, Provis JM, Langmann T. Retinal microglia: just bystander or target for therapy? *Prog Retin Eye Res.* 2015;45:30–57. https://doi.org/10.1016/j.preteyeres.2014.11.004.

48. Krady JK, Basu A, Allen CM, et al. Minocycline reduces proinflammatory cytokine expression, microglial activation, and caspase-3 activation in a rodent model of diabetic retinopathy. *Diabetes.* 2005;54(5):1559–1565. https://doi.org/10.2337/diabetes.54.5.1559.

49. Jiang M, Xie H, Zhang C, et al. Enhancing fractalkine/CX3CR1 signalling pathway can reduce neuroinflammation by attenuating microglia activation in experimental diabetic retinopathy. *J Cell Mol Med.* 2022;26(4):1229–1244. https://doi.org/10.1111/jcmm.17179.

50. Xie H, Zhang C, Liu D, et al. Erythropoietin protects the inner blood-retinal barrier by inhibiting microglia phagocytosis via Src/Akt/cofilin signalling in experimental diabetic retinopathy. *Diabetologia.* 2021;64(1):211–225. https://doi.org/10.1007/s00125-020-05299-x.

51. Takeda A, Shinozaki Y, Kashiwagi K, et al. Microglia mediate non-cell-autonomous cell death of retinal ganglion cells. *Glia.* 2018;66(11):2366–2384. https://doi.org/10.1002/glia.23475.

52. Goto Y, Kakizaki M, Masaki N. Production of spontaneous diabetic rats by repetition of selective breeding. *Tohoku J Exp Med.* 1976;119(1):85–90. https://doi.org/10.1620/tjem.119.85.

53. Omri S, Behar-Cohen F, de Kozak Y, et al. Microglia/macrophages migrate through retinal epithelium barrier by a transcellular route in diabetic retinopathy: role of PKCζ in the Goto Kakizaki rat model. *Am J Pathol.* 2011;179(2):942–953. https://doi.org/10.1016/j.ajpath.2011.04.018.

54. Zeng HY, Green WR, Tso MO. Microglial activation in human diabetic retinopathy. *Arch Ophthalmol Chic Ill 1960.* 2008;126(2):227–232. https://doi.org/10.1001/archophthalmol.2007.65.

55. Scholz R, Sobotka M, Caramoy A, Stempfl T, Moehle C, Langmann T. Minocycline counter-regulates pro-inflammatory microglia responses in the retina and protects from degeneration. *J Neuroinflammation.* 2015;12:209. https://doi.org/10.1186/s12974-015-0431-4.

56. Grotegut P, Perumal N, Kuehn S, et al. Minocycline reduces inflammatory response and cell death in a S100B retina degeneration model. *J Neuroinflammation.* 2020;17(1):375. https://doi.org/10.1186/s12974-020-02012-y.

57. Gao W, Du J, Chi Y, Zhu R, Gao X, Yang L. Minocycline prevents the inflammatory response after retinal detachment, where microglia phenotypes being regulated through A20. *Exp Eye Res.* 2021;203:108403. https://doi.org/10.1016/j.exer.2020.108403.

58. Bosco A, Inman DM, Steele MR, et al. Reduced retina microglial activation and improved optic nerve integrity with minocycline treatment in the DBA/2J mouse model of glaucoma. *Invest Ophthalmol Vis Sci.* 2008;49(4):1437–1446. https://doi.org/10.1167/iovs.07-1337.

59. Cukras CA, Petrou P, Chew EY, Meyerle CB, Wong WT. Oral minocycline for the treatment of diabetic macular edema (DME): results of a phase I/II clinical study. *Invest Ophthalmol Vis Sci*. 2012;53(7):3865−3874. https://doi.org/10.1167/iovs.11-9413.

60. Taghavi Y, Hassanshahi G, Kounis NG, Koniari I, Khorramdelazad H. Monocyte chemoattractant protein-1 (MCP-1/CCL2) in diabetic retinopathy: latest evidence and clinical considerations. *J Cell Commun Signal*. 2019;13(4):451−462. https://doi.org/10.1007/s12079-018-00500-8.

61. Noma H, Mimura T, Yasuda K, Shimura M. Role of inflammation in diabetic macular edema. *Ophthalmol J Int Ophthalmol Int J Ophthalmol Z Augenheilkd*. 2014;232(3):127−135. https://doi.org/10.1159/000364955.

62. Funatsu H, Yamashita H, Noma H, et al. Aqueous humor levels of cytokines are related to vitreous levels and progression of diabetic retinopathy in diabetic patients. *Graefes Arch Clin Exp Ophthalmol Albrecht Von Graefes Arch Klin Exp Ophthalmol*. 2005;243(1):3−8. https://doi.org/10.1007/s00417-004-0950-7.

63. Hernández C, Segura RM, Fonollosa A, Carrasco E, Francisco G, Simó R. Interleukin-8, monocyte chemoattractant protein-1 and IL-10 in the vitreous fluid of patients with proliferative diabetic retinopathy. *Diabet Med J Br Diabet Assoc*. 2005;22(6):719−722. https://doi.org/10.1111/j.1464-5491.2005.01538.x.

64. Funatsu H, Noma H, Mimura T, Eguchi S, Hori S. Association of vitreous inflammatory factors with diabetic macular edema. *Ophthalmology*. 2009;116(1):73−79. https://doi.org/10.1016/j.ophtha.2008.09.037.

65. Arjamaa O, Nikinmaa M. Oxygen-dependent diseases in the retina: role of hypoxia-inducible factors. *Exp Eye Res*. 2006;83(3):473−483. https://doi.org/10.1016/j.exer.2006.01.016.

66. Amadio M, Scapagnini G, Lupo G, Drago F, Govoni S, Pascale A. PKCbetaII/HuR/VEGF: a new molecular cascade in retinal pericytes for the regulation of VEGF gene expression. *Pharmacol Res*. 2008;57(1):60−66. https://doi.org/10.1016/j.phrs.2007.11.006.

67. Lin M, Chen Y, Jin J, et al. Ischaemia-induced retinal neovascularisation and diabetic retinopathy in mice with conditional knockout of hypoxia-inducible factor-1 in retinal Müller cells. *Diabetologia*. 2011;54(6):1554−1566. https://doi.org/10.1007/s00125-011-2081-0.

68. Boulton M, Foreman D, Williams G, McLeod D. VEGF localisation in diabetic retinopathy. *Br J Ophthalmol*. 1998;82(5):561−568. https://doi.org/10.1136/bjo.82.5.561.

69. Simó R, Sundstrom JM, Antonetti DA. Ocular Anti-VEGF therapy for diabetic retinopathy: the role of VEGF in the pathogenesis of diabetic retinopathy. *Diabetes Care*. 2014;37(4):893−899. https://doi.org/10.2337/dc13-2002.

70. Peach CJ, Mignone VW, Arruda MA, et al. Molecular pharmacology of VEGF-A isoforms: binding and signalling at VEGFR2. *Int J Mol Sci*. 2018;19(4):E1264. https://doi.org/10.3390/ijms19041264.

71. Shibuya M. VEGF-VEGFR system as a target for suppressing inflammation and other diseases. *Endocr Metab Immune Disord Drug Targets*. 2015;15(2):135−144. https://doi.org/10.2174/1871530315666150316121956.

72. Zachary I. VEGF signalling: integration and multi-tasking in endothelial cell biology. *Biochem Soc Trans*. 2003;31(Pt 6):1171−1177. https://doi.org/10.1042/bst0311171.

73. Shibuya M, Claesson-Welsh L. Signal transduction by VEGF receptors in regulation of angiogenesis and lymphangiogenesis. *Exp Cell Res*. 2006;312(5):549−560. https://doi.org/10.1016/j.yexcr.2005.11.012.

74. Bai Y, Ma JX, Guo J, et al. Müller cell-derived VEGF is a significant contributor to retinal neovascularization: Müller cell-derived VEGF in retinal neovascularization. *J Pathol*. 2009;219(4):446−454. https://doi.org/10.1002/path.2611.

75. Hu J, Li T, Du X, Wu Q, Le YZ. G protein-coupled receptor 91 signaling in diabetic retinopathy and hypoxic retinal diseases. *Vision Res*. 2017;139:59−64. https://doi.org/10.1016/j.visres.2017.05.001.

76. Brancato SK, Albina JE. Wound macrophages as key regulators of repair: origin, phenotype, and function. *Am J Pathol*. 2011;178(1):19−25. https://doi.org/10.1016/j.ajpath.2010.08.003.

77. Nürnberg C, Kociok N, Brockmann C, et al. Myeloid cells contribute indirectly to VEGF expression upon hypoxia via activation of Müller cells. *Exp Eye Res*. 2018;166:56−69. https://doi.org/10.1016/j.exer.2017.10.011.

78. Liu Y, Shen J, Fortmann SD, Wang J, Vestweber D, Campochiaro PA. Reversible retinal vessel closure from VEGF-induced leukocyte plugging. *JCI Insight*. 2017;2(18):e95530. https://doi.org/10.1172/jci.insight.95530.

79. Aiello LP, Avery RL, Arrigg PG, et al. Vascular endothelial growth factor in ocular fluid of patients with diabetic retinopathy and other retinal disorders. *N Engl J Med*. 1994;331(22):1480−1487. https://doi.org/10.1056/NEJM199412013312203.

80. Bressler NM, Beaulieu WT, Glassman AR, et al. Persistent macular thickening following intravitreous aflibercept, bevacizumab, or ranibizumab for central-involved diabetic macular edema with vision impairment: a secondary analysis of a randomized clinical trial. *JAMA Ophthalmol*. 2018;136(3):257−269. https://doi.org/10.1001/jamaophthalmol.2017.6565.

81. Bromberg-White JL, Glazer L, Downer R, Furge K, Boguslawski E, Duesbery NS. Identification of VEGF-independent cytokines in proliferative diabetic retinopathy vitreous. *Invest Ophthalmol Vis Sci*. 2013;54(10):6472−6480. https://doi.org/10.1167/iovs.13-12518.

82. Van Bergen T, Etienne I, Cunningham F, et al. The role of placental growth factor (PlGF) and its receptor system in retinal vascular diseases. *Prog Retin Eye Res*. 2019;69:116−136. https://doi.org/10.1016/j.preteyeres.2018.10.006.

83. DiPalma T, Tucci M, Russo G, et al. The placenta growth factor gene of the mouse. *Mamm Genome*. 1996;7(1):6−12. https://doi.org/10.1007/s003359900003.

84. Shibuya M. Vascular endothelial growth factor (VEGF) and its receptor (VEGFR) signaling in angiogenesis: a crucial target for anti- and pro-angiogenic therapies. *Genes Cancer*. 2011;2(12):1097−1105. https://doi.org/10.1177/1947601911423031.

85. Perelman N, Selvaraj SK, Batra S, et al. Placenta growth factor activates monocytes and correlates with sickle cell disease severity. *Blood*. 2003;102(4):1506−1514. https://doi.org/10.1182/blood-2002-11-3422.

86. Ribatti D. The discovery of the placental growth factor and its role in angiogenesis: a historical review. *Angiogenesis*. 2008;11(3):215−221. https://doi.org/10.1007/s10456-008-9114-4.

87. Bellik L, Vinci MC, Filippi S, Ledda F, Parenti A. Intracellular pathways triggered by the selective FLT-1-agonist placental growth factor in vascular smooth muscle cells exposed to hypoxia. *Br J Pharmacol*. 2005;146(4):568−575. https://doi.org/10.1038/sj.bjp.0706347.

88. Ando R, Noda K, Namba S, Saito W, Kanda A, Ishida S. Aqueous humour levels of placental growth factor in diabetic retinopathy. *Acta Ophthalmol.* 2014;92(3): e245−e246. https://doi.org/10.1111/aos.12251.

89. Kovacs K, Marra KV, Yu G, et al. Angiogenic and inflammatory vitreous biomarkers associated with increasing levels of retinal ischemia. *Invest Ophthalmol Vis Sci.* 2015;56(11):6523−6530. https://doi.org/10.1167/iovs.15-16793.

90. Rangasamy S, McGuire PG, Franco Nitta C, Monickaraj F, Oruganti SR, Das A. Chemokine mediated monocyte trafficking into the retina: role of inflammation in alteration of the blood-retinal barrier in diabetic retinopathy. *PLoS One.* 2014;9(10):e108508. https://doi.org/10.1371/journal.pone.0108508.

91. Funatsu H, Yamashita H, Sakata K, et al. Vitreous levels of vascular endothelial growth factor and intercellular adhesion molecule 1 are related to diabetic macular edema. *Ophthalmology.* 2005;112(5):806−816. https://doi.org/10.1016/j.ophtha.2004.11.045.

92. Yao Y, Du J, Li R, et al. Association between ICAM-1 level and diabetic retinopathy: a review and meta-analysis. *Postgrad Med J.* 2019;95(1121):162−168. https://doi.org/10.1136/postgradmedj-2018-136102.

93. Gharaee-Kermani M, Denholm EM, Phan SH. Costimulation of fibroblast collagen and transforming growth factor beta1 gene expression by monocyte chemoattractant protein-1 via specific receptors. *J Biol Chem.* 1996;271(30):17779−17784. https://doi.org/10.1074/jbc.271.30.17779.

94. Ueda A, Okuda K, Ohno S, et al. NF-kappa B and Sp1 regulate transcription of the human monocyte chemoattractant protein-1 gene. *J Immunol Baltim Md 1950.* 1994; 153(5):2052−2063.

95. Harada C, Mitamura Y, Harada T. The role of cytokines and trophic factors in epiretinal membranes: involvement of signal transduction in glial cells. *Prog Retin Eye Res.* 2006; 25(2):149−164. https://doi.org/10.1016/j.preteyeres.2005.09.001.

96. Harada C, Okumura A, Namekata K, et al. Role of monocyte chemotactic protein-1 and nuclear factor kappa B in the pathogenesis of proliferative diabetic retinopathy. *Diabetes Res Clin Pract.* 2006;74(3):249−256. https://doi.org/10.1016/j.diabres.2006.04.017.

97. Eastlake K, Banerjee PJ, Angbohang A, Charteris DG, Khaw PT, Limb GA. Müller glia as an important source of cytokines and inflammatory factors present in the gliotic retina during proliferative vitreoretinopathy. *Glia.* 2016;64(4):495−506. https://doi.org/10.1002/glia.22942.

98. Hong KH, Ryu J, Han KH. Monocyte chemoattractant protein-1-induced angiogenesis is mediated by vascular endothelial growth factor-A. *Blood.* 2005;105(4):1405−1407. https://doi.org/10.1182/blood-2004-08-3178.

99. Abu El-Asrar AM, Struyf S, Kangave D, Geboes K, Van Damme J. Chemokines in proliferative diabetic retinopathy and proliferative vitreoretinopathy. *Eur Cytokine Netw.* 2006;17(3):155−165.

100. Dong N, Li X, Xiao L, Yu W, Wang B, Chu L. Upregulation of retinal neuronal MCP-1 in the rodent model of diabetic retinopathy and its function in vitro. *Invest Ophthalmol Vis Sci.* 2012;53(12):7567−7575. https://doi.org/10.1167/iovs.12-9446.

101. Bian ZM, Elner SG, Strieter RM, Kunkel SL, Lukacs NW, Elner VM. IL-4 potentiates IL-1beta- and TNF-alpha-stimulated IL-8 and MCP-1 protein production in human retinal pigment epithelial cells. *Curr Eye Res.* 1999;18(5):349−357. https://doi.org/10.1076/ceyr.18.5.349.5353.

102. Harkness KA, Sussman JD, Davies-Jones GaB, Greenwood J, Woodroofe MN. Cytokine regulation of MCP-1 expression in brain and retinal microvascular endothelial cells. *J Neuroimmunol*. 2003;142(1−2):1−9. https://doi.org/10.1016/s0165-5728(03)00251-0.

103. Dong N, Xu B, Wang B, Chu L. Study of 27 aqueous humor cytokines in patients with type 2 diabetes with or without retinopathy. *Mol Vis*. 2013;19:1734−1746.

104. Murugeswari P, Shukla D, Rajendran A, Kim R, Namperumalsamy P, Muthukkaruppan V. Proinflammatory cytokines and angiogenic and anti-angiogenic factors in vitreous of patients with proliferative diabetic retinopathy and eale's disease. *Retina Phila Pa*. 2008;28(6):817−824. https://doi.org/10.1097/IAE.0b013e31816576d5.

105. Mitamura Y, Takeuchi S, Matsuda A, Tagawa Y, Mizue Y, Nishihira J. Monocyte chemotactic protein-1 in the vitreous of patients with proliferative diabetic retinopathy. *Ophthalmol J Int Ophtalmol Int J Ophthalmol Z Augenheilkd*. 2001; 215(6):415−418. https://doi.org/10.1159/000050900.

106. Tashimo A, Mitamura Y, Nagai S, et al. Aqueous levels of macrophage migration inhibitory factor and monocyte chemotactic protein-1 in patients with diabetic retinopathy. *Diabet Med J Br Diabet Assoc*. 2004;21(12):1292−1297. https://doi.org/10.1111/j.1464-5491.2004.01334.x.

107. Demircan N, Safran BG, Soylu M, Ozcan AA, Sizmaz S. Determination of vitreous interleukin-1 (IL-1) and tumour necrosis factor (TNF) levels in proliferative diabetic retinopathy. *Eye Lond Engl*. 2006;20(12):1366−1369. https://doi.org/10.1038/sj.eye.6702138.

108. Limb GA, Chignell AH, Green W, LeRoy F, Dumonde DC. Distribution of TNF alpha and its reactive vascular adhesion molecules in fibrovascular membranes of proliferative diabetic retinopathy. *Br J Ophthalmol*. 1996;80(2):168−173. https://doi.org/10.1136/bjo.80.2.168.

109. Joussen AM, Doehmen S, Le ML, et al. TNF-alpha mediated apoptosis plays an important role in the development of early diabetic retinopathy and long-term histopathological alterations. *Mol Vis*. 2009;15:1418−1428.

110. Behl Y, Krothapalli P, Desta T, DiPiazza A, Roy S, Graves DT. Diabetes-enhanced tumor necrosis factor-alpha production promotes apoptosis and the loss of retinal microvascular cells in type 1 and type 2 models of diabetic retinopathy. *Am J Pathol*. 2008; 172(5):1411−1418. https://doi.org/10.2353/ajpath.2008.071070.

111. Huang H, Gandhi JK, Zhong X, et al. TNFalpha is required for late BRB breakdown in diabetic retinopathy, and its inhibition prevents leukostasis and protects vessels and neurons from apoptosis. *Invest Ophthalmol Vis Sci*. 2011;52(3):1336−1344. https://doi.org/10.1167/iovs.10-5768.

112. Mohr S, Xi X, Tang J, Kern TS. Caspase activation in retinas of diabetic and galactosemic mice and diabetic patients. *Diabetes*. 2002;51(4):1172−1179. https://doi.org/10.2337/diabetes.51.4.1172.

113. Sui A, Chen X, Shen J, et al. Inhibiting the NLRP3 inflammasome with MCC950 ameliorates retinal neovascularization and leakage by reversing the IL-1β/IL-18 activation pattern in an oxygen-induced ischemic retinopathy mouse model. *Cell Death Dis*. 2020; 11(10):901. https://doi.org/10.1038/s41419-020-03076-7.

114. Kowluru RA, Odenbach S. Role of interleukin-1beta in the development of retinopathy in rats: effect of antioxidants. *Invest Ophthalmol Vis Sci*. 2004;45(11):4161−4166. https://doi.org/10.1167/iovs.04-0633.

115. Vincent JA, Mohr S. Inhibition of caspase-1/interleukin-1beta signaling prevents degeneration of retinal capillaries in diabetes and galactosemia. *Diabetes.* 2007; 56(1):224−230. https://doi.org/10.2337/db06-0427.

116. Funatsu H, Yamashita H, Noma H, Mimura T, Yamashita T, Hori S. Increased levels of vascular endothelial growth factor and interleukin-6 in the aqueous humor of diabetics with macular edema. *Am J Ophthalmol.* 2002;133(1):70−77. https://doi.org/10.1016/s0002-9394(01)01269-7.

117. Yao Y, Li R, Du J, Long L, Li X, Luo N. Interleukin-6 and diabetic retinopathy: a systematic review and meta-analysis. *Curr Eye Res.* 2019;44(5):564−574. https://doi.org/10.1080/02713683.2019.1570274.

118. Sonoda S, Sakamoto T, Shirasawa M, Yamashita T, Otsuka H, Terasaki H. Correlation between reflectivity of subretinal fluid in OCT images and concentration of intravitreal VEGF in eyes with diabetic macular edema. *Invest Ophthalmol Vis Sci.* 2013;54(8): 5367−5374. https://doi.org/10.1167/iovs.13-12382.

119. Chung YR, Kim YH, Ha SJ, et al. Role of inflammation in classification of diabetic macular edema by optical coherence tomography. *J Diabetes Res.* 2019;2019: 8164250. https://doi.org/10.1155/2019/8164250.

120. Vujosevic S, Torresin T, Berton M, Bini S, Convento E, Midena E. Diabetic macular edema with and without subfoveal neuroretinal detachment: two different morphologic and functional entities. *Am J Ophthalmol.* 2017;181:149−155. https://doi.org/10.1016/j.ajo.2017.06.026.

121. Puri MC, Rossant J, Alitalo K, Bernstein A, Partanen J. The receptor tyrosine kinase TIE is required for integrity and survival of vascular endothelial cells. *EMBO J.* 1995;14(23):5884−5891.

122. Augustin HG, Koh GY, Thurston G, Alitalo K. Control of vascular morphogenesis and homeostasis through the angiopoietin-Tie system. *Nat Rev Mol Cell Biol.* 2009;10(3): 165−177. https://doi.org/10.1038/nrm2639.

123. Scholz A, Plate KH, Reiss Y. Angiopoietin-2: a multifaceted cytokine that functions in both angiogenesis and inflammation. *Ann N Y Acad Sci.* 2015;1347:45−51. https://doi.org/10.1111/nyas.12726.

124. Joussen AM, Ricci F, Paris LP, Korn C, Quezada-Ruiz C, Zarbin M. Angiopoietin/Tie2 signalling and its role in retinal and choroidal vascular diseases: a review of preclinical data. *Eye Lond Engl.* 2021;35(5):1305−1316. https://doi.org/10.1038/s41433-020-01377-x.

125. Oh H, Takagi H, Suzuma K, Otani A, Matsumura M, Honda Y. Hypoxia and vascular endothelial growth factor selectively up-regulate angiopoietin-2 in bovine microvascular endothelial cells. *J Biol Chem.* 1999;274(22):15732−15739. https://doi.org/10.1074/jbc.274.22.15732.

126. Ohashi H, Takagi H, Koyama S, et al. Alterations in expression of angiopoietins and the Tie-2 receptor in the retina of streptozotocin induced diabetic rats. *Mol Vis.* 2004;10: 608−617.

127. Rangasamy S, Srinivasan R, Maestas J, McGuire PG, Das A. A potential role for angiopoietin 2 in the regulation of the blood-retinal barrier in diabetic retinopathy. *Invest Ophthalmol Vis Sci.* 2011;52(6):3784−3791. https://doi.org/10.1167/iovs.10-6386.

128. Park SW, Yun JH, Kim JH, Kim KW, Cho CH, Kim JH. Angiopoietin 2 induces pericyte apoptosis via α3β1 integrin signaling in diabetic retinopathy. *Diabetes.* 2014;63(9): 3057−3068. https://doi.org/10.2337/db13-1942.

129. Lee SG, Lee CG, Yun IH, Hur DY, Yang JW, Kim HW. Effect of lipoic acid on expression of angiogenic factors in diabetic rat retina. *Clin Exp Ophthalmol.* 2012;40(1): e47−e57. https://doi.org/10.1111/j.1442-9071.2011.02695.x.

130. Wykoff CC, Abreu F, Adamis AP, et al. Efficacy, durability, and safety of intravitreal faricimab with extended dosing up to every 16 weeks in patients with diabetic macular oedema (YOSEMITE and RHINE): two randomised, double-masked, phase 3 trials. *Lancet Lond Engl.* January 21, 2022;S0140-S6736(22):00018-6. https://doi.org/10.1016/S0140-6736(22)00018-6.

131. Shirley M. Faricimab: first approval. *Drugs.* April 26, 2022. https://doi.org/10.1007/s40265-022-01713-3.

132. Silva PS, Sun JK, Aiello LP. Role of steroids in the management of diabetic macular edema and proliferative diabetic retinopathy. *Semin Ophthalmol.* 2009;24(2):93−99. https://doi.org/10.1080/08820530902800355.

133. Tamura H, Miyamoto K, Kiryu J, et al. Intravitreal injection of corticosteroid attenuates leukostasis and vascular leakage in experimental diabetic retina. *Invest Ophthalmol Vis Sci.* 2005;46(4):1440−1444. https://doi.org/10.1167/iovs.04-0905.

134. Wang K, Wang Y, Gao L, Li X, Li M, Guo J. Dexamethasone inhibits leukocyte accumulation and vascular permeability in retina of streptozotocin-induced diabetic rats via reducing vascular endothelial growth factor and intercellular adhesion molecule-1 expression. *Biol Pharm Bull.* 2008;31(8):1541−1546. https://doi.org/10.1248/bpb.31.1541.

135. Kodjikian L, Bellocq D, Bandello F, et al. First-line treatment algorithm and guidelines in center-involving diabetic macular edema. *Eur J Ophthalmol.* 2019;29(6):573−584. https://doi.org/10.1177/1120672119857511.

136. Rosenblatt A, Udaondo P, Cunha-Vaz J, et al. A collaborative retrospective study on the efficacy and safety of intravitreal dexamethasone implant (Ozurdex) in patients with diabetic macular edema: the European DME registry study. *Ophthalmology.* 2020; 127(3):377−393. https://doi.org/10.1016/j.ophtha.2019.10.005.

137. Boyer DS, Yoon YH, Belfort R, et al. Three-year, randomized, sham-controlled trial of dexamethasone intravitreal implant in patients with diabetic macular edema. *Ophthalmology.* 2014;121(10):1904−1914. https://doi.org/10.1016/j.ophtha.2014.04.024.

138. Campochiaro PA, Brown DM, Pearson A, et al. Sustained delivery fluocinolone acetonide vitreous inserts provide benefit for at least 3 years in patients with diabetic macular edema. *Ophthalmology.* 2012;119(10):2125−2132. https://doi.org/10.1016/j.ophtha.2012.04.030.

139. Cunha-Vaz J, Ashton P, Iezzi R, et al. Sustained delivery fluocinolone acetonide vitreous implants: long-term benefit in patients with chronic diabetic macular edema. *Ophthalmology.* 2014;121(10):1892−1903. https://doi.org/10.1016/j.ophtha.2014.04.019.

140. Bressler SB, Ayala AR, Bressler NM, et al. Persistent macular thickening after ranibizumab treatment for diabetic macular edema with vision impairment. *JAMA Ophthalmol.* 2016;134(3):278−285. https://doi.org/10.1001/jamaophthalmol.2015.5346.

141. Sadhukhan K, Naskar S. Role of combined therapy of intravitreal ranibizumab and dexamethasone in refractory diabetic macular edema: a retrospective study. *Maedica.* 2021;16(4):615−619. https://doi.org/10.26574/maedica.2021.16.4.615.

142. Busch C, Zur D, Fraser-Bell S, et al. Shall we stay, or shall we switch? Continued anti-VEGF therapy versus early switch to dexamethasone implant in refractory diabetic

macular edema. *Acta Diabetol.* 2018;55(8):789−796. https://doi.org/10.1007/s00592-018-1151-x.

143. Yolcu Ü, Sobaci G. The effect of combined treatment of bevacizumab and triamcinolone for diabetic macular edema refractory to previous intravitreal mono-injections. *Int Ophthalmol.* 2015;35(1):73−79. https://doi.org/10.1007/s10792-014-0019-5.

144. Du Y, Sarthy VP, Kern TS. Interaction between NO and COX pathways in retinal cells exposed to elevated glucose and retina of diabetic rats. *Am J Physiol Regul Integr Comp Physiol.* 2004;287(4):R735−R741. https://doi.org/10.1152/ajpregu.00080.2003.

145. Johnson EI, Dunlop ME, Larkins RG. Increased vasodilatory prostaglandin production in the diabetic rat retinal vasculature. *Curr Eye Res.* 1999;18(2):79−82. https://doi.org/10.1076/ceyr.18.2.79.5386.

146. Ayalasomayajula SP, Amrite AC, Kompella UB. Inhibition of cyclooxygenase-2, but not cyclooxygenase-1, reduces prostaglandin E2 secretion from diabetic rat retinas. *Eur J Pharmacol.* 2004;498(1−3):275−278. https://doi.org/10.1016/j.ejphar.2004.07.046.

147. Joussen AM, Poulaki V, Mitsiades N, et al. Nonsteroidal anti-inflammatory drugs prevent early diabetic retinopathy via TNF-alpha suppression. *FASEB J.* 2002;16(3):438−440. https://doi.org/10.1096/fj.01-0707fje.

148. Sfikakis PP, Markomichelakis N, Theodossiadis GP, Grigoropoulos V, Katsilambros N, Theodossiadis PG. Regression of sight-threatening macular edema in type 2 diabetes following treatment with the anti-tumor necrosis factor monoclonal antibody infliximab. *Diabetes Care.* 2005;28(2):445−447. https://doi.org/10.2337/diacare.28.2.445.

149. Stahel M, Becker M, Graf N, Michels S. Systemic interleukin 1β inhibition in proliferative diabetic retinopathy: a prospective open-label study using canakinumab. *Retina Phila Pa.* 2016;36(2):385−391. https://doi.org/10.1097/IAE.0000000000000701.

150. Tang D, Kang R, Coyne CB, Zeh HJ, Lotze MT. PAMPs and DAMPs: signal 0s that spur autophagy and immunity. *Immunol Rev.* 2012;249(1):158−175. https://doi.org/10.1111/j.1600-065X.2012.01146.x.

151. Takahashi H, Okayama N, Yamaguchi N, et al. Associations of interactions between NLRP3 SNPs and HLA mismatch with acute and extensive chronic graft-versus-host diseases. *Sci Rep.* 2017;7(1):13097. https://doi.org/10.1038/s41598-017-13506-w.

152. Yang Y, Wang H, Kouadir M, Song H, Shi F. Recent advances in the mechanisms of NLRP3 inflammasome activation and its inhibitors. *Cell Death Dis.* 2019;10(2):128. https://doi.org/10.1038/s41419-019-1413-8.

153. Jo EK, Kim JK, Shin DM, Sasakawa C. Molecular mechanisms regulating NLRP3 inflammasome activation. *Cell Mol Immunol.* 2016;13(2):148−159. https://doi.org/10.1038/cmi.2015.95.

154. Chaurasia SS, Lim RR, Parikh BH, et al. The NLRP3 inflammasome may contribute to pathologic neovascularization in the advanced stages of diabetic retinopathy. *Sci Rep.* 2018;8(1):2847. https://doi.org/10.1038/s41598-018-21198-z.

155. Hao J, Zhang H, Yu J, Chen X, Yang L. Methylene blue attenuates diabetic retinopathy by inhibiting NLRP3 inflammasome activation in STZ-induced diabetic rats. *Ocul Immunol Inflamm.* 2019;27(5):836−843. https://doi.org/10.1080/09273948.2018.1450516.

156. Thankam FG, Roesch ZK, Dilisio MF, et al. Association of inflammatory responses and ECM disorganization with HMGB1 upregulation and NLRP3 inflammasome activation

in the injured rotator cuff tendon. *Sci Rep*. 2018;8(1):8918. https://doi.org/10.1038/s41598-018-27250-2.

157. Sun H, Zhao H, Yan Z, Liu X, Yin P, Zhang J. Protective role and molecular mechanism of action of Nesfatin-1 against high glucose-induced inflammation, oxidative stress and apoptosis in retinal epithelial cells. *Exp Ther Med*. 2021;22(2):833. https://doi.org/10.3892/etm.2021.10265.

158. Karmakar M, Katsnelson MA, Dubyak GR, Pearlman E. Neutrophil P2X7 receptors mediate NLRP3 inflammasome-dependent IL-1β secretion in response to ATP. *Nat Commun*. 2016;7:10555. https://doi.org/10.1038/ncomms10555.

159. Fu Q, Wu J, Zhou XY, et al. NLRP3/Caspase-1 pathway-induced pyroptosis mediated cognitive deficits in a mouse model of sepsis-associated encephalopathy. *Inflammation*. 2019;42(1):306−318. https://doi.org/10.1007/s10753-018-0894-4.

160. Zhang Y, Lv X, Hu Z, et al. Protection of Mcc950 against high-glucose-induced human retinal endothelial cell dysfunction. *Cell Death Dis*. 2017;8(7):e2941. https://doi.org/10.1038/cddis.2017.308.

161. Trotta MC, Maisto R, Guida F, et al. The activation of retinal HCA2 receptors by systemic beta-hydroxybutyrate inhibits diabetic retinal damage through reduction of endoplasmic reticulum stress and the NLRP3 inflammasome. *PLoS One*. 2019;14(1):e0211005. https://doi.org/10.1371/journal.pone.0211005.

162. Whitaker CM, Cooper NGF. Differential distribution of exchange proteins directly activated by cyclic AMP within the adult rat retina. *Neuroscience*. 2010;165(3):955−967. https://doi.org/10.1016/j.neuroscience.2009.10.054.

163. Jiang Y, Liu L, Curtiss E, Steinle JJ. Epac1 blocks NLRP3 inflammasome to reduce IL-1β in retinal endothelial cells and mouse retinal vasculature. *Mediat Inflamm*. 2017;2017:2860956. https://doi.org/10.1155/2017/2860956.

164. Jiang Y, Steinle JJ. Epac1 requires AMPK phosphorylation to regulate HMGB1 in the retinal vasculature. *Invest Ophthalmol Vis Sci*. 2020;61(11):33. https://doi.org/10.1167/iovs.61.11.33.

165. Hombrebueno JR, Chen M, Penalva RG, Xu H. Loss of synaptic connectivity, particularly in second order neurons is a key feature of diabetic retinal neuropathy in the Ins2Akita mouse. *PLoS One*. 2014;9(5):e97970. https://doi.org/10.1371/journal.pone.0097970.

166. Sohn EH, van Dijk HW, Jiao C, et al. Retinal neurodegeneration may precede microvascular changes characteristic of diabetic retinopathy in diabetes mellitus. *Proc Natl Acad Sci U S A*. 2016;113(19):E2655−E2664. https://doi.org/10.1073/pnas.1522014113.

167. Simó R, Stitt AW, Gardner TW. Neurodegeneration in diabetic retinopathy: does it really matter? *Diabetologia*. 2018;61(9):1902−1912. https://doi.org/10.1007/s00125-018-4692-1.

168. Forrester JV, Xu H, Lambe T, Cornall R. Immune privilege or privileged immunity? *Mucosal Immunol*. 2008;1(5):372−381. https://doi.org/10.1038/mi.2008.27.

169. Xu Y, Cheng Q, Yang B, et al. Increased sCD200 levels in vitreous of patients with proliferative diabetic retinopathy and its correlation with VEGF and proinflammatory cytokines. *Invest Ophthalmol Vis Sci*. 2015;56(11):6565−6572. https://doi.org/10.1167/iovs.15-16854.

170. Nebbioso M, Lambiase A, Armentano M, et al. Diabetic retinopathy, oxidative stress, and sirtuins: an in depth look in enzymatic patterns and new therapeutic horizons. *Surv Ophthalmol*. 2022;67(1):168−183. https://doi.org/10.1016/j.survophthal.2021.04.003.

171. Kobayashi Y, Yoshida S, Nakama T, et al. Overexpression of CD163 in vitreous and fibrovascular membranes of patients with proliferative diabetic retinopathy: possible involvement of periostin. *Br J Ophthalmol*. 2015;99(4):451−456. https://doi.org/10.1136/bjophthalmol-2014-305321.

172. Abu El-Asrar AM, Ahmad A, Allegaert E, et al. Interleukin-11 overexpression and M2 macrophage density are associated with angiogenic activity in proliferative diabetic retinopathy. *Ocul Immunol Inflamm*. 2020;28(4):575−588. https://doi.org/10.1080/09273948.2019.1616772.

173. Geng P, Ding Y, Qiu L, Lu Y. Serum mannose-binding lectin is a strong biomarker of diabetic retinopathy in Chinese patients with diabetes. *Diabetes Care*. 2015;38(5):868−875. https://doi.org/10.2337/dc14-1873.

174. Zhang J, Gerhardinger C, Lorenzi M. Early complement activation and decreased levels of glycosylphosphatidylinositol-anchored complement inhibitors in human and experimental diabetic retinopathy. *Diabetes*. 2002;51(12):3499−3504. https://doi.org/10.2337/diabetes.51.12.3499.

175. Muramatsu D, Wakabayashi Y, Usui Y, Okunuki Y, Kezuka T, Goto H. Correlation of complement fragment C5a with inflammatory cytokines in the vitreous of patients with proliferative diabetic retinopathy. *Graefes Arch Clin Exp Ophthalmol Albrecht Von Graefes Arch Klin Exp Ophthalmol*. 2013;251(1):15−17. https://doi.org/10.1007/s00417-012-2024-6.

176. Wang H, Feng L, Hu J, Xie C, Wang F. Differentiating vitreous proteomes in proliferative diabetic retinopathy using high-performance liquid chromatography coupled to tandem mass spectrometry. *Exp Eye Res*. 2013;108:110−119. https://doi.org/10.1016/j.exer.2012.11.023.

177. Ahn BY, Song ES, Cho YJ, Kwon OW, Kim JK, Lee NG. Identification of an anti-aldolase autoantibody as a diagnostic marker for diabetic retinopathy by immunoproteomic analysis. *Proteomics*. 2006;6(4):1200−1209. https://doi.org/10.1002/pmic.200500457.

178. Li Y, Smith D, Li Q, et al. Antibody-mediated retinal pericyte injury: implications for diabetic retinopathy. *Invest Ophthalmol Vis Sci*. 2012;53(9):5520−5526. https://doi.org/10.1167/iovs.12-10010.

179. Nakaizumi A, Fukumoto M, Kida T, et al. Measurement of serum and vitreous concentrations of anti-type II collagen antibody in diabetic retinopathy. *Clin Ophthalmol Auckl NZ*. 2015;9:543−547. https://doi.org/10.2147/OPTH.S75422.

180. Ponsioen TL, van Luyn MJA, van der Worp RJ, van Meurs JC, Hooymans JMM, Los LI. Collagen distribution in the human vitreoretinal interface. *Invest Ophthalmol Vis Sci*. 2008;49(9):4089−4095. https://doi.org/10.1167/iovs.07-1456.

181. Obasanmi G, Lois N, Armstrong D, et al. Circulating leukocyte alterations and the development/progression of diabetic retinopathy in type 1 diabetic patients—a pilot study. *Curr Eye Res*. 2020;45(9):1144−1154. https://doi.org/10.1080/02713683.2020.1718165.

182. Falavarjani KG, Golabi S, Modarres M. Intravitreal injection of methotrexate in persistent diabetic macular edema: a 6-month follow-up study. *Graefes Arch Clin Exp Ophthalmol Albrecht Von Graefes Arch Klin Exp Ophthalmol*. 2016;254(11):2159−2164. https://doi.org/10.1007/s00417-016-3374-2.

183. Kahan BD. Sirolimus: a comprehensive review. *Expert Opin Pharmacother*. 2001;2(11):1903−1917. https://doi.org/10.1517/14656566.2.11.1903.

184. Krishnadev N, Forooghian F, Cukras C, et al. Subconjunctival sirolimus in the treatment of diabetic macular edema. *Graefes Arch Clin Exp Ophthalmol Albrecht Von Graefes Arch Klin Exp Ophthalmol.* 2011;249(11):1627−1633. https://doi.org/10.1007/s00417-011-1694-9.

185. Sfikakis PP, Grigoropoulos V, Emfietzoglou I, et al. Infliximab for diabetic macular edema refractory to laser photocoagulation: a randomized, double-blind, placebo-controlled, crossover, 32-week study. *Diabetes Care.* 2010;33(7):1523−1528. https://doi.org/10.2337/dc09-2372.

186. Eklund L, Saharinen P. Angiopoietin signaling in the vasculature. *Exp Cell Res.* 2013;319(9):1271−1280. https://doi.org/10.1016/j.yexcr.2013.03.011.

Neurodegeneration and microangiopathy in diabetic retina and choroid

6

Distinct pathophysiologic mechanisms in diabetic retinal neurons, glial cells, and vascular cells

Recent advances in retinal biology have led to the emergence of the concept that the retinal dysfunction in diabetes is associated with changes of the retinal neurovascular unit (NVU).[1] In this book, the retinal NVU is divided into inner and outer NVU (see Chapter 3). This concept that DR is a disorder of the NVU emphasizes the intimate relationship among retinal neurons, glial cells, vascular cells, retinal pigment epithelial (RPE) cells, and the retinal immune cells (microglia and perivascular macrophages).[1,2] Proper functioning of all elements of the NVU is essential if the neural retina is to adapt successfully to various physiological conditions. For the inner retina, endothelial cells recruit pericytes by platelet-derived growth factor subunit B signaling and then pericytes promote the barrier properties of the endothelium.[3] Macroglia cells, that is, astrocytes and Müller cells, provide the Norrin signaling that is required for inner blood–retinal barrier (iBRB) integrity. For the outer retina, RPE-derived cytokines, such as pigment epithelium-derived factor (PEDF), insulin-like growth factor-1, brain-derived growth factor, and ciliary neurotrophic factor, support the survival of photoreceptors and ensure structural integrity for optimal circulation and nutrient supply.[4]

The relationships among retinal vascular cells, glial cells, and neuronal cells are interdependent.[2] In diabetic retina, all the cellular components may be affected. Hyperglycemia can cause endothelial cell dysfunction and cell death, and pericyte loss, resulting in microaneurysm and acellular capillaries. Loss of pericytes leads to hyperresponsiveness of endothelial cells to vascular endothelial growth factor (VEGF) signaling, which promotes proliferation, migration, and tube formation of endothelial cells, eventually culminating in retinal neovascularization. The retinal neurodegeneration manifesting as reduced thickness of retinal layers such as retinal nerve fiber layer (NFL) and the ganglion cell layer/inner plexiform layer (GCL/IPL) was also documented by both experimental and clinical studies.[5] Müller glia and microglia become activated and increased in number with diabetes progression,[2,6,7] while astrocytes undergo degeneration and decrease in number.[8,9] Recent work of our laboratory showed that microglia became activated under diabetic conditions, penetrating the basement membranes of retinal capillaries and phagocytosing endothelial cells, thus contributing to the leakage of the retinal blood vessels and acellular capillary formation.[7] All these changes disrupt the integrity of the blood−retinal barrier (BRB) and alter normal functioning of the NVU in diabetic retina.

Under diabetic conditions, Müller glia and astrocytes increase the production of vasoactive substances such as VEGF-A and the associated Delta-like protein 4 (Dll4), angiopoietin-related protein 4 (ANGPTL4), and leucine-rich α2-glycoprotein 1 (LRG1) that promote vascular permeability and angiogenesis.[3] Activated microglia and other retinal cells increase the production of inflammatory cytokines, including tumor necrosis factor α (TNF-α), interleukin-1β (IL-1β), and chemokine (C−C motif) ligand 2 (CCL2, also known as MCP-1), which participate in the pathogenesis of diabetic retinopathy (DR) and aggravate the disease severity. Meanwhile, hyperglycemia can cause RPE dysfunction and disrupt tight junctions (TJs), resulting in RPE degeneration and the breakdown of the outer BRB (oBRB).[10,11] Evidence exists that inner and outer retina undergo different pathogenic mechanisms under diabetic insults. Several questions remain to be discussed. For example, as for neurodegeneration and microangiopathy, which initiates the disease process first after diabetic onset? Do these two entities initiate the disease independently or in tandem during diabetes progression? Is there a common underlying molecular mechanism of these two entities?

The European Consortium for the Early Treatment of Diabetic Retinopathy (EUROCONDOR) study assessed 449 patients with type 2 diabetes mellitus for both functional change by multifocal electroretinography (mfERG) and structural changes in the retina using spectral domain optical coherence tomography (SD-OCT).[12] Diabetic patients with no vascular defects were compared with patients with mild vascular defects. It showed that 61% of patients without microvascular disease showed neurodegenerative abnormalities detected by mfERG or SD-OCT, while 32% of patients with visible microvascular disease did not show any signs of neurodegeneration.[12] Therefore, the microvascular abnormalities are not necessarily parallel to the neurodegenerative changes in DR, suggesting that these two pathological events are interdependent but result from distinct mechanistic pathways. Moving forward, the relation between diabetic vasculopathy and neurodegeneration requires further exploration.[13,14] In exploration of this relation, observable clinical biomarkers that can sensitively detect vascular and neuronal defects are essential. In this regard, DR may be categorized as diabetic retinal microangiopathy and diabetic retinal neuronopathy, that is, neurodegeneration. The former can be further categorized as inner and outer retinal microangiopathy.

Diabetic retinal neuronopathy

Diabetic retinal neuronopathy is also called diabetic retinal neurodegeneration (DRN). DRN involves degenerative alterations in retinal neurons and glia, including retinal ganglion cells (RGCs), photoreceptors, amacrine cells, bipolar cells, and glial cells. DRN is thought to be driven by glutamate, oxidative stress, and dysregulation of neuroprotective factors in the retina. As discussed above, DRN and diabetic retinal microangiopathy are distinct but interdependent components of DR.[15–18] Chronic hyperglycemia causes DRN, which manifests early in the retina and progresses throughout the disease.[5] The hallmark features of DRN are neuronal cell apoptosis, reactive gliosis, and reduced retinal neuronal function. Possible mechanisms for DRN include inflammation, oxidative stress, and altered balance of neurotrophic factors.

Neuronal dysfunction and cell loss

Several clinical tools are available to detect neuronal dysfunction at early stages of diabetic retinal disease. Many functional changes in the neural retina can be identified before the overt vascular pathology develops. The functional changes of DRN have been demonstrated such as altered retinal sensitivity by microperimetric and perimetric testing,[19,20] increased implicit times and reduction in oscillatory potentials in the mfERG,[21,22] and abnormal contrast sensitivity and color vision.[23,24] These functional alterations correlate with laboratory findings containing thinning of the retinal neuronal layers, increased apoptosis of neurons and activation of glial cells.[25] In the clinic, people with diabetic macular edema (DME) complain of a variety of symptoms of visual impairment, which include decreased visual acuity and visual field loss.[26] These visual impairments can also be documented subjectively by using National Eye Institute Visual Function Questionnaire, in conjunction with self-reported symptoms, including cloudy or blurred vision, impaired color vision, reduced peripheral vision, poor night vision, etc.[27–29] Nittala et al. reported reduced retinal sensitivity in diabetic patients without DR.[19,30,31] It was also noticed that the thickness of retinal neuronal layers is reduced in eyes with no apparent clinical DR.[19,31,32] These findings indicate that retinal neurodegeneration may precede the established clinical and morphometric vascular changes caused by diabetes. In a prospective longitudinal study including 45 patients with type 1 diabetes mellitus with no or minimal DR, OCT showed thinning of the inner retinal layers of the macula, that is, NFL, ganglion cell layer (GCL), and IPL decreased significantly over time.[5] In this study, after adjustment for duration of diabetes mellitus before inclusion, sex, age, hemoglobin A_{1c}, presence of DR at inclusion, and progression of DR after inclusion, a significant, progressive loss of NFL (0.25 μm/year) both parafoveally and perifoveally and the GCL+IPL (0.29 μm/year) parafoveally was detected in patients with type 1 diabetes mellitus.[5] In a separate observation including 5 donor eyes with diabetes mellitus and no or minimal DR and 5 age-matched donor eyes without diabetes mellitus, the NFL was significantly thinner (17.3 μm) in the donors with diabetes mellitus than the control group (30.4 μm), while the retinal capillary density did not differ between the two groups.[5] All these observations strongly suggest that diabetes directly affects the neuroretina rather than being solely secondary to BRB breakdown.

Neurodegeneration characterized by an increase in neural cell apoptosis could be detected in the early stage of DR.[33] In diabetic retina, RGCs are the earliest cells affected and have the highest rate of apoptosis (see Chapters 3 and 4).[33,34] In diabetic donors, RGCs showed cytoplasmic immunoreactivity for caspase-3, Fas, and Bax.[35] An elevated rate of apoptosis has been also observed in the outer nuclear layer, with a reduction in photoreceptors seen between 4 and 24 weeks after diabetes onset in diabetic rats.[36,37] In the eyes of patients with nonproliferative diabetic retinopathy (NPDR), the immunohistochemistry showed the association of upregulation of Bax, caspase-9 and -3 expression with neuronal degeneration.[38] Amacrine cells are also affected in DR. Dopaminergic and cholinergic amacrine cells are lost during the early stages of retinal neuropathy in diabetes.[39] Dopamine and acetylcholine-dependent amacrine cells exhibit reduced enzyme activity for tyrosine hydroxylase and acetylcholinesterase in the early stages of diabetes.[40,41] Activation of caspase-3 increases the apoptosis of dopaminergic amacrine cells in retinas of mice within 2 weeks after the onset of hyperglycemia.[39] The mitochondria- and caspase-dependent cell death pathways are associated with neuronal degeneration in diabetic retinas.

In diabetes, hyperglycemia leads to neuron vulnerability and apoptosis through many mechanisms. Glutamate excitotoxicity is indicated as one of the mechanisms by which RGCs undergo apoptosis via oxidative stress-mediated pathways in diabetes. Increasing evidence suggests that glutamate excitotoxicity also plays a role in degeneration of other retinal neurons in the diabetic retina. Experimental studies with diabetic models have revealed increased levels of glutamate in retinal extracellular space[42,43] and an association between increased glutamate levels and neurotoxicity in the retina.[44] Elevated glutamate and over activation of the glutamate N-methyl-D-aspartate (NMDA) receptor lead to an increased intracellular influx of calcium and sequential activation of a cascade finally resulting in the death of retinal neurons.[45]

Retinal glial reactivity and microinflammation

Retinal glial reactivity, also called reactive gliosis, is an early pathological event in DR. This reactivity is characterized by increased expression of glial fibrillar acidic protein (GFAP) by Müller cells, impaired function of astrocytes, and activation of microglial cells.[46] Under pathological conditions, Müller cells exhibit three important nonspecific gliotic responses: increase in cell number, change in cell shape, and upregulation of GFAP.[47] The reactive glia continuously produce and release various cytokines and proinflammatory mediators, leading to microinflammation and accelerated neuronal cell death. Microinflammation, a low-grade inflammation accompanied by activated inflammatory cells and inflammation-related cytokines, was defined in Chapter 5.

Müller cells are a significant source of numerous factors and play a pivotal role in the onset of the inflammatory process.[48] Under hyperglycemia, Müller cells are activated and release many cytokines and factors, including VEGF, PEDF, IL-1β, IL-6,

TNF-α, and CCL2.[49–52] Evidence exists that most of these growth factors, cytokines, and chemokines found in the vitreous of diabetic patients are synthesized by activated Müller cells.[53–56] For example, cluster of differentiation 40 (CD40), a tumor necrosis factor receptor superfamily member, expressed on various hematopoietic and nonhematopoietic cells, is also expressed by retinal endothelial cells and Müller cells.[57–59] Interaction of CD40 with its ligand CD154 regulates cellular and humoral immunity[60] and potentiates inflammation by activating macrophages/microglia.[59] By using mice with CD40 expression restricted to Müller cells, it is reported that Müller cells specifically trigger proinflammatory cytokine expression via CD40-ATP-P2X7 pathway. These proinflammatory cytokines include TNF-α, IL-1β, intercellular adhesion molecule 1 (ICAM-1), and inducible nitric oxide synthase 2 (NOS2). The diabetic mice expressing CD40 in their Müller cells were shown to have developed key elements of inflammatory pathology including leukostasis and capillary degeneration.[59]

Microglia, the resident immunocompetent cells in retina and central nervous system (CNS), become activated in early stages of DR. In CNS, microglia with their highly motile processes extending into the capillary wall are assumed to be the first detector of metabolic changes in diabetes.[61] Microglia sense dyslipidemia, increased reactive oxygen species (ROS) and cytokines, and accumulated advanced glycation end products (AGEs). For instance, AGEs-stimulated microglia can secret TNF-α in early stages of DR.[62] Once activated, microglia become mobile and migrate to the site of inflammation. Under hyperglycemic conditions, microglia are continuously stimulated to secret numerous products including IL-1β, IL-3, IL-6, TNF-α, VEGF, lymphotoxin, macrophage inflammatory protein-1α (MIP-1α), matrix metalloproteinases (MMPs), inducible nitric oxide synthase (iNOS), nitric oxide (NO), ROS, complement factors, and proteases. With long-term stimulus, the factors produced by activated microglia are extremely toxic to retinal neurons, including RGCs, greatly exacerbating neuronal cell dysfunction and death.[63–65] The mechanism by which cytokines contribute to neural apoptosis is not completely clear but may involve the induction of excitotoxicity, oxidative stress, and mitochondrial dysfunction.[66,67] A representative example of a neuron–microglia interaction is the fractalkine (FKN or CX3CL1)/CX3CR1 system, which illustrates a mechanism to modulate microglial activation by neurons. FKN is located on neuronal membranes and functions by signaling through its unique receptor CX3CR1 present on microglia. Several reports support the notion that FKN exerts an inhibitory signal on microglia.[68,69] It has been demonstrated that increased inflammatory microglial responses in the absence of the FKN receptor contribute to inflammation-mediated damage to neurons in the diabetic retina.[70] In our recent study, exogenous FKN deactivated microglia via inhibiting the nuclear factor-kappa B (NF-κB) pathway and activating the nuclear factor E2-related factor 2 (Nrf2) pathway. The deactivated microglia reduce the production of inflammation-related cytokines, such as ICAM-1, TNF-α, IL-1β, and ROS, resulting in the protection of the retina from diabetes insult.[69] Thus, targeting FKN/CX3CR1 appears to be a promising pharmacologic strategy for treating neuroinflammation in diabetic retina.

Altered balance of neurotrophic factors

Besides the activated Müller glia and microglia, the altered balance of neurotrophic factors is also involved in retinal neurodegeneration. This includes increased VEGF and erythropoietin (EPO), as well as decreased PEDF, somatostatin, and interphotoreceptor retinoid-binding protein (IRBP). Increased VEGF plays a key role in disrupting the BRB and causes neovascularization in DR.[71] PEDF has an inverse function, that is, anti-angiogenesis and against VEGF. The increased levels of VEGF in DR result in downregulation of PEDF through increased activity of MMPs.[72] Decreased PEDF level was reported in vitreous samples in diabetic patients.[73] The protective effects of PEDF consist of anti-oxidative, anti-inflammatory, and neuroprotective properties in diabetic retina.[74] Somatostatin, an endogenous peptide secreted by the RPE, shows antiangiogenic and neuroprotective properties in the human retina.[75] Decreased somatostatin is associated with glial activation and neural death in diabetic retina.[75] Decreased levels of somatostatin have been detected in the vitreous of diabetic patients.[76,77] IRBP, a glycoprotein synthesized by photoreceptors has significant impact on the survival of photoreceptors.[78] A low expression of IRBP in early DR has been demonstrated, which is associated with an impairment of photoreceptor functions.[78,79] EPO and its receptor are expressed by many types of retinal cells and is associated with neuroprotection and angiogenesis, depending on the stage of DR. High levels of EPO were reported in vitreous samples of diabetic patients.[80,81] The "double-edged sword" function of EPO for patients with DR is discussed in depth in Chapter 10.

Diabetic retinal microangiopathy

Diabetic retinal microangiopathy consisting of vasoregressive and proliferative stages is a long-term sequela of diabetes mellitus. Nearly 63% persons with over 30-year type 2 diabetic history develop some degree of microangiopathy.[82] On the other hand, diabetic retinal microangiopathy essentially represents ischemia-driven pathologic events in the microvasculature. Two clinical endpoints, that is, DME and proliferative diabetic retinopathy (PDR) are blinding disorders. DME can occur at any stage of the disease, while PDR is the end stage of microangiopathy. Diabetic retinal microangiopathy is no longer considered as a mere vascular disease of the inner retina, with the relationship between DRN and the circulation of inner and outer retina gradually being clarified (see Chapter 3).

Inner BRB breakdown

Both iBRB and oBRB breakdown occur early in experimental DR.[10,83,84] The central mechanism of altered BRB function is the change in the permeability of retinal endothelial cells and RPE cells.[84,85] For iBRB, paracellular and transcellular transport across the vascular wall relies on opening of endothelial intercellular junctions and changing endothelial caveolar transcellular transport. For oBRB, paracellular and transcellular transport are concentrated at the apical surface of RPE cells. This anatomic feature helps separate the choriocapillaris and subretinal space.[86] In inner retinal NVU, functional changes in pericytes and astrocytes, as well as compositional changes of the endothelial glycocalyx (EG) and the basal lamina around iBRB together determine iBRB permeability. Pericyte loss, dysfunctional endothelial cells, thickened basement membrane, and glial cell activation contribute to disruption of iBRB in the early stages of diabetes.[87] In contrast, study of the oBRB is limited. Accumulating evidence indicates that in DR, TJ complexes between RPE cells including ZO-1 and occludin proteins become disassembled. This molecular event is determined by interaction between microglia and RPE cells, in which IL-6 is a key player.[84]

Endothelial glycocalyx loss

Here, we specifically discuss diabetic changes in the retinal endothelial barrier, that is, iBRB. The endothelial barrier comprises intercellular junctions between cells, which is covered by the glycocalyx. EG is the inner stratum of the vessel. Proteoglycans are the major components of EG. Another important constituent, the polysaccharide hyaluronic acid, is embedded in EG on the endothelial cell membrane.[88] Endothelial cells are connected by intercellular junctions, that is, the adherens junction providing mechanical anchorage, the TJ sealing the intercellular space to limit paracellular permeability, and the gap junction forming connexin-mediated transmembrane channels.[89] Decreased glycocalyx density has been observed in diabetic animal models.[86] A recent report confirmed high glucose-induced changes in expression and shedding of various components of EG (Fig. 6.1), including an increased shedding of the TJ protein occludin.[86,90,91]

EG is a crucial regulator of vascular permeability. The integrity of EG limits the passage of molecules from the plasma through endothelial cells because the glycocalyx is negatively charged. Enzymatic degradation of the glycocalyx has been shown to increase retinal vascular leakage in animal models of DR. For instance, both diabetes and exogenous hyaluronidase that can degrade hyaluronic acid on the endothelial surface result in reduction of EG thickness.[92] Moreover, the glycocalyx affects interactions between blood cells and the vessel wall, such as adhesion of platelets and leukocytes to the endothelium. Adherent leukocytes, an early sign of inflammation, have been associated with retinal endothelial cell injury and death in an animal model of diabetes (Fig. 6.1).[93] In addition to EG affecting vessel permeability and leukocyte adhesion, the impaired EG contributes to changes in shear stress-induced endothelial nitric oxide synthase activation, angiogenesis, and anchoring of blood borne factors.[91]

Taken together, chronic hyperglycemia leads to glycocalyx-mediated endothelial cell injury, causing impaired junctional capacity, impaired capillary function, and vasoregression in DR.[94,95] Therefore, protection of the EG is a reasonable strategy for the prevention and treatment of DR. Although clinical therapeutic strategies that specifically target the glycocalyx are not currently available,[96] preclinical studies on

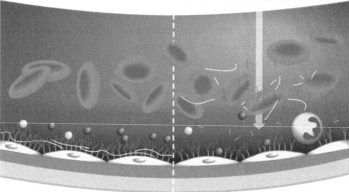

Atherosclerosis   Sepsis
Ischemia-reperfusion
Kidney injury   Diabetes

Syndecan-1
Heparan sulfate
Hyaluronan
CD44

FIGURE 6.1

Schematic representation of the endothelial glycocalyx covering endothelial cells in the lumen of a vessel, under physiological conditions (*left of the white dashed line*) and during various diseases inducing shedding of its components (*right of the white dashed line*). Hyaluronan is shown in *light green*; heparan sulfate in *blue*; syndecan-1 in *yellow*. These molecules are main components of endothelial glycocalyx.

Modified from Dogné and Flamion[90]

regulation of EG expression and subsequent endothelial functions are underway. For example, endomucin, an anti-inflammatory membrane glycoprotein is mainly expressed in endothelial cells, including retinal endothelial cells. Since it has been shown that endomucin levels are decreased during hyperglycemia in vitro and in vivo, overexpression of endomucin with adeno-associated virus was used to treat streptozotocin (STZ)-induced diabetic rat retinas. The increase in endomucin restored the endothelium coverage to the control level. Most convincingly, the restored EG was validated by an increase in syndecan-1, a biomarker of glycocalyx synthesis. In addition, endomucin could prevent leukocyte-endothelial cell adhesion by decreasing the effect of adhesion molecules in diabetic retinas, leading to stabilization of the BRB.[97]

Outer BRB breakdown

As noted above, diabetic retinal microangiopathy comprises both inner and outer retinal components. The oBRB is formed by RPE and maintained by the TJs between RPE cells. RPE is a specialized epithelium located at the interface between the neurosensory retina and the choriocapillaris.[4] The main functions of the RPE are the following: (1) transport of nutrients, ions, and water; (2) absorption of light and protection against photooxidation; (3) reisomerization of all-trans-retinal into 11-cis-retinal, which is crucial for the visual cycle; (4) phagocytosis of shed photoreceptor outer segments; and (5) secretion of essential factors for the functional and structural integrity of the retina. In DR, hyperglycemia alters the functions of the RPE,[4] causing the breakdown of oBRB and RPE secretory function. The disruptions of oBRB have been studied and documented in diabetic patients[4,98−100], diabetic animals,[101,102] and diabetic cell models.[10,103−106] For instance, the presence of albumin detected by immunostaining was found in the outer retina and RPE in donor diabetic eyes, suggesting RPE cell injury and oBRB breakdown.[98] Fluorescein angiograms in NPDR patients showed diffuse RPE leakage spreading around the macular area in late phase, suggesting the breakdown of oBRB.[99] The clinical observations showed that oBRB breakdown is likely to contribute to the development of DME. In our previous study, RPE degeneration, disruption of Bruch's membrane, and the accumulation of collagen were observed in STZ-induced diabetic rats as early as 7−10 days after diabetes onset, with a widened space between Bruch's membrane and the RPE.[83] In experimental diabetic animals, longitudinal electron microscopy showed deepened hollows in the basal infoldings of RPE after 1-month of diabetes and larger concavities into the cytoplasm after 6 months in STZ-induced diabetic rats.[101,107] In the type 2 diabetes Goto-Kakizaki rat model, hyperglycemia-induced overactivation of PKCζ was associated with oBRB breakdown and photoreceptor degeneration.[108] Short-term inhibition of PKCζ restored the outer barrier structure and reduced photoreceptor cell death, indicating PKCζ is a potential target for inhibiting early diabetes-induced RPE pathology.[108]

The underlying mechanisms of RPE dysfunction in both in vitro and in vivo diabetic models have been studied. Evidence exists that the RPE dysfunction following glycated-albumin treatment was mediated via receptor for AGEs and vascular endothelial growth factor receptor 2 (VEGFR2) signaling.[103] ARPE-19 cells, a human RPE cell line, when exposed to hyperglycemia, increased the levels of TNF-α and iNOS, forming nitrosative stress and S-nitrosylation of caveolin-1 (CAV-1).[104] The S-nitrosylation of CAV-1 triggers endocytosis of claudin-1 and occludin, leading to the breakdown of oBRB.[104] Furthermore, hyperglycemia plus hypoxia (hyperglycemia/hypoxia) exposure increases fluorescein isothiocyanate-dextran permeability and decreases transepithelial electrical resistance of ARPE-19 cells, resulting in reduction and disorganization of occludin and ZO-1.[105] Other studies with ARPE-19 cells showed that the activity-dependent neuroprotective protein− derived peptide could counteract hyperglycemia/hypoxia induced RPE barrier breakdown through modulation of hypoxia inducible factors (HIFs) and VEGF expression.[106] In our recent study using diabetic rat models, the breakdown of oBRB was observed in early onset of diabetes.[10] The expression of ZO-1 and occludin proteins in the RPE−Bruch's membrane choriocapillaris complex were significantly decreased, whereas the HIF-1α and JNK pathways were activated, in 4-week diabetic rats. These findings have provided new information on molecular mechanisms of oBRB breakdown in diabetes.[10] This mechanism can also help explain the neuroprotective function of EPO because EPO maintains the oBRB integrity through downregulation of HIF-1α and JNK signaling, and upregulation of ZO-1 and occludin expression in RPE cells.[10] In addition, other molecules that may be protective to the RPE barrier in experimental DR, for example, metformin, resveratrol, and melatonin, merit further investigation.[109−112]

Diabetic choroidopathy

Diabetic choroidopathy, a form of microangiopathy in diabetes, was first reported in 1997.[113] The choroid is the vascular system responsible for the blood supply to the outer layers of the retina, including RPE and photoreceptors. The choroidal circulation is the only source of metabolic exchange for the avascular fovea.[114] Since the nourishment of the macula is provided by the choroid, there is growing interest in studying the role of the choroid in the pathogenesis of DR, particularly DME.[114] Accumulating studies showed that the risk factors for diabetic choroidopathy are the existence of severe DR, poor diabetic control, and the nature of the treatment regimen.[115] On the other hand, clinical and experimental findings suggest that choroidal vasculopathy (diabetic choroidopathy) plays an independent role in the pathogenesis of DR. A prospective, observational, and case-control study showed that diabetic choroidopathy seems to be strongly associated with photoreceptor damage.[116] In this study, compared with normal control, patients with NPDR displayed macular hypoperfusion and photoreceptor damage, the latter indicated by a lower "normalized" reflectivity of ellipsoid zone on OCT (0.96 ± 0.25 in controls and 0.73 ± 0.19 in the NPDR group, $P < .0001$).[116]

Early histopathological changes in the diabetic choroid include choriocapillaris loss, tortuous blood vessels, microaneurysms, and drusenoid deposits on Bruch's membrane. The histopathological studies also showed intrachoroidal microvascular abnormality, choriocapillaris degeneration, and choroidal neovascularization.[117−119] By using color Doppler imaging, the subfoveal choroidal blood flow can be assessed in patients with diabetes. Foveolar choroidal blood volume and blood flow are significantly reduced in PDR patients compared with that in normal controls.[120] Subfoveal choroidal blood flow is also decreased significantly in diabetic patients without DR or with NPDR compared with normal controls examined with laser Doppler flowmetry. This phenomenon became more prominent in patients with DME.[121] Using swept-source optical coherence tomography angiography, choriocapillaris flow deficits (FDs) in eyes with DR were objectively and quantitatively assessed with the percentage of choriocapillaris flow deficits (FD%) and FD size determined. The clinical findings showed that both choriocapillaris FD% and FD size are increased in the macular region of eyes with DR.[122] Meta-analysis showed that the ratio of luminal areas, corresponding to the choroidal vascular lumens, in total choroidal areas was significantly lower in diabetic eyes with no DR than in healthy control eyes, suggesting that choroidal vascular structures are affected before the onset of retinopathy.[123] By using indocyanine green angiography and enhanced depth imaging spectral-domain optical coherence tomography, Hua et al. reported multiple biomarkers for studying diabetic choroidopathy.[124] These biomarkers consist of early hypofluorescent spots, late choroidal nonperfusion regions, inverted inflow phenomena, higher subfoveal choroidal thickness (SFCT), and larger choroidal area. The choroidal area was defined by the authors as the region between the outer RPE and inner scleral borders.[124] Among these biomarkers, the changes of SFCT in diabetic choroidopathy may serve as a predictor for DR progression.

In one study, DME patients with thicker baseline SFCT have better short-term anatomic and functional responses to anti-VEGF treatment.[125] However, the changes of choroidal thickness in DR remains controversial when examined by OCT measurement.[114] Several studies found correlations between decreases in choroidal thickness and the progressing stages of DR. However, some studies showed that the choroidal thinning is unrelated to the stage of DR,[126,127] while others found choroidal thinning is related to the stage of DR, but no difference between diabetic eyes without retinopathy and controls.[128−131] For example, an overall thinning of the choroid was reported among diabetic patients, suggesting that decreased choroidal blood flow is the primary event in the development of DR and diabetic choroidopathy.[127,132] It was proposed that the decreased choroidal thickness may lead to the reduction of oxygen supply, leading to an increase in the level of VEGF and resultant breakdown of BRB and development of DME.[127] In another study, choroidal thickness was increased in patients with DR, increased significantly as the severity worsened from mild/moderate NPDR to PDR.[133] The correlation between choroidal thickness and DME remains uncertain and variable. Some authors reported a thinner choroid in clinically significant macular edema than in controls.[127,134] However, one study reported that the subfoveal choroid is thicker in eyes with DME than in those without DME. The thickest subfoveal choroid was found in DME with subretinal detachment.[133] This discrepancy reflects the complex pathophysiology of the choroid in diabetic choroidopathy. In future studies, more sensitive and reliable parameters to quantify choroid pathology are required.

It is important to know that the choroid is characterized as a branching vascular network receiving abundant autonomic innervation. Therefore, the term diabetic choroidopathy might encompass both neuronopathy and microangiopathy. Yamamoto et al. found parasympathetic nitric oxide synthase (NOS) innervation to the choroid in rats.[135] Evidence exists that in STZ-induced diabetic rats, the activity and the amount of choroidal NOS is lowered 6 weeks after diabetic onset, correlating with decreased choroidal blood flow. The reduced NOS is mainly the neuronal NOS isoform (nNOS), indicating the decrease in nNOS is attributable to a neural disorder of the diabetic choroid.[136]

In diabetes, the choroid behaves as a proinflammatory environment. Diabetic choroidopathy is regarded as an inflammatory disease, in which leukocyte adhesion molecules are elevated.[137] In fact, inflammatory cell trafficking, glial cell activation, and migration from the retina to the choroid are observed in diabetic animals.[65,138] By using Goto-Kakizaki rats, a model for spontaneous type 2 diabetes, sparse microglia/macrophages are detected in the subretinal space. In addition, numerous pores in RPE, allowing inflammatory cell traffic between the retina and choroid were found at 5 months of hyperglycemia, which was mediated by PKCζ.[138] Dropout of choriocapillaris was shown in diabetic choroid, and there was a direct correlation between the number of polymorphonuclear leukocytes or neutrophils (PMNs) and the area of choriocapillaris dropout.[118,137] There was about 4.4-fold greater area of acellular capillaries in diabetic choroid compared with the control subjects.[113,122] A previous study demonstrated that ICAM-1 and P-selectin are constitutively expressed in the normal choroid and upregulated in the choroidal vasculature in diabetes.[139] Both upregulated ICAM-1 and P-selectin could mediate increased cell adhesion, contributing to the choroidal microangiopathy observed in diabetics. The relationship between diabetic choroidopathy and DR remains largely unknown. With the advent of advanced imaging technologies, diabetic choroidopathy needs further investigation. The information obtained may be translated into clinical biomarkers for predicting and regulating microangiopathy in diabetic retina and choroid.

Potential therapeutic targets in diabetic retina and choroid

Diabetes affects the inner and outer retinal NVU because it disrupts communication among neurons, glial cells, and vascular cells. Understanding the pathophysiology of the diabetic retina and choroid has provided insight into potential prevention and management strategies. Several potential therapeutic targets and approaches to the diabetic retina and choroid are highlighted below.

First, based on current data, occurrence of DRN preceding retinal microangiopathy is the earliest pathologic event of DR. Therefore, more sensitive and specific biomarkers are required to reveal early structural and functional alterations of diabetic neurosensory retina, RPE, and choroid. Meanwhile, systemic control of the early biochemical and metabolic disturbances of diabetes, particularly glycemic control, is imperative to benefit physiologic functions of both retina and choroid. In addition, several interconnected biochemical pathways discussed in Chapter 2 are activated during diabetes, which increase the expression of angiogenic and inflammatory mediators and induce aberrant downstream signaling. All of these systemic and local diabetic events have delineated an architecture for understanding neurodegeneration and vasculopathy in retina and choroid.

Second, increased oxidative stress and lipid peroxidation due to diabetes contribute to the physiological photooxidation at the level of the neural retina because of direct exposure of the retina to light.[140] In fact, oxidative stress plays a crucial role in both retinal neurodegeneration and vasculopathy.[141,142] Since oxidative stress is involved in diverse molecular mechanisms, combating oxidative stress is a strategy that is disease-context dependent and cell-specific. For example, oxidation resistance 1 (*OXR1*) gene is reported as a key player in the pathology of neurodegenerative diseases including diabetic neurodegeneration. In the Akita diabetic mouse model, miR-200b was used to destabilize *OXR1* mRNA and protein.[143] As the *OXR1* mRNA and protein levels declined, the retinal neurons presented an excess of oxidative DNA damage, resulting in the initiation of apoptosis of retinal neurons. Furthermore, when miR-200b was introduced into cultured retinal Müller cells, a similar phenomenon occurred, that is, increased oxidative damage and Müller cell death. Most significantly, when using a miR-200b resistant form of *OXR1* along with the miR-200b, Müller cells demonstrated therapeutic results, that is, reduced oxidative damage and decreased apoptosis. Thus, restoration of the *OXR1* gene product is a neuron-glial cell specific antioxidative therapy against neurodegeneration.[144]

Third, in diabetic retina, neurons such as RGCs undergo apoptosis, whereas glia cells become reactive. The glia cell—specific reaction is noteworthy although retinal neurons, glial cells, and vascular cells are all under the diabetic stress. Individual glial cell types react differentially to the diabetic stress. One of the first structural alterations in experimental and human DR is reactive gliosis of Müller cells in the initial stages of diabetes.[46] Reactive gliosis may be interpreted as an effort to limit the extension of tissue damage, but the resulting sustained inflammation in DR leads to more severe forms of reactive gliosis.[145] Müller cells undergo further hypertrophy, lose their functionality, ultimately forming glial scars that are inhibitory to axonal regeneration and neuronal survival.[145,146] In the study of a murine Müller cell injury model, the reactive gliosis can be considered as a fibrotic-like process.[147] Therefore, regulation of reactive gliosis of Müller cells may be a cell-specific approach for the prevention of neurodegeneration.

Fourth, in DR, glutamate is increased in the vitreous of diabetic patients.[148,149] Excessive glutamate results in neuronal cell death via activation of the NMDA receptor in retinal neurons, especially the RGCs.[45] Even though similar studies have not been reported in the context of DR, it has been demonstrated that microglia activation leads to increased tau phosphorylation and decreased expression of the synaptic protein synaptophysin in degenerative neurons. These molecular events are associated with the release of high levels of glutamate that increase excitotoxicity.[150] In a recent study, experimental mice were treated with intravitreal NMDA to induce excitotoxic damage in the retina including neuronal death, microglial reactivity, and upregulation of proinflammatory cytokines.[151] Biochemical ablation of microglia resulted in aggravated cell death in excitotoxin-damaged retina. Exogenous IL-1β stimulated the proliferation and reactivity of microglia in normal retina, and reduced numbers of dying cells in damaged retinas. These findings indicate that reactive microglia cells are necessary for neuronal survival because they provide a neuroprotective function in excitotoxin-damaged retina.[151] In other words, specific types of glial cells such as microglia could play a "double-edged sword" role in combating diabetic neurodegeneration in a disease-specific context.

Fifth, diabetes affects not only the retinal vasculature but also that of the choroid. The essential pathophysiology of diabetic choroidopathy is reflective of an inflammatory disease. The diabetes-induced inflammatory disease is able to activate leukocytes. It is known that more leukocytes, especially PMNs, circulate in diabetics than in nondiabetics.[118] Once PMNs are firmly adherent to the vascular wall, they can undergo an oxidative burst damaging choroidal endothelial cells. Subsequent closure of choroidal vessels and loss of blood supply to outer retina can damage RPE—photoreceptor complex. Therefore, diabetic choroidopathy needs to be diagnosed early. Development of sensitive biomarkers and new imaging modalities for choroidal circulation are imperative for the diagnosis of diabetic choroidopathy. The antiinflammatory approach as the mainstay for treating diabetic choroidopathy is a future direction.[117]

References

1. Antonetti DA, Klein R, Gardner TW. Diabetic retinopathy. *N Engl J Med*. 2012;366(13): 1227—1239. https://doi.org/10.1056/NEJMra1005073.
2. Simó R, Stitt AW, Gardner TW. Neurodegeneration in diabetic retinopathy: does it really matter? *Diabetologia*. 2018;61(9):1902—1912. https://doi.org/10.1007/s00125-018-4692-1.
3. Antonetti DA, Silva PS, Stitt AW. Current understanding of the molecular and cellular pathology of diabetic retinopathy. *Nat Rev Endocrinol*. 2021;17(4):195—206. https://doi.org/10.1038/s41574-020-00451-4.
4. Simó R, Villarroel M, Corraliza L, Hernández C, Garcia-Ramírez M. The retinal pigment epithelium: something more than a constituent of the blood-retinal barrier-implications for the pathogenesis of diabetic retinopathy. *J Biomed Biotechnol*. 2010; 2010. https://doi.org/10.1155/2010/190724, 190724.
5. Sohn EH, van Dijk HW, Jiao C, et al. Retinal neurodegeneration may precede microvascular changes characteristic of diabetic retinopathy in diabetes mellitus. *Proc Natl Acad Sci U S A*. 2016;113(19):E2655—E2664. https://doi.org/10.1073/pnas.1522014113.
6. Hu LM, Luo Y, Zhang J, et al. EPO reduces reactive gliosis and stimulates neurotrophin expression in Muller cells. *Front Biosci Elite Ed*. 2011;3:1541—1555. https://doi.org/10.2741/e355.
7. Xie H, Zhang C, Liu D, et al. Erythropoietin protects the inner blood-retinal barrier by inhibiting microglia phagocytosis via Src/Akt/cofilin signalling in experimental diabetic retinopathy. *Diabetologia*. 2021;64(1):211—225. https://doi.org/10.1007/s00125-020-05299-x.
8. Ly A, Yee P, Vessey KA, Phipps JA, Jobling AI, Fletcher EL. Early inner retinal astrocyte dysfunction during diabetes and development of hypoxia, retinal stress, and neuronal functional loss. *Invest Ophthalmol Vis Sci*. 2011;52(13):9316—9326. https://doi.org/10.1167/iovs.11-7879.
9. Barber AJ, Antonetti DA, Gardner TW. Altered expression of retinal occludin and glial fibrillary acidic protein in experimental diabetes. The Penn State Retina Research Group. *Invest Ophthalmol Vis Sci*. 2000;41(11):3561—3568.

10. Zhang C, Xie H, Yang Q, et al. Erythropoietin protects outer blood-retinal barrier in experimental diabetic retinopathy by up-regulating ZO-1 and occludin. *Clin Exp Ophthalmol*. 2019;47(9):1182−1197. https://doi.org/10.1111/ceo.13619.

11. Xu HZ, Le YZ. Significance of outer blood-retina barrier breakdown in diabetes and ischemia. *Invest Ophthalmol Vis Sci*. 2011;52(5):2160−2164. https://doi.org/10.1167/iovs.10-6518.

12. Santos AR, Ribeiro L, Bandello F, et al. Functional and structural findings of neurodegeneration in early stages of diabetic retinopathy: cross-sectional analyses of baseline data of the EUROCONDOR project. *Diabetes*. 2017;66(9):2503−2510. https://doi.org/10.2337/db16-1453.

13. Duh EJ, Sun JK, Stitt AW. Diabetic retinopathy: current understanding, mechanisms, and treatment strategies. *JCI Insight*. 2017;2(14):93751. https://doi.org/10.1172/jci.insight.93751.

14. Antonetti DA, Barber AJ, Bronson SK, et al. Diabetic retinopathy: seeing beyond glucose-induced microvascular disease. *Diabetes*. 2006;55(9):2401−2411. https://doi.org/10.2337/db05-1635.

15. Abcouwer SF, Gardner TW. Diabetic retinopathy: loss of neuroretinal adaptation to the diabetic metabolic environment. *Ann N Y Acad Sci*. 2014;1311:174−190. https://doi.org/10.1111/nyas.12412.

16. Simó R, Hernández C, European Consortium for the Early Treatment of Diabetic Retinopathy (EUROCONDOR). Neurodegeneration in the diabetic eye: new insights and therapeutic perspectives. *Trends Endocrinol Metab TEM*. 2014;25(1):23−33. https://doi.org/10.1016/j.tem.2013.09.005.

17. Simó R, Hernández C. Novel approaches for treating diabetic retinopathy based on recent pathogenic evidence. *Prog Retin Eye Res*. 2015;48:160−180. https://doi.org/10.1016/j.preteyeres.2015.04.003.

18. Stitt AW, Curtis TM, Chen M, et al. The progress in understanding and treatment of diabetic retinopathy. *Prog Retin Eye Res*. 2016;51:156−186. https://doi.org/10.1016/j.preteyeres.2015.08.001.

19. Verma A, Rani PK, Raman R, et al. Is neuronal dysfunction an early sign of diabetic retinopathy? Microperimetry and spectral domain optical coherence tomography (SD-OCT) study in individuals with diabetes, but no diabetic retinopathy. *Eye Lond Engl*. 2009;23(9):1824−1830. https://doi.org/10.1038/eye.2009.184.

20. Gardner TW, Abcouwer SF, Barber AJ, Jackson GR. An integrated approach to diabetic retinopathy research. *Arch Ophthalmol Chic Ill 1960*. 2011;129(2):230−235. https://doi.org/10.1001/archophthalmol.2010.362.

21. Li X, Sun X, Hu Y, Huang J, Zhang H. Electroretinographic oscillatory potentials in diabetic retinopathy. An analysis in the domains of time and frequency. *Doc Ophthalmol Adv Ophthalmol*. 1992;81(2):173−179. https://doi.org/10.1007/BF00156006.

22. Bearse MA, Adams AJ, Han Y, et al. A multifocal electroretinogram model predicting the development of diabetic retinopathy. *Prog Retin Eye Res*. 2006;25(5):425−448. https://doi.org/10.1016/j.preteyeres.2006.07.001.

23. Sokol S, Moskowitz A, Skarf B, Evans R, Molitch M, Senior B. Contrast sensitivity in diabetics with and without background retinopathy. *Arch Ophthalmol Chic Ill 1960*. 1985;103(1):51−54. https://doi.org/10.1001/archopht.1985.01050010055018.

24. Roy MS, Gunkel RD, Podgor MJ. Color vision defects in early diabetic retinopathy. *Arch Ophthalmol Chic Ill 1960*. 1986;104(2):225−228. https://doi.org/10.1001/archopht.1986.01050140079024.

25. de Moraes G, Layton CJ. Therapeutic targeting of diabetic retinal neuropathy as a strategy in preventing diabetic retinopathy. *Clin Exp Ophthalmol*. 2016;44(9):838−852. https://doi.org/10.1111/ceo.12795.

26. Chen XD, Gardner TW. A critical review: psychophysical assessments of diabetic retinopathy. *Surv Ophthalmol*. 2021;66(2):213−230. https://doi.org/10.1016/j.survophthal.2020.08.003.

27. Akkaya S, Düzova S, Şahin Ö, Kazokoğlu H, Bavbek T. National Eye Institute Visual function scale in type 2 diabetes patients. *J Ophthalmol*. 2016;2016. https://doi.org/10.1155/2016/1549318, 1549318.

28. Cusick M, SanGiovanni JP, Chew EY, et al. Central visual function and the NEI-VFQ-25 near and distance activities subscale scores in people with type 1 and 2 diabetes. *Am J Ophthalmol*. 2005;139(6):1042−1050. https://doi.org/10.1016/j.ajo.2005.01.008.

29. Klein R, Moss SE, Klein BE, Gutierrez P, Mangione CM. The NEI-VFQ-25 in people with long-term type 1 diabetes mellitus: the Wisconsin Epidemiologic Study of Diabetic Retinopathy. *Arch Ophthalmol Chic Ill 1960*. 2001;119(5):733−740. https://doi.org/10.1001/archopht.119.5.733.

30. Nittala MG, Gella L, Raman R, Sharma T. Measuring retinal sensitivity with the microperimeter in patients with diabetes. *Retina Phila Pa*. 2012;32(7):1302−1309. https://doi.org/10.1097/IAE.0b013e3182365a24.

31. Neriyanuri S, Pardhan S, Gella L, et al. Retinal sensitivity changes associated with diabetic neuropathy in the absence of diabetic retinopathy. *Br J Ophthalmol*. 2017;101(9):1174−1178. https://doi.org/10.1136/bjophthalmol-2016-309641.

32. Verma A, Raman R, Vaitheeswaran K, et al. Does neuronal damage precede vascular damage in subjects with type 2 diabetes mellitus and having no clinical diabetic retinopathy? *Ophthalmic Res*. 2012;47(4):202−207. https://doi.org/10.1159/000333220.

33. Barber AJ, Lieth E, Khin SA, Antonetti DA, Buchanan AG, Gardner TW. Neural apoptosis in the retina during experimental and human diabetes. Early onset and effect of insulin. *J Clin Invest*. 1998;102(4):783−791. https://doi.org/10.1172/JCI2425.

34. Kern TS, Barber AJ. Retinal ganglion cells in diabetes. *J Physiol*. 2008;586(18):4401−4408. https://doi.org/10.1113/jphysiol.2008.156695.

35. Abu-El-Asrar AM, Dralands L, Missotten L, Al-Jadaan IA, Geboes K. Expression of apoptosis markers in the retinas of human subjects with diabetes. *Invest Ophthalmol Vis Sci*. 2004;45(8):2760−2766. https://doi.org/10.1167/iovs.03-1392.

36. Park SH, Park JW, Park SJ, et al. Apoptotic death of photoreceptors in the streptozotocin-induced diabetic rat retina. *Diabetologia*. 2003;46(9):1260−1268. https://doi.org/10.1007/s00125-003-1177-6.

37. Énzsöly A, Szabó A, Kántor O, et al. Pathologic alterations of the outer retina in streptozotocin-induced diabetes. *Invest Ophthalmol Vis Sci*. 2014;55(6):3686−3699. https://doi.org/10.1167/iovs.13-13562.

38. Oshitari T, Yamamoto S, Hata N, Roy S. Mitochondria- and caspase-dependent cell death pathway involved in neuronal degeneration in diabetic retinopathy. *Br J Ophthalmol*. 2008;92(4):552−556. https://doi.org/10.1136/bjo.2007.132308.

39. Gastinger MJ, Singh RSJ, Barber AJ. Loss of cholinergic and dopaminergic amacrine cells in streptozotocin-diabetic rat and Ins2Akita-diabetic mouse retinas. *Invest Ophthalmol Vis Sci*. 2006;47(7):3143−3150. https://doi.org/10.1167/iovs.05-1376.

40. Nishimura C, Kuriyama K. Alterations in the retinal dopaminergic neuronal system in rats with streptozotocin-induced diabetes. *J Neurochem*. 1985;45(2):448−455. https://doi.org/10.1111/j.1471-4159.1985.tb04008.x.

41. Sánchez-Chávez G, Salceda R. Acetyl- and butyrylcholinesterase in normal and diabetic rat retina. *Neurochem Res*. 2001;26(2):153−159. https://doi.org/10.1023/a:1011098829378.

42. Lieth E, Barber AJ, Xu B, et al. Glial reactivity and impaired glutamate metabolism in short-term experimental diabetic retinopathy. Penn State Retina Research Group. *Diabetes*. 1998;47(5):815−820. https://doi.org/10.2337/diabetes.47.5.815.

43. Lieth E, LaNoue KF, Antonetti DA, Ratz M. Diabetes reduces glutamate oxidation and glutamine synthesis in the retina. The Penn State Retina Research Group. *Exp Eye Res*. 2000;70(6):723−730. https://doi.org/10.1006/exer.2000.0840.

44. Vorwerk CK, Lipton SA, Zurakowski D, Hyman BT, Sabel BA, Dreyer EB. Chronic low-dose glutamate is toxic to retinal ganglion cells. Toxicity blocked by memantine. *Invest Ophthalmol Vis Sci*. 1996;37(8):1618−1624.

45. Carvajal FJ, Mattison HA, Cerpa W. Role of NMDA receptor-mediated glutamatergic signaling in chronic and acute neuropathologies. *Neural Plast*. 2016;2016:2701526. https://doi.org/10.1155/2016/2701526.

46. Rungger-Brändle E, Dosso AA, Leuenberger PM. Glial reactivity, an early feature of diabetic retinopathy. *Invest Ophthalmol Vis Sci*. 2000;41(7):1971−1980.

47. Bringmann A, Pannicke T, Grosche J, et al. Müller cells in the healthy and diseased retina. *Prog Retin Eye Res*. 2006;25(4):397−424. https://doi.org/10.1016/j.preteyeres.2006.05.003.

48. Rübsam A, Parikh S, Fort PE. Role of inflammation in diabetic retinopathy. *Int J Mol Sci*. 2018;19(4):E942. https://doi.org/10.3390/ijms19040942.

49. Mu H, Zhang XM, Liu JJ, Dong L, Feng ZL. Effect of high glucose concentration on VEGF and PEDF expression in cultured retinal Müller cells. *Mol Biol Rep*. 2009;36(8):2147−2151. https://doi.org/10.1007/s11033-008-9428-8.

50. Liu X, Ye F, Xiong H, et al. IL-1β induces IL-6 production in retinal Müller cells predominantly through the activation of p38 MAPK/NF-κB signaling pathway. *Exp Cell Res*. 2015;331(1):223−231. https://doi.org/10.1016/j.yexcr.2014.08.040.

51. Wang J, Xu X, Elliott MH, Zhu M, Le YZ. Müller cell-derived VEGF is essential for diabetes-induced retinal inflammation and vascular leakage. *Diabetes*. 2010;59(9):2297−2305. https://doi.org/10.2337/db09-1420.

52. Lei X, Zhang J, Shen J, et al. EPO attenuates inflammatory cytokines by Muller cells in diabetic retinopathy. *Front Biosci Elite Ed*. 2011;3:201−211. https://doi.org/10.2741/e234.

53. Abu el Asrar AM, Maimone D, Morse PH, Gregory S, Reder AT. Cytokines in the vitreous of patients with proliferative diabetic retinopathy. *Am J Ophthalmol*. 1992;114(6):731−736. https://doi.org/10.1016/s0002-9394(14)74052-8.

54. Brooks HL, Caballero S, Newell CK, et al. Vitreous levels of vascular endothelial growth factor and stromal-derived factor 1 in patients with diabetic retinopathy and cystoid macular edema before and after intraocular injection of triamcinolone. *Arch Ophthalmol Chic Ill 1960*. 2004;122(12):1801−1807. https://doi.org/10.1001/archopht.122.12.1801.

55. Demircan N, Safran BG, Soylu M, Ozcan AA, Sizmaz S. Determination of vitreous interleukin-1 (IL-1) and tumour necrosis factor (TNF) levels in proliferative diabetic

retinopathy. *Eye Lond Engl*. 2006;20(12):1366−1369. https://doi.org/10.1038/sj.eye.6702138.

56. Hernández C, Segura RM, Fonollosa A, Carrasco E, Francisco G, Simó R. Interleukin-8, monocyte chemoattractant protein-1 and IL-10 in the vitreous fluid of patients with proliferative diabetic retinopathy. *Diabet Med J Br Diabet Assoc*. 2005;22(6):719−722. https://doi.org/10.1111/j.1464-5491.2005.01538.x.

57. Portillo JAC, Schwartz I, Zarini S, et al. Proinflammatory responses induced by CD40 in retinal endothelial and Müller cells are inhibited by blocking CD40-Traf2,3 or CD40-Traf6 signaling. *Invest Ophthalmol Vis Sci*. 2014;55(12):8590−8597. https://doi.org/10.1167/iovs.14-15340.

58. Peters AL, Stunz LL, Bishop GA. CD40 and autoimmunity: the dark side of a great activator. *Semin Immunol*. 2009;21(5):293−300. https://doi.org/10.1016/j.smim.2009.05.012.

59. Portillo JAC, Lopez Corcino Y, Miao Y, et al. CD40 in retinal Müller cells induces P2X7-dependent cytokine expression in macrophages/microglia in diabetic mice and development of early experimental diabetic retinopathy. *Diabetes*. 2017;66(2):483−493. https://doi.org/10.2337/db16-0051.

60. van Kooten C, Banchereau J. CD40-CD40 ligand. *J Leukoc Biol*. 2000;67(1):2−17. https://doi.org/10.1002/jlb.67.1.2.

61. Graeber MB, Li W, Rodriguez ML. Role of microglia in CNS inflammation. *FEBS Lett*. 2011;585(23):3798−3805. https://doi.org/10.1016/j.febslet.2011.08.033.

62. Ibrahim AS, El-Remessy AB, Matragoon S, et al. Retinal microglial activation and inflammation induced by amadori-glycated albumin in a rat model of diabetes. *Diabetes*. 2011;60(4):1122−1133. https://doi.org/10.2337/db10-1160.

63. Yang LP, Sun HL, Wu LM, et al. Baicalein reduces inflammatory process in a rodent model of diabetic retinopathy. *Invest Ophthalmol Vis Sci*. 2009;50(5):2319−2327. https://doi.org/10.1167/iovs.08-2642.

64. Zeng HY, Green WR, Tso MOM. Microglial activation in human diabetic retinopathy. *Arch Ophthalmol Chic Ill 1960*. 2008;126(2):227−232. https://doi.org/10.1001/archophthalmol.2007.65.

65. Grigsby JG, Cardona SM, Pouw CE, et al. The role of microglia in diabetic retinopathy. *J Ophthalmol*. 2014;2014:705783. https://doi.org/10.1155/2014/705783.

66. Fogal B, Hewett SJ. Interleukin-1beta: a bridge between inflammation and excitotoxicity? *J Neurochem*. 2008;106(1):1−23. https://doi.org/10.1111/j.1471-4159.2008.05315.x.

67. Abcouwer SF, Shanmugam S, Gomez PF, et al. Effect of IL-1beta on survival and energy metabolism of R28 and RGC-5 retinal neurons. *Invest Ophthalmol Vis Sci*. 2008;49(12):5581−5592. https://doi.org/10.1167/iovs.07-1032.

68. Sheridan GK, Murphy KJ. Neuron-glia crosstalk in health and disease: fractalkine and CX3CR1 take centre stage. *Open Biol*. 2013;3(12):130181. https://doi.org/10.1098/rsob.130181.

69. Jiang M, Xie H, Zhang C, et al. Enhancing fractalkine/CX3CR1 signalling pathway can reduce neuroinflammation by attenuating microglia activation in experimental diabetic retinopathy. *J Cell Mol Med*. 2022;26(4):1229−1244. https://doi.org/10.1111/jcmm.17179.

70. Cardona SM, Mendiola AS, Yang YC, Adkins SL, Torres V, Cardona AE. Disruption of fractalkine signaling leads to microglial activation and neuronal damage in the diabetic

retina. *ASN Neuro*. 2015;7(5). https://doi.org/10.1177/1759091415608204, 1759091415608204.

71. Aiello LP, Avery RL, Arrigg PG, et al. Vascular endothelial growth factor in ocular fluid of patients with diabetic retinopathy and other retinal disorders. *N Engl J Med*. 1994; 331(22):1480−1487. https://doi.org/10.1056/NEJM199412013312203.

72. Becerra SP. Focus on molecules: pigment epithelium-derived factor (PEDF). *Exp Eye Res*. 2006;82(5):739−740. https://doi.org/10.1016/j.exer.2005.10.016.

73. Barnstable CJ, Tombran-Tink J. Neuroprotective and antiangiogenic actions of PEDF in the eye: molecular targets and therapeutic potential. *Prog Retin Eye Res*. 2004;23(5): 561−577. https://doi.org/10.1016/j.preteyeres.2004.05.002.

74. Elahy M, Baindur-Hudson S, Cruzat VF, Newsholme P, Dass CR. Mechanisms of PEDF-mediated protection against reactive oxygen species damage in diabetic retinopathy and neuropathy. *J Endocrinol*. 2014;222(3):R129−R139. https://doi.org/10.1530/JOE-14-0065.

75. Carrasco E, Hernández C, Miralles A, Huguet P, Farrés J, Simó R. Lower somatostatin expression is an early event in diabetic retinopathy and is associated with retinal neurodegeneration. *Diabetes Care*. 2007;30(11):2902−2908. https://doi.org/10.2337/dc07-0332.

76. Simó R, Lecube A, Sararols L, et al. Deficit of somatostatin-like immunoreactivity in the vitreous fluid of diabetic patients: possible role in the development of proliferative diabetic retinopathy. *Diabetes Care*. 2002;25(12):2282−2286. https://doi.org/10.2337/diacare.25.12.2282.

77. Simó R, Carrasco E, Fonollosa A, García-Arumí J, Casamitjana R, Hernández C. Deficit of somatostatin in the vitreous fluid of patients with diabetic macular edema. *Diabetes Care*. 2007;30(3):725−727. https://doi.org/10.2337/dc06-1345.

78. Garcia-Ramírez M, Hernández C, Villarroel M, et al. Interphotoreceptor retinoid-binding protein (IRBP) is downregulated at early stages of diabetic retinopathy. *Diabetologia*. 2009;52(12):2633−2641. https://doi.org/10.1007/s00125-009-1548-8.

79. Gonzalez-Fernandez F, Ghosh D. Focus on molecules: interphotoreceptor retinoid-binding protein (IRBP). *Exp Eye Res*. 2008;86(2):169−170. https://doi.org/10.1016/j.exer.2006.09.003.

80. Watanabe D, Suzuma K, Matsui S, et al. Erythropoietin as a retinal angiogenic factor in proliferative diabetic retinopathy. *N Engl J Med*. 2005;353(8):782−792. https://doi.org/10.1056/NEJMoa041773.

81. Hernández C, Fonollosa A, García-Ramírez M, et al. Erythropoietin is expressed in the human retina and it is highly elevated in the vitreous fluid of patients with diabetic macular edema. *Diabetes Care*. 2006;29(9):2028−2033. https://doi.org/10.2337/dc06-0556.

82. Voigt M, Schmidt S, Lehmann T, et al. Prevalence and progression rate of diabetic retinopathy in type 2 diabetes patients in correlation with the duration of diabetes. *Exp Clin Endocrinol Diabetes*. 2018;126(9):570−576. https://doi.org/10.1055/s-0043-120570.

83. Zhang J, Wu Y, Jin Y, et al. Intravitreal injection of erythropoietin protects both retinal vascular and neuronal cells in early diabetes. *Invest Ophthalmol Vis Sci*. 2008;49(2): 732−742. https://doi.org/10.1167/iovs.07-0721.

84. Jo DH, Yun JH, Cho CS, Kim JH, Kim JH, Cho CH. Interaction between microglia and retinal pigment epithelial cells determines the integrity of outer blood-retinal barrier in diabetic retinopathy. *Glia*. 2019;67(2):321−331. https://doi.org/10.1002/glia.23542.

85. Klaassen I, Van Noorden CJF, Schlingemann RO. Molecular basis of the inner blood-retinal barrier and its breakdown in diabetic macular edema and other pathological conditions. *Prog Retin Eye Res.* 2013;34:19–48. https://doi.org/10.1016/j.preteyeres.2013.02.001.

86. O'Leary F, Campbell M. The blood-retina barrier in health and disease. *FEBS J.* December 18, 2021. https://doi.org/10.1111/febs.16330.

87. Cunha-Vaz J, Bernardes R, Lobo C. Blood-retinal barrier. *Eur J Ophthalmol.* 2011; 21(Suppl 6):S3–S9. https://doi.org/10.5301/EJO.2010.6049.

88. Jedlicka J, Becker BF, Chappell D. Endothelial glycocalyx. *Crit Care Clin.* 2020;36(2): 217–232. https://doi.org/10.1016/j.ccc.2019.12.007.

89. Radeva MY, Waschke J. Mind the gap: mechanisms regulating the endothelial barrier. *Acta Physiol Oxf Engl.* 2018;222(1). https://doi.org/10.1111/apha.12860.

90. Dogné S, Flamion B. Endothelial glycocalyx impairment in disease: focus on hyaluronan shedding. *Am J Pathol.* 2020;190(4):768–780. https://doi.org/10.1016/j.ajpath.2019.11.016.

91. Kaur G, Rogers J, Rashdan NA, et al. Hyperglycemia-induced effects on glycocalyx components in the retina. *Exp Eye Res.* 2021;213:108846. https://doi.org/10.1016/j.exer.2021.108846.

92. Leskova W, Pickett H, Eshaq RS, Shrestha B, Pattillo CB, Harris NR. Effect of diabetes and hyaluronidase on the retinal endothelial glycocalyx in mice. *Exp Eye Res.* 2019; 179:125–131. https://doi.org/10.1016/j.exer.2018.11.012.

93. Joussen AM, Murata T, Tsujikawa A, Kirchhof B, Bursell SE, Adamis AP. Leukocyte-mediated endothelial cell injury and death in the diabetic retina. *Am J Pathol.* 2001; 158(1):147–152. https://doi.org/10.1016/S0002-9440(10)63952-1.

94. Chou J, Rollins S, Fawzi AA. Role of endothelial cell and pericyte dysfunction in diabetic retinopathy: review of techniques in rodent models. *Adv Exp Med Biol.* 2014;801: 669–675. https://doi.org/10.1007/978-1-4614-3209-8_84.

95. Hammes HP. Diabetic retinopathy: hyperglycaemia, oxidative stress and beyond. *Diabetologia.* 2018;61(1):29–38. https://doi.org/10.1007/s00125-017-4435-8.

96. Pillinger NL, Kam P. Endothelial glycocalyx: basic science and clinical implications. *Anaesth Intensive Care.* 2017;45(3):295–307. https://doi.org/10.1177/0310057X1704500305.

97. Niu T, Zhao M, Jiang Y, et al. Endomucin restores depleted endothelial glycocalyx in the retinas of streptozotocin-induced diabetic rats. *FASEB J.* 2019;33(12): 13346–13357. https://doi.org/10.1096/fj.201901161R.

98. Vinores SA, Gadegbeku C, Campochiaro PA, Green WR. Immunohistochemical localization of blood-retinal barrier breakdown in human diabetics. *Am J Pathol.* 1989; 134(2):231–235.

99. Weinberger D, Fink-Cohen S, Gaton DD, Priel E, Yassur Y. Non-retinovascular leakage in diabetic maculopathy. *Br J Ophthalmol.* 1995;79(8):728–731. https://doi.org/10.1136/bjo.79.8.728.

100. Xu HZ, Song Z, Fu S, Zhu M, Le YZ. RPE barrier breakdown in diabetic retinopathy: seeing is believing. *J Ocul Biol Dis Infor.* 2011;4(1–2):83–92. https://doi.org/10.1007/s12177-011-9068-4.

101. Aizu Y, Oyanagi K, Hu J, Nakagawa H. Degeneration of retinal neuronal processes and pigment epithelium in the early stage of the streptozotocin-diabetic rats. *Neuropathol.* 2002;22(3):161–170. https://doi.org/10.1046/j.1440-1789.2002.00439.x.

102. Kirber WM, Nichols CW, Grimes PA, Winegrad AI, Laties AM. A permeability defect of the retinal pigment epithelium. Occurrence in early streptozocin diabetes. *Arch Ophthalmol Chic Ill 1960*. 1980;98(4):725−728. https://doi.org/10.1001/archopht.1980.01020030719015.

103. Dahrouj M, Desjardins DM, Liu Y, Crosson CE, Ablonczy Z. Receptor mediated disruption of retinal pigment epithelium function in acute glycated-albumin exposure. *Exp Eye Res*. 2015;137:50−56. https://doi.org/10.1016/j.exer.2015.06.004.

104. Rosales MAB, Silva KC, Duarte DA, Rossato FA, Lopes de Faria JB, Lopes de Faria JM. Endocytosis of tight junctions caveolin nitrosylation dependent is improved by cocoa via opioid receptor on RPE cells in diabetic conditions. *Invest Ophthalmol Vis Sci*. 2014;55(9):6090−6100. https://doi.org/10.1167/iovs.14-14234.

105. Wang S, Du S, Wu Q, Hu J, Li T. Decorin prevents retinal pigment epithelial barrier breakdown under diabetic conditions by suppressing p38 MAPK activation. *Invest Ophthalmol Vis Sci*. 2015;56(5):2971−2979. https://doi.org/10.1167/iovs.14-15874.

106. D'Amico AG, Maugeri G, Rasà DM, et al. NAP counteracts hyperglycemia/hypoxia induced retinal pigment epithelial barrier breakdown through modulation of HIFs and VEGF expression. *J Cell Physiol*. 2018;233(2):1120−1128. https://doi.org/10.1002/jcp.25971.

107. Desjardins DM, Yates PW, Dahrouj M, Liu Y, Crosson CE, Ablonczy Z. Progressive early breakdown of retinal pigment epithelium function in hyperglycemic rats. *Invest Ophthalmol Vis Sci*. 2016;57(6):2706−2713. https://doi.org/10.1167/iovs.15-18397.

108. Omri S, Behar-Cohen F, Rothschild PR, et al. PKCζ mediates breakdown of outer blood-retinal barriers in diabetic retinopathy. *PLoS One*. 2013;8(11):e81600. https://doi.org/10.1371/journal.pone.0081600.

109. Amin SV, Khanna S, Parvar SP, et al. Metformin and retinal diseases in preclinical and clinical studies: insights and review of literature. *Exp Biol Med Maywood NJ*. 2022;247(4):317−329. https://doi.org/10.1177/15353702211069986.

110. Popescu M, Bogdan C, Pintea A, Rugină D, Ionescu C. Antiangiogenic cytokines as potential new therapeutic targets for resveratrol in diabetic retinopathy. *Drug Des Dev Ther*. 2018;12:1985−1996. https://doi.org/10.2147/DDDT.S156941.

111. Qu S, Zhang C, Liu D, et al. Metformin protects ARPE-19 cells from glyoxal-induced oxidative stress. *Oxid Med Cell Longev*. 2020;2020:1740943. https://doi.org/10.1155/2020/1740943.

112. Lai YH, Hu DN, Rosen R, et al. Hypoxia-induced vascular endothelial growth factor secretion by retinal pigment epithelial cells is inhibited by melatonin via decreased accumulation of hypoxia-inducible factors-1α protein. *Clin Exp Ophthalmol*. 2017;45(2):182−191. https://doi.org/10.1111/ceo.12802.

113. Lutty GA. Effects of diabetes on the eye. *Invest Ophthalmol Vis Sci*. 2013;54(14):ORSF81−87. https://doi.org/10.1167/iovs.13-12979.

114. Campos A, Campos EJ, Martins J, Ambrósio AF, Silva R. Viewing the choroid: where we stand, challenges and contradictions in diabetic retinopathy and diabetic macular oedema. *Acta Ophthalmol*. 2017;95(5):446−459. https://doi.org/10.1111/aos.13210.

115. Shiragami C, Shiraga F, Matsuo T, Tsuchida Y, Ohtsuki H. Risk factors for diabetic choroidopathy in patients with diabetic retinopathy. *Graefes Arch Clin Exp Ophthalmol Albrecht Von Graefes Arch Klin Exp Ophthalmol*. 2002;240(6):436−442. https://doi.org/10.1007/s00417-002-0451-5.

116. Borrelli E, Palmieri M, Viggiano P, Ferro G, Mastropasqua R. Photoreceptor damage in diabetic choroidopathy. *Retina Phila Pa*. 2020;40(6):1062−1069. https://doi.org/10.1097/IAE.0000000000002538.

117. Lutty GA. Diabetic choroidopathy. *Vision Res*. 2017;139:161−167. https://doi.org/10.1016/j.visres.2017.04.011.

118. Cao J, McLeod S, Merges CA, Lutty GA. Choriocapillaris degeneration and related pathologic changes in human diabetic eyes. *Arch Ophthalmol Chic Ill 1960*. 1998;116(5):589−597. https://doi.org/10.1001/archopht.116.5.589.

119. Fukushima I, McLeod DS, Lutty GA. Intrachoroidal microvascular abnormality: a previously unrecognized form of choroidal neovascularization. *Am J Ophthalmol*. 1997;124(4):473−487. https://doi.org/10.1016/s0002-9394(14)70863-3.

120. Schocket LS, Brucker AJ, Niknam RM, Grunwald JE, DuPont J, Brucker AJ. Foveolar choroidal hemodynamics in proliferative diabetic retinopathy. *Int Ophthalmol*. 2004;25(2):89−94. https://doi.org/10.1023/b:inte.0000031744.93778.60.

121. Nagaoka T, Kitaya N, Sugawara R, et al. Alteration of choroidal circulation in the foveal region in patients with type 2 diabetes. *Br J Ophthalmol*. 2004;88(8):1060−1063. https://doi.org/10.1136/bjo.2003.035345.

122. Dai Y, Zhou H, Zhang Q, et al. Quantitative assessment of choriocapillaris flow deficits in diabetic retinopathy: a swept-source optical coherence tomography angiography study. *PLoS One*. 2020;15(12):e0243830. https://doi.org/10.1371/journal.pone.0243830.

123. Kase S, Endo H, Takahashi M, et al. Choroidal vascular structures in diabetic patients: a meta-analysis. *Graefes Arch Clin Exp Ophthalmol Albrecht Von Graefes Arch Klin Exp Ophthalmol*. 2021;259(12):3537−3548. https://doi.org/10.1007/s00417-021-05292-z.

124. Hua R, Liu L, Wang X, Chen L. Imaging evidence of diabetic choroidopathy in vivo: angiographic pathoanatomy and choroidal-enhanced depth imaging. *PLoS One*. 2013;8(12):e83494. https://doi.org/10.1371/journal.pone.0083494.

125. Rayess N, Rahimy E, Ying GS, et al. Baseline choroidal thickness as a predictor for response to anti-vascular endothelial growth factor therapy in diabetic macular edema. *Am J Ophthalmol*. 2015;159(1):85−91.e1-3. https://doi.org/10.1016/j.ajo.2014.09.033.

126. Esmaeelpour M, Brunner S, Ansari-Shahrezaei S, et al. Choroidal thinning in diabetes type 1 detected by 3-dimensional 1060 nm optical coherence tomography. *Invest Ophthalmol Vis Sci*. 2012;53(11):6803−6809. https://doi.org/10.1167/iovs.12-10314.

127. Querques G, Lattanzio R, Querques L, et al. Enhanced depth imaging optical coherence tomography in type 2 diabetes. *Invest Ophthalmol Vis Sci*. 2012;53(10):6017−6024. https://doi.org/10.1167/iovs.12-9692.

128. Vujosevic S, Martini F, Cavarzeran F, Pilotto E, Midena E. Macular and peripapillary choroidal thickness in diabetic patients. *Retina Phila Pa*. 2012;32(9):1781−1790. https://doi.org/10.1097/IAE.0b013e31825db73d.

129. Adhi M, Brewer E, Waheed NK, Duker JS. Analysis of morphological features and vascular layers of choroid in diabetic retinopathy using spectral-domain optical coherence tomography. *JAMA Ophthalmol*. 2013;131(10):1267−1274. https://doi.org/10.1001/jamaophthalmol.2013.4321.

130. Lee HK, Lim JW, Shin MC. Comparison of choroidal thickness in patients with diabetes by spectral-domain optical coherence tomography. *Korean J Ophthalmol KJO*. 2013;27(6):433−439. https://doi.org/10.3341/kjo.2013.27.6.433.

131. Unsal E, Eltutar K, Zirtiloğlu S, Dinçer N, Ozdoğan Erkul S, Güngel H. Choroidal thickness in patients with diabetic retinopathy. *Clin Ophthalmol Auckl NZ*. 2014;8: 637−642. https://doi.org/10.2147/OPTH.S59395.

132. Esmaeelpour M, Považay B, Hermann B, et al. Mapping choroidal and retinal thickness variation in type 2 diabetes using three-dimensional 1060-nm optical coherence tomography. *Invest Ophthalmol Vis Sci*. 2011;52(8):5311−5316. https://doi.org/ 10.1167/iovs.10-6875.

133. Kim JT, Lee DH, Joe SG, Kim JG, Yoon YH. Changes in choroidal thickness in relation to the severity of retinopathy and macular edema in type 2 diabetic patients. *Invest Ophthalmol Vis Sci*. 2013;54(5):3378−3384. https://doi.org/10.1167/iovs.12-11503.

134. Gerendas BS, Waldstein SM, Simader C, et al. Three-dimensional automated choroidal volume assessment on standard spectral-domain optical coherence tomography and correlation with the level of diabetic macular edema. *Am J Ophthalmol*. 2014;158(5): 1039−1048. https://doi.org/10.1016/j.ajo.2014.08.001.

135. Yamamoto R, Bredt DS, Snyder SH, Stone RA. The localization of nitric oxide synthase in the rat eye and related cranial ganglia. *Neuroscience*. 1993;54(1):189−200. https:// doi.org/10.1016/0306-4522(93)90393-t.

136. Sakurai M, Higashide T, Takeda H, Shirao Y. Characterization and diabetes-induced impairment of nitric oxide synthase in rat choroid. *Curr Eye Res*. 2002;24(2): 139−146. https://doi.org/10.1076/ceyr.24.2.139.8163.

137. Lutty GA, Cao J, McLeod DS. Relationship of polymorphonuclear leukocytes to capillary dropout in the human diabetic choroid. *Am J Pathol*. 1997;151(3):707−714.

138. Omri S, Behar-Cohen F, de Kozak Y, et al. Microglia/macrophages migrate through retinal epithelium barrier by a transcellular route in diabetic retinopathy: role of PKCζ in the Goto Kakizaki rat model. *Am J Pathol*. 2011;179(2):942−953. https:// doi.org/10.1016/j.ajpath.2011.04.018.

139. McLeod DS, Lefer DJ, Merges C, Lutty GA. Enhanced expression of intracellular adhesion molecule-1 and P-selectin in the diabetic human retina and choroid. *Am J Pathol*. 1995;147(3):642−653.

140. Nita M, Grzybowski A. The role of the reactive oxygen species and oxidative stress in the pathomechanism of the age-related ocular diseases and other pathologies of the anterior and posterior eye segments in adults. *Oxid Med Cell Longev*. 2016;2016: 3164734. https://doi.org/10.1155/2016/3164734.

141. Xiao C, He M, Nan Y, et al. Physiological effects of superoxide dismutase on altered visual function of retinal ganglion cells in db/db mice. *PLoS One*. 2012;7(1):e30343. https://doi.org/10.1371/journal.pone.0030343.

142. Fukumoto M, Nakaizumi A, Zhang T, Lentz SI, Shibata M, Puro DG. Vulnerability of the retinal microvasculature to oxidative stress: ion channel-dependent mechanisms. *Am J Physiol Cell Physiol*. 2012;302(9):C1413−C1420. https://doi.org/10.1152/ ajpcell.00426.2011.

143. Murray AR, Chen Q, Takahashi Y, Zhou KK, Park K, Ma JX. MicroRNA-200b downregulates oxidation resistance 1 (Oxr1) expression in the retina of type 1 diabetes model. *Invest Ophthalmol Vis Sci*. 2013;54(3):1689−1697. https://doi.org/10.1167/ iovs.12-10921.

144. Volkert MR, Crowley DJ. Preventing neurodegeneration by controlling oxidative stress: the role of OXR1. *Front Neurosci*. 2020;14:611904. https://doi.org/10.3389/ fnins.2020.611904.

145. Bringmann A, Iandiev I, Pannicke T, et al. Cellular signaling and factors involved in Müller cell gliosis: neuroprotective and detrimental effects. *Prog Retin Eye Res*. 2009;28(6):423—451. https://doi.org/10.1016/j.preteyeres.2009.07.001.

146. Roy S, Amin S, Roy S. Retinal fibrosis in diabetic retinopathy. *Exp Eye Res*. 2016;142: 71—75. https://doi.org/10.1016/j.exer.2015.04.004.

147. Conedera FM, Quintela Pousa AM, Presby DM, Mercader N, Enzmann V, Tschopp M. Diverse signaling by TGFβ isoforms in response to focal injury is associated with either retinal regeneration or reactive gliosis. *Cell Mol Neurobiol*. 2021;41(1):43—62. https://doi.org/10.1007/s10571-020-00830-5.

148. Ambati J, Chalam KV, Chawla DK, et al. Elevated gamma-aminobutyric acid, glutamate, and vascular endothelial growth factor levels in the vitreous of patients with proliferative diabetic retinopathy. *Arch Ophthalmol Chic Ill 1960*. 1997;115(9): 1161—1166. https://doi.org/10.1001/archopht.1997.01100160331011.

149. Pulido JE, Pulido JS, Erie JC, et al. A role for excitatory amino acids in diabetic eye disease. *Exp Diabetes Res*. 2007;2007:36150. https://doi.org/10.1155/2007/36150.

150. Barger SW, Basile AS. Activation of microglia by secreted amyloid precursor protein evokes release of glutamate by cystine exchange and attenuates synaptic function. *J Neurochem*. 2001;76(3):846—854. https://doi.org/10.1046/j.1471-4159.2001.00075.x.

151. Todd L, Palazzo I, Suarez L, et al. Reactive microglia and IL1β/IL-1R1-signaling mediate neuroprotection in excitotoxin-damaged mouse retina. *J Neuroinflammation*. 2019;16(1):118. https://doi.org/10.1186/s12974-019-1505-5.

Proliferative diabetic retinopathy, a disease of pathologic angiogenesis and vasculogenesis

Proliferative diabetic retinopathy (PDR) is a late complication of diabetic retinopathy (DR). PDR along with diabetic macular edema (DME) are the two major causes of vision loss in diabetic patients. PDR contributes 12,000 to 24,000 new cases of blindness each year among working-age adults in the United States.[1,2] Pathologic processes in DR start with vasoregression leading to vessel closure and hence retinal ischemia. The compromised blood–retinal barrier (BRB) results in excessive vascular leakage. The continuation of severe retinal ischemia accelerates retinal neovascularization that grows along the vitreoretinal interface and causes tractional retinal detachment and vitreous hemorrhage. Most importantly, these new vessels are unable to cover the nonperfused area for amelioration of retinal ischemia. Overall, PDR is clinically characterized by the presence of abnormal growth of new retinal blood vessels together with retinal neurodegeneration. In the diabetic retina, microvascular cells, glial cells, and neurons work interdependently to delineate PDR as a disease of the neurovascular unit (NVU). During disease progression, multiple cellular components of the NVU produce more pro-angiogenic than anti-angiogenic factors, tipping the balance toward pathologic angiogenesis. In addition, inflammatory molecules produced by cellular components of the diabetic NVU trigger and accelerate angiogenesis. The cross talk between inflammation and angiogenesis involves biochemical, hemodynamic, and immunological mechanisms, by which pathological angiogenesis and defected vasculogenesis lead to the progression of PDR. Vasculogenesis is defined as new capillary formation by de novo production of endothelial cells (ECs). Therefore, PDR is a paradigm of both pathological angiogenesis and defected vasculogenesis, in which normalization of angiogenic and vasculogenic events could be potential therapeutic approaches.

Angiogenesis and vasculogenesis in physiological and diabetic retina

Vascular endothelial growth factor and sprouting angiogenesis

Angiogenesis occurs in two principal types. First type, sprouting angiogenesis is a dense, immature, evenly spaced network of new vessels, which develops by recursive

Therapeutic Targets for Diabetic Retinopathy. https://doi.org/10.1016/B978-0-323-93064-2.00004-4

sprouting and fusion of sprouts. Second type, intussusceptive angiogenesis is the process in which preexisting blood vessels split, expand, and remodel during postnatal development through the formation of transluminal pillars and folds when spanning opposite vessel walls.[3] The new sprout is oriented by a specialized EC, which responds to angiogenic growth factors by extending filopodia, that is, the slender cytoplasmic projections from the nascent sprout and migrating toward the signal.[4]

Among the angiogenic growth factors, VEGF is the central signal as well as regulator. In humans, the VEGF family comprises five secreted protein ligands, including VEGF-A, B, C, D and placental growth factor (PlGF). The five ligands have different binding affinities for three tyrosine kinase receptors, that is, VEGF receptor (VEGFR)-1, -2 and -3.[5] VEGF-A, B and PlGF bind to VEGFR-1; VEGF-A binds to VEGFR-2; VEGF-C and -D bind to VEGFR-3 (Fig. 7.1).[6]

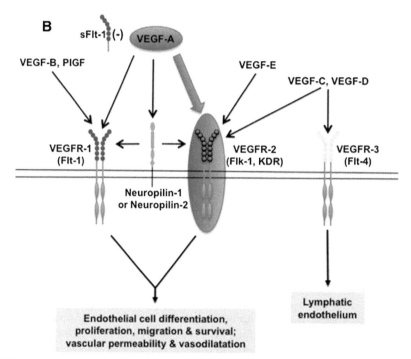

FIGURE 7.1

Simplified schematic of the VEGF system. Illustrating the principal ligand–receptor interactions between the VEGF family members. VEGF exerts its effect via its receptor VEGFR-1, VEGFR-2, and VEGFR-3. sFlt-1 is a soluble, truncated form of VEGFR-1 and functions, at least in part, as an antagonist of VEGF-A. Neuropilin-1 (NRP-1) and Neuropilin-2 (NRP-2) act as coreceptors that form homo- or heterodimers and that can form a holoreceptor complex with VEGFR-2. VEGFR-3 is expressed almost exclusively by the lymphatic endothelium in adults. Other proteins, like integrin and vascular endothelial-protein tyrosine phosphorylase (VE-PTP) are accessory proteins that facilitate VEGF/VEGFR signaling.

Modified from Majumder et al.[6]

VEGF-A interacts with VEGFR-2, also known as fetal liver kinase-1/kinase-insert domain receptor (Flk-1/KDR), and VEGFR-1, also known as Fms-like tyrosine kinase-1 (Flt-1) (Fig. 7.1), which regulate endothelial responses, such as the proliferation and migration of ECs, vascular permeability, and induction of tip cell filopodia (Fig. 7.2 & Fig. 7.5).[7] Flt-1 is a high-affinity receptor for VEGF-A, but it undergoes only weak tyrosine autophosphorylation in response to the ligand.[8] A soluble form of Flt-1 (sFlt-1) synthesized by ECs, truncated form of VEGFR-1 and as a decoy receptor of VEGFR-1, is capable of binding VEGF-A, thereby inhibiting the proangiogenic functions of the ligand vide infra.[6,9]

VEGF-A is constitutively expressed at low levels in many normal adult tissues. It is expressed at high levels in developmental angiogenesis and pathological angiogenesis. During pathological angiogenesis, for example, hypoxia-activated ECs in diabetic retina start a new blood vessel sprout from existing damaged vessel. A

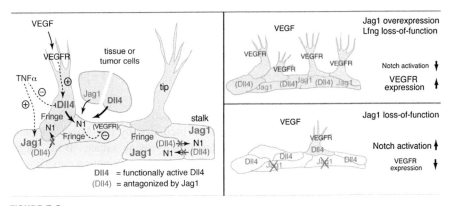

FIGURE 7.2

The key role of VEGF in a model of sprouting angiogenesis. In this model, the modulation of Dll4-Notch signaling by Jagged-1 (*left*) and alterations in the Jag1 and Lfng mutant vasculature (*right*) are presented. Lfng refers to Lunatic Fringe genes that are expressed in the developing vasculature. VEGF signaling in tip endothelial cells induces (+) the expression of Dll4. Fringe modification of Notch (most probably Notch1; N1) in stalk endothelial cells enhances Notch signaling by Dll4-presenting tip cells, which reduces VEGF receptor expression and maintains the stalk phenotype. Dll4 is antagonized by Jag1, which promotes angiogenesis and increases tip cell numbers by lowering Notch activation levels, while VEGF signaling is enhanced. Angiogenic sprouting might be positively (+) or negatively (−) modulated by differential regulation of Jag1 and Dll4 in endothelial cells as well as in adjacent nonendothelial cells, such as the tumor cells shown in this figure. TNF-α upregulates (+) Jag1 but lowers (−) Dll4 transcript levels. Dll4 but not Jag1 is induced by Notch signaling. Jag1 in stalk cells prevents activation of Notch in neighboring (stalk or tip) endothelial cells that coexpress Dll4. This activity of Jag1 depends on Fringe, which reduces Notch activation by Jag1 and thereby leads to competition between a strong agonist (Dll4) and antagonistically acting Jag1.

Modified from Benedito et al.[10]

specialized tip cell, instructing many adjacent stalk cells to follow, guides vessel sprouting toward growth factor gradients, for example, gradients of VEGF (Fig. 7.2). The interaction between the tip and stalk cells is regulated by endothelial Notch signaling through the Notch ligand Delta-like 4 (Dll4) expressed in tip cells. In stalk cells, Dll4 signals activate Notch downstream targets and reduce VEGFR expression levels, thereby preventing stalk cell transformation into tip cell. By using loss-of-function and gain-of-function mouse models, Benedito et al. demonstrated the role of Jagged-1 (Jag1), which is a ligand in the Notch signaling pathway, in sprouting angiogenesis.[10] This study suggests that Jag1, a ligand that interacts with Dll4-mediated Notch signaling, negatively regulates Notch activity and antagonizes Dll4-mediated Notch activation (Fig. 7.2). Overall, Jag1 is expressed in stalk cells but is absent or minimally expressed in tip cells. In contrast, Dll4 is strongly expressed in tip cells, but only at lower levels in stalk cells. Fringe proteins, named β3-N-acetylglucosaminyltransferases, modulate Notch activity by modifying O-fucose residues on epidermal growth factor (EGF)-like repeats of Notch (Fig. 7.2).[11]

Angiopoietin (Ang)/tyrosine kinase with immunoglobulin-like and EGF-like domains (Tie) system interacts with VEGF in sprouting angiogenesis

The angiopoietins (Ang-1 and Ang-2) are growth factors that regulate a dynamic balance between vascular stability and growth mediated by the Ang/Tie ligand/receptor system. Tie2 is an EC-specific receptor tyrosine kinase. Both Ang-1 and Ang-2 ligands interact with the Tie2. Loss- and gain-of-function experiments have demonstrated the critical contributions of the Ang/Tie2 system to vascular development and vascular diseases (Fig. 7.3).[12,13] Ang-1/Tie2 binding regulates the phosphoinositide 3 (PI3) kinase (PI3K)/Akt signal transduction pathway. Ang-2 is a weaker agonist when competing with Ang-1 for binding and reducing phosphorylation of Tie2. Thus, Ang-2 is considered as a natural Ang-1/Tie2 inhibitor.[14] In other words, Ang-2 has been characterized as a weak Tie-2 agonist that competitively inhibits Ang-1/Tie2 signaling. Structural studies have identified an agonistic domain in Ang-1 that is capable of converting chimeric ligands of Ang-2 such as Ang-2-TAG into full agonists,[15] indicating the close structural relationship between Ang-1 and Ang-2. Overall, the data suggest that Ang-1 protects from pathological angiogenesis potentiating a quiescent, mature vessel formation, whereas Ang-2 promotes vascular leakage and abnormally activated vessels (Fig. 7.3).[12,16] Ang-2 also amplifies proapoptotic signals in pericytes under stresses such as proinflammatory cytokines,[17] contributing to destabilization of vessels. Regula et al. studied the interplay of VEGF-A and Angs in an in vitro model of EC barrier breakdown.[16] The data showed that VEGF-A increases the amount of Ang-2, whereas Ang-1 reduces the secretion of Ang-2. Endothelial barrier breakdown is mainly done by VEGF-A. When adding anti-Ang-2 together with VEGF-A, barrier breakdown was alleviated. This suggests that VEGF-A

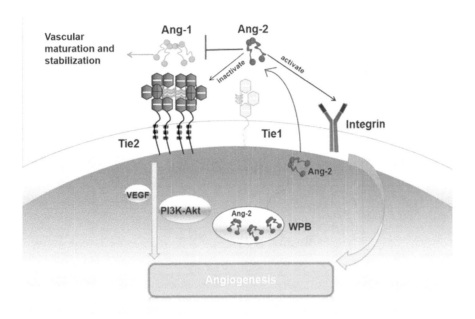

FIGURE 7.3

Ang-Tie ligand receptor system. Tie2 is activated by Ang-1 and its expression is highly enriched in endothelial cells. Tie1 is an orphan receptor homolog of Tie2 whose intact expression enhances Tie2 activation. Weibel—Palade bodies (WPBs) are the storage granules of endothelial cells.

Modified from Wu et al.[12]

triggers EC barrier breakdown, at least in part via Ang-2.[16] The function of Ang-2 for new blood vessel formation is VEGF-A concentration-dependent. For example, in a genetically modified mouse model with ischemic retinopathy, Ang-2 accelerates new vessel formation in response to high VEGF-A levels; however, if VEGF-A levels are low, Ang-2 promotes regression of angiogenesis.[18]

Notably, ligand-stimulated activation of Tie2 leads to tyrosine phosphorylation of the intracellular domain of the receptor and ultimately signal transduction. Dephosphorylation of receptor tyrosine kinases by protein tyrosine phosphatases (PTPs) is a common mechanism by which downstream cellular events such as growth arrest, apoptosis, and migration are regulated. Tie2 is also regulated by a phosphatase, vascular endothelial protein tyrosine phosphatase (VE-PTP).[19] VE-PTP is associated with Tie2 and deactivates it via dephosphorylation (Fig. 7.4). Therefore, biochemically VE-PTP acts like Ang-2 when binding to Tie2.[20] Like Ang-2, VE-PTP is increased in hypoxic retina.[18,21]

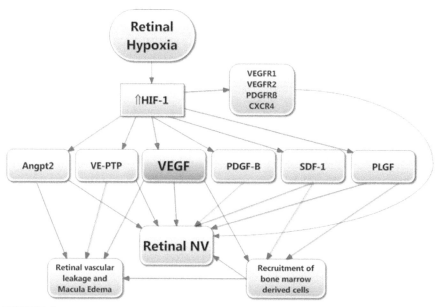

FIGURE 7.4

Molecular pathogenesis of retinal neovascularization (NV). A simplified version of the molecular pathogenesis of retinal NV illustrates several important molecular signals. It highlights soluble mediators and omits cell—cell and cell—matrix signaling. Retinal NV occurs in diabetic retinopathy and other ischemic retinopathies. The underlying disease process (e.g., high glucose in diabetic retinopathy) damages retinal vessels causing vessel closure and retinal ischemia, which results in elevated HIF-1 levels. HIF-1 upregulates several vasoactive gene products including angiopoietin-2 (Ang-2), vascular endothelial-protein tyrosine phosphatase (VE-PTP), vascular endothelial growth factor (VEGF), platelet-derived growth factor B (PDGF-B), stromal-derived growth factor (SDF-1), placental growth factor (PlGF), and several of their receptors. VEGF causes vascular leakage and in combination with Ang-2 and VE-PTP causes sprouting of new vessels. VEGF, SDF-1, and PlGF recruit bone marrow—derived cells which provide paracrine stimulation. PDGF-B recruits pericytes which also provide paracrine stimulation.

Modified from Campochiaro[18]

Pathological angiogenesis in PDR

From vasoregression to angiogenesis in PDR progression

From nonproliferative to proliferative stage, the retinal vasculature in diabetes undergoes a distinct process from vasoregression to neovascularization. First of all, DR is part of a systemic vascular disease in which vasoregression is the primary evolutionary process. In the milieu of diabetic retina, persistent hyperglycemia upregulates Ang-2 level, which has been found to be associated with accelerated pericyte loss.[22] As described in Chapter 4, pericyte dropout and acellular capillaries (ACs) are characteristics of early clinical pathology of diabetic retina. However, the precise mechanisms by which pericytes undergo apoptosis under hyperglycemia are still not completely elucidated. Hammes et al. reported that in diabetic rats 3 weeks after onset, Ang-2 protein was upregulated 37-fold compared with nondiabetic controls and remained 2.5-fold elevated after 3 months of diabetes.[23] Yao et al. reported that high glucose induces Ang-2 expression in early diabetes. For example, in mouse kidney ECs, high glucose causes increased methylglyoxal modification of the core-pressor mSin3A, a transcriptional regulatory protein. Methylglyoxal modification of mSin3A results in the activation of hexosamine biosynthetic pathway and advanced glycation end products accumulation, with consequently increased modification of transcription factor specificity protein 3 (Sp3) by O-linked N-acetylglucosamine. This modification of Sp3 causes decreased binding to a glucose-responsive GC-box in the Ang-2 promoter, leading to upregulation of Ang-2 expression. Increased Ang-2 expression induced by high glucose increased expression of intercellular adhesion molecule 1 (ICAM-1) and vascular cell adhesion molecule 1 (VCAM-1) in kidneys from diabetic mice and sensitized microvascular ECs to the proinflammatory effects of tumor necrosis factor-α (TNF-α).[24,25] When Ang-2 functions as an autocrine regulator of endothelial inflammatory responses, it also plays a key role in the induction of pericyte apoptosis via the p53 pathway. Retinal endothelial and glial cells (Müller cells) express Ang-2 as a dominant negative ligand blocking Tie2 phosphorylation.[22] Notably, aside from Tie2 receptor, integrin is also important as a receptor for Ang-2 in both ECs and pericytes (Fig. 7.3). Evidence exists that high glucose levels increase integrin $\alpha 3 \beta 1$ in pericytes.[25] Consequently, Ang-2 promotes pericyte apoptosis. This finding is corroborated by using integrin $\alpha 3 \beta 1$ blocker, which effectively attenuated Ang2-induced pericyte apoptosis in vivo and in vitro.[25] Overall, the pericyte dropout, endothelial degeneration, and ACs formation lead to vasoregression in the nonproliferative stage of DR.

In contrast, Ang-1 plays a substantial role in the formation of the retinal vascular network during development. Ang-1 can rescue microangiopathy by simultaneously promoting healthy vascular network formation and inhibiting subsequent abnormal angiogenesis, vascular leakage, and neuronal dysfunction in the ischemic retina.[26] Ang-1 can affect dual signaling pathways, that is, Tie2 signaling in the vascular cells and integrin $\alpha v \beta 5$ signaling in the astrocytes. The activation of integrin $\alpha v \beta 5$ signaling promoted fibronectin accumulation and radial distribution along the sprouting ECs, which consequently stimulated guided angiogenesis in the retina (Fig. 7.5). At the non-PDR (NPDR) stage, upregulation of Ang-2 induced by hyperglycemia dominates in the vasoregression process, whereas Ang-1 plays a substantial role in the recovery of devascularized areas. At NPDR stage, ischemia is not a predominant event and VEGF production does not reach the critical point inducing aberrant angiogenesis.[27] Following the natural course from NPDR to PDR, the resultant pericyte loss, endothelial degeneration, glial activation, capillary occlusion, and BRB breakdown together gradually lead to regional hypoxia in diabetic retina. Moving forward, expansion of retinal nonperfusion further leads to upregulation of

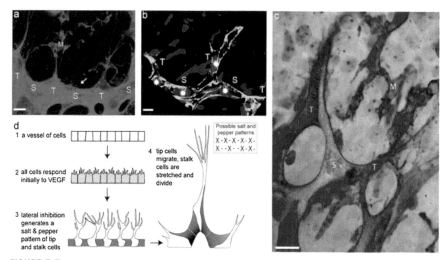

FIGURE 7.5

(A) Representative image of the growing and stabilizing vascular front in a mouse retina. Endothelial cells visualized by Isolectin B4 conjugated to AlexaFluor 568 (*red*). Alternating stretches of leading membrane, with and without filopodia extension, correspond to an alternating pattern of tip (*T*) and stalk cells (*S*). *Red* macrophage above the vessel labeled *M. Arrow* points to filopodia still visible on stalk cell, as it is not yet fully inhibited. (B) Combined nuclear DAPI labeling (*blue*) and endothelial cell junction labeling with VE-cadherin antibodies (*green*) illustrate that a limited number of endothelial nuclei (*stars*), which correspond to either tip cells (*T*) or stalk cells (*S*), constitute the sprouting front. Nuclei outside the vessel belong to astrocytes. (C) High magnification of the tip cell region of a mouse retina from the transgenic notch reporter line (TNR1).[33] Active notch signaling in the stalk cell (S) between two tip cells (*T*) is indicated by the green GFP signal. Cell nuclei are counterstained with DAPI (*blue*). Dll4 protein labeled red is prominent in the tip cells. Macrophage is labeled M. All scale bars are 10 μm. (D) Schematic of tip cell selection initiating sprouting.

Modified from Bentley[34]

hypoxia-inducible factor-1 (HIF-1), a key transcription factor. HIF-1 is a heterodimeric protein composed of an exquisitely oxygen-sensitive α-subunit and a ubiquitous β-subunit. The α-β heterodimeric transcription factors are stabilized by decreased cellular O_2 concentration, thereby functioning as intracellular oxygen sensors. Under hypoxic conditions, degradation of the oxygen-sensitive HIF-1α subunit is reduced, whereas its transcriptional activity is enhanced.[28] HIF-1 mediates increased expression of hypoxia-regulated genes, such as VEGF, platelet-derived growth factor-B (PDGF-B), PlGF, stromal-derived growth factor-1 (SDF-1) and their receptors, as well as other hypoxia-regulated gene products including Ang-2.[29] Among these proangiogenic factors, VEGF-A is the major regulator of blood vessel formation and function at subsequent ischemia-driven stages of DR. With the progression of ischemia, HIF-1-mediated VEGF expression leads to abundance of VEGF without a succinct gradient. ECs, in turn, stimulate expansion and activation of the pericyte precursor cell population. Existing data show that pericytes express Notch3, whereas ECs express Notch1 and Notch4 receptors. Activated Notch signaling induces Ang-2 upregulation in both ECs and pericytes.[30] Therefore, VEGF and Ang-2 synergistically cooperate to induce angiogenesis and destabilization of new vessels, as a result of endothelial proliferation and pericyte activation.[30–32]

At the initiation of sprouting angiogenesis in the diabetic retina, tip cells in sprouting vessels guide the vessel along a gradient of heparin-bound VEGF-A sensed by VEGFR-2 expressed on cell extrusions (filopodia) that extend and retract (Fig. 7.5).[35] Tip cells are incapable of proliferation. In contrast, endothelial stalk cells do proliferate. Notch ligand Dll4 in tip cells and the ligand Jag1 in stalk cells together regulate the angiogenic process.[36] The proliferative activity of stalk cells is determined by the availability of VEGF and other growth factors such as Ang-2.[13] The transition from a proliferating to a mature quiescent EC, that is, the transition from a stalk cell to a so-called phalanx cell, is determined by the expression of Ang-1 and the dense coverage by pericytes. In mature retinal vessels, pericyte-derived Ang-1 causes Tie2 phosphorylation in ECs. Activation of Ang-1/Tie2 controls EC proliferation and induces intercellular contacts and junctions, thereby stabilizing retinal vasculature and promoting the formation of the BRB.

Crosstalk between inflammation and angiogenesis in NVU during PDR progression

In the early stage of DR, communication and interplay among ECs, pericytes, and glia cells are disturbed. Late stage of DR, such as PDR, is a sequela of this disturbance.[30,37] For example, a key feature of DR is the increased expression of inflammatory cytokines and growth factors from various cell sources. The proinflammatory peptide VEGF is well-recognized as a major player in DR, including its role in promoting retinal vascular permeability and new vessel formation. During disease progression, VEGF overexpression is stimulated by persistent hyperglycemia and long-lasting tissue hypoxia. Meanwhile, proinflammatory mediators regulated by cytokines, such as TNF-α and interleukin-1β (IL-1β), and growth factors, lead to increase in vascular permeability and/or pathological angiogenesis.[30,38] Recently, Nawaz et al. demonstrated cross talk between inflammation and angiogenesis through biochemical characterization of vitreous from eyes with PDR. PDR vitreous can induce endothelial responses in vitro, ex vivo, and in vivo (Fig. 7.6). The novelty of this study was recapitulation of biochemical and molecular events, in which ECs, pericytes, glial cells, and neurons are involved because vitreous represents a reservoir of reactants and products of these cells. Both pro- and anti-angiogenic proteins are detected in the vitreous of patients with PDR. Because of the combination of upregulation of proangiogenic factors and downregulation of antiangiogenic factors,

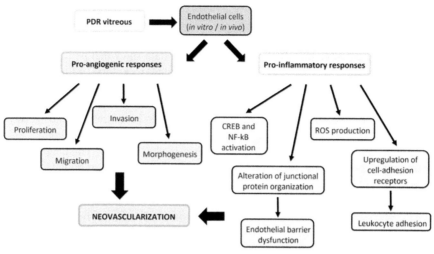

FIGURE 7.6

The vitreous of patients with PDR induces proangiogenic and proinflammatory response in endothelial cells. The vitreous of patients with PDR exerts a series of proangiogenic and proinflammatory responses that induce new vessel formation by endothelial cells in vitro and in vivo.

Modified from Nawaz et al.[47]

the balance is tipped to a proangiogenic state. In addition to VEGF, numerous pro-angiogenic factors are upregulated in the vitreous of patients with PDR, including Ang-1 and Ang-2,[39] PDGF-B,[40] erythropoietin (EPO),[41] SDF-1, and PlGF.[42,43] Notably, in the vitreous of PDR patients, the levels of several anti-angiogenic mediators are decreased. These include endostatin,[44] thrombospondin-1,[45] and pigment epithelium-derived factor.[46]

The expression of inflammatory proteins is regulated by pro-inflammatory transcription factors, such as nuclear factor kappa B (NF-κB), HIF-1, and cyclic adenosine monophosphate (cAMP) response element-binding protein (CREB), which are activated by hyperglycemia (Fig. 7.6).[48] This leads to the synthesis of pro-inflammatory cytokines, chemokines, acute-phase proteins, and other pro-inflammatory molecules in the diabetic eye.[48–50] Elevated TNF-α has been observed in vitreous, serum, and ocular fibrovascular membranes from patients with PDR and in retinas from rodent model of diabetes mellitus.[51,52] IL-1β and its downstream signaling molecule caspase 1 are significantly increased in vitreous, retinas, and serum from diabetic patients and rats.[52–54] Chemokines such as C—C motif chemokine ligand (CCL) 2 (CCL2), CCL5, C-X-C motif chemokine ligand (CXCL) 8 (CXCL8), CXCL10, and CXCL12 are also upregulated in vitreous samples from DR patients.[55–57] Increases in IL-6, ICAM-1, and VCAM-1 have been shown to be related to the progression of DR.[48,57,58] Because the vitreous concentrations of major pro-angiogenic and pro-inflammatory mediators are markedly upregulated in eyes with PDR,[48,59] PDR vitreous is viewed as a platform of neurovascular activities, on which angiogenic and inflammatory events cooperate (Fig. 7.6).

Intussusceptive angiogenesis in PDR

As described above, intussusceptive angiogenesis is an alternative and complementary form of sprouting angiogenesis.[3] Intussusception is a form of vascular remodeling and growth, starting from the splitting of vessels by extending cellular processes into the vascular lumen. As these processes anastomose, they form transluminal, intussusceptive pillars. The pillars that extend and fuse with other intussusceptive pillars remodel into extravascular columns of interstitial tissue. Eventually, this leads to the original vessel transformed into vascular loops or by longitudinal intussusception into duplicated vessels.[60]

The molecular mechanisms of intussusceptive angiogenesis involve many growth factors. In addition to Angs and their Tie receptors,[61] PDGF-B,[62] monocyte chemoattractant protein-1 (MCP-1),[63] ephrins, and Eph-B receptors[64,65] are mediators of endothelial to endothelial and endothelial to pericyte interactions. They all participate in the process of intussusceptive angiogenesis.[66] In a transgenic mouse model overexpressing Ang-1, or Ang-1 in combination with VEGF, the presence of abundant small holes in the capillary plexus is a symptomatic finding of intussusception.[67] For instance, hypoxia is also a regulator of intussusceptive angiogenesis. Thus, hypoxia-inducible factors (e.g., HIF-2 alpha) stimulate the expression of EPO, which can enhance intussusceptive angiogenesis.[68] In addition, ischemia and Notch inhibition facilitate the recruitment and extravasation of mononuclear cells.[3]

Beside the molecular mechanisms of intussusceptive angiogenesis, hemodynamic forces play an essential role in the vascular network formation and remodeling. Shear stress (to ECs) and wall stress (in smooth muscle cells and pericytes) of vessels activate different biochemical cascades, beginning with the activation of an ion channel (within seconds) and resulting in rearrangements of cytoskeletal components and adaptations in gap-junction complexes after as soon as minutes to as long as hours. Interactions among the ECs, pericytes, and macrophages appear to be involved in the adaptive mechanisms to physiological or pathophysiological changes in shear stress, for example, in arteriogenesis.[66,69] Intussusceptive angiogenesis under hypoxic condition is represented histologically in Fig. 7.7.[70]

In animal models and isolated human vascular ECs from donor eyes, hypoxia-induced intussusceptive angiogenesis was studied.[60] The hypoxia-induced intussusception, that is regulated by HIF-1α-VEGF-A-VEGFR2 signaling axis, is initially regulated mainly by luminal endothelial sprouting without involvement of basolateral or perivascular structures, suggesting a role for intussusception in endothelial priming before neovascularization.[60] The temporal sequence of intussusception remodeling as an initial step and neovascularization formation as the outcome has shed new light on a potential regulatory window for preventing pathological neovascularization at early stage. Mentzer and Konerding raised inspiring questions for further studies on the contribution of intussusceptive angiogenesis to PDR, as

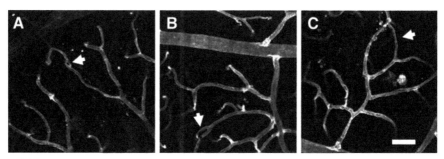

FIGURE 7.7

Exposure to whole-body hypoxia for 3 weeks results in vascular loop formation in the superficial networks of the adult mouse retina. High magnification (20×) confocal images obtained from retinal whole-mounts labeled with lectin (*white*) were used to examine the presence of vascular loops (*arrows*). Representative vascular loops illustrate the wide range of loop sizes observed in hypoxia-exposed retinas, which appear to correspond to the progressive stages of intussusceptive microvascular growth,[66] from the initial formation of a tissue pillar (A) to its subsequent elongation (B) and expansion to form larger vascular loops (C). The smallest loops detected (A) corresponded to the size and morphology of early tissue pillars previously identified in the developing amphibian retina. Scale bar, 50 μm.

Modified from Taylor et al.[70]

follows: (1) What are the physiologic and pathologic signals that trigger pillar formation? (2) What endothelial and blood flow conditions specify pillar location? (3) How do pillars respond to the mechanical influence of blood flow and diabetic proangiogenic impact? (4) What do pathophysiologic factors contribute to pillar extension? The answers to these questions should provide insights into the regulation of pathologic intussusception in diabetic retina.[71]

Translational approach for anti-angiogenesis in PDR
Anti-sprouting angiogenesis for PDR and beyond the surface

PDR and DME treatment have been revolutionized with the development of inhibitors of VEGF. However, a significant number of patients failed to achieve clinically significant visual improvement.[72] Therefore, there is an urgent need for the development of new treatments. As described above, based on the understanding of the HIF-1/VEGF/VEGFR system in diabetic retina, a soluble form of VEGF receptor-1 (sFlt-1) synthesized by ECs is capable of binding VEGF-A. In addition to the pharmacological approach to suppress VEGF, intravitreal adeno-associated virus–delivered sFlt-1 shows effective inhibition of VEGF in a choroidal neovascularization model. This kind of gene therapy may be used for sustained VEGF suppression (see Chapter 9 for more details).[73] Notably, endogenous VEGF also plays a neuroprotective role in the retina because the permanent loss of VEGF by targeted deletion of *vegfa* gene in experimental animals could cause retinal neurodegeneration. Therefore, novel therapies that conditionally target VEGF upstream rather than using higher dose and longer lasting anti-VEGF per se may keep physiological expressions of angiogenic genes.[74]

Though anti-VEGF therapy with diverse mechanisms of pathological angiogenesis is critical, it is not the only treatment for neovascularization of PDR. Herein, several anti-VEGF independent approaches are selected. More detailed discussion of these approaches is presented in Chapters 5, 9 and 10. In Fig. 7.2, the opposing roles of Dll4 and Jag1 in regulation of sprouting angiogenesis are demonstrated. Both Dll4 and Jag1 are ligands of Notch receptors. The opposing effects of these two ligands are due to their different cellular distributions on ECs. Namely, Dll4 is the ligand expressed in tip cells at the end of the growing vascular sprouts, whereas Jag1 is in stalk cells of the leading vasculature, a site where Dll4 is absent.[75] Based on these findings, selective inhibition of Dll4 or Jag1 is possible to control tumor angiogenesis. In addition to inhibition of Dll4 or Jag1, it is proposed that Notch receptor could be a therapeutic target because the downstream ligand−Notch interaction can be modulated by various posttranslational modifications. Whether these translational approaches can be used clinically for PDR requires further study.[10]

Clearly, the VEGF pathway is vitally important in retinal vascular diseases. Another vascular tyrosine kinase pathway, the Ang/Tie2 pathway is also critical in diabetic retinal microvascular disease. Activation of Tie2 receptor via Ang-1 maintains vascular stability to limit exudation. Ang-2, a competitive antagonist to Ang-1, and VE-PTP, interferes with the Ang-1/Tie2 axis, resulting in vascular leakage (Fig. 7.3 & Fig. 7.4). A bispecific antibody that inhibits both VEGF-A and Ang-2, namely faricimab, is a US Food and Drug Administration (FDA) newly approved agent for DME and neovascular age-related macular degeneration (see Chapters 9 and 10).[76,77]

AXT107 is a collagen IV-derived synthetic peptide with a dual mechanism of action that involves suppression of VEGF signaling and activation of the Tie2 pathway. Currently, an AXT107 trial is in the preclinical phase. ARP-1536 is an intravitreally administered VE-PTP inhibitor undergoing preclinical studies. AKB-9778 is a subcutaneously administered VE-PTP inhibitor that, when combined with monthly ranibizumab, reduced DME more effectively than ranibizumab monotherapy in a phase 2 study. The development of Ang/Tie2 pathway modulators show promise in reducing the anti-VEGF treatment burden and improving visual outcomes in patients with DR, of which details are discussed in Chapter 9.[21,77]

Pathogenesis of PDR is heavily dependent on pathological sprouting angiogenesis. The complex cellular components, multiple pro- and anti-angiogenic factors and signaling pathways participate in pathological events leading to neovascularization. Each angiogenic event could be viewed as a step of PDR progression as well as a potential therapeutic target. PDR is characterized as ischemia-driven pathological neovascularization at the vitreoretinal interface. PDR progression involves a complex interplay of biochemical, immunological, and inflammatory factors, but the exact mechanisms remain unclear. Currently, some surgical procedures, pan-retinal photocoagulation, and intravitreal anti-VEGF therapy can offer transient effect.[78] Systematic strategies for halting PDR progression are still lacking. Therefore, PDR-specific angiogenic mechanisms and potential translational strategies for PDR management are the focus of the following sections.

The recent study by Korhonen et al. on global gene expression of retinal fibrovascular tissue of eyes with PDR is a significant achievement for understanding angiogenesis mechanisms in PDR.[79] The fibrovascular membranes were excised from 11 vitrectomized PDR eyes of 11 patients. Purified mRNA was evaluated and analyzed with high-throughput sequencing. There were 1447 differentially expressed genes (DEGs) in PDR. Of these, 910 were upregulated and 537 downregulated in the PDR cohort. Gene ontology enrichment analysis (GOEA) of the top principal component genes revealed vasculature-related biological processes (BPs). Based on the DEGs upregulated in PDR, 701 BPs, 53 CCs, and 37 molecular functions (MFs) were significant in GOEA. The top BPs, enriched CCs, and enriched MFs, gene expression of PDR-specific processes are summarized in Table 7.1.[79]

The upregulated, differentially expressed vasculature-related mRNA in PDR has made tremendous advances in understanding and determining the importance of antiangiogenic therapy including both anti-VEGF−dependent and non-VEGF−dependent modulators. The current anti-VEGF modulators for PDR and DME have been introduced previously. Herein, several anti-VEGF−independent modulators in Table 7.1, which should have captured more attention, are explained as follows: (1) all angiopoietins can bind to Tie2, but no ligand binds to Tie1 (Fig. 7.3). However, the orphan receptor Tie1 is able to modulate Ang-1/Tie2-mediated signaling and plays antiangiogenic roles in ECs.[80] Therefore, Tie1 could be a target for anti-angiogenic therapy. (2) VEGF-A activates endothelial nitric oxide synthase (eNOS) via the Akt pathway. eNOS regulates EC function and blood vessel maturation in retinal angiogenesis.[81] Since PI3K/Akt/mTOR pathway is a convergent pathway for a variety of growth factors, pro-inflammatory mediators, and downstream substrates, inhibition of this pathway may regulate cellular survival processes and prevent progression of DR.[82] (3) A possible target is activin receptor-like kinase (ALK)-1, a transforming growth factor (TGF)-β type-I receptor, which binds bone morphogenetic protein (BMP)-9 and -10 with high affinity and has an important role in regulating angiogenesis. Therefore, inhibition of ALK-1 signaling is a strategy for anti-angiogenesis.[83] (4) Hepatocyte growth factor (HGF) binding to c-MET results in receptor homodimerization and phosphorylation of two tyrosine residues (Y1234 and Y1235) located within the catalytic loop of the tyrosine kinase domain. HGF signaling involves activation of both protein kinase C and PI3K, which is critical for migration and growth of ECs. It is noteworthy that VEGF does not mediate these initial HGF effects. The initial HGF effects act as VEGFA-independent angiogenic mechanisms. Therefore, inhibition of HGF/cMet pathway appears to overcome anti-VEGF escape mechanisms.[84] (5) Gucciardo et al. created a three-dimensional patient-derived PDR neovascular tissue model which contains lymphatic EC sprouting and lymphatic-like capillaries.[85] The main lymphangiogenic growth factors VEGF-C and −D are not DEGs, but their receptor

Table 7.1 Regulatory mechanisms of angiogenesis in PDR based on mRNA sequencing.

	DEGs in PDR	Activated signaling pathways and functions by DEGs	Therapeutic targets
VEGF-A ligand-dependent mechanisms	VEGF family ligand—receptor interactions	VEGF-A/VEGFR1 and VEGFR2: angiogenesis, vasculature development, and cell motility	VEGF-A, VEGFR1, VEGFR2
	eNOS and NO	VEGFA-activated eNOS via Akt pathway and eNOS: EC function and blood vessel maturation	eNOS, NO, Akt pathway
VEGF-A ligand-independent mechanisms	Ang-1/Tie2 signaling	Vessel maturation and stability; Anti-VEGF-A therapy escape mechanisms including Dll4/Notch-1 via Wnt/β-catenin pathway	Ang-1, Ang-2, Tie1, and Tie2
	Ang-2/Tie-2 signaling	Vessel destabilization	
	ALK-1/receptor	EC proliferating	ALK-1/receptor
	TGF-β	Neovascularization	TGF-β
	HGF	HGF/cMet pathway	HGF/cMet
Overrepresented lymphatic development	Lymphangiogenic growth factors, VEGF-C and -D receptor VEGFR3 (FLT4)	Lymph vessel development and lymphangiogenesis	VEGF-C, VEGF-D, and VEGFR3
Inflammation and wound healing responses	Genes related to chemotaxis, leukocyte migration, response to wounding, immune system development, inflammatory response, coagulation and platelet activation, KEGG pathways	Leukocyte extravasation signaling, leukocyte migration, cell movement of mononuclear leukocytes, migration of mononuclear leukocytes, binding of leukocytes, and	Up-reg. 50 DEGs/ 637 GO-term inflammatory response

Continued

Table 7.1 Regulatory mechanisms of angiogenesis in PDR based on mRNA sequencing.—*cont'd*

	DEGs in PDR	Activated signaling pathways and functions by DEGs	Therapeutic targets
	platelet activation, and leukocyte transendothelial migration	cell movement of lymphocytes	
EMT overrepresented	Genes related to mesenchyme development, mesenchymal cell development, mesenchymal cell differentiation, mesenchyme morphogenesis, and EMT	Regulation of the EMT	Up-reg. 19 DEGs/ 104 genes in EMT, TGF-β, SMAD2, −3, and −4
ECM related genes	Genes related to KEGG pathway ECM −receptor interaction	Determination of ECM composition in PDR	Up-reg. 132 DEGs/ 1013 mmatrisome genes
Inhibition of angiogenesis	TSP-1 and genes related to eIF2 signaling, visual cycle	Antiangiogenesis	TSP1 and eIF2

Abbreviations: Akt, also known as protein kinase B, belongs to the AGC family of protein kinases; ALK-1, activin receptor-like kinase 1; Ang-1, angiopoietin 1; Ang-2, angiopoietin 2; cMet, a receptor tyrosine kinase; DEGs, differentially expressed genes; Dll4, delta-like ligand 4; EC, endothelial cell; ECM, extracellular matrix; eIF2, eukaryotic initiation factor 2, a complex cell signaling that regulates both global and specific mRNA translation; EMT, epithelial to mesenchymal transition; eNOS, endothelial nitric oxide synthase; FLT4, Fms-related tyrosine kinase 4; GO-term, Gene ontology term; HGF, hepatocyte growth factor; IPAs, Ingenuity Pathway Analysis; KEGGs, Kyoto Encyclopedia of Genes and Genomes; Matrisome, the ensemble of >1000 genes encoding ECM and ECM-associated proteins; NO, nitric oxide; PDR, proliferative diabetic retinopathy; SMAD, small mothers against decapentaplegic; TGF-β, transforming growth factor β; Tie, tyrosine kinase with immunoglobulin and epidermal growth factor homology domains; TSP1, trombospondin-1; Up-reg., Up-regulated; VEGF, vascular endothelial growth factor; VEGFR, vascular endothelial growth factor receptor.

VEGFR-3 (FLT4) is upregulated (Fig. 7.1). Cioffi et al. reported that Tbx1, a transcription factor, activates VEGFR-3 in ECs under ischemic condition. The interaction between Tbx1 and VEGFR-3 is critical for the development of the lymphatic vasculature.[86] These findings indicate that the PDR microenvironment supports pathological neolymphovascularization, suggesting that lymphatics can emerge in the posterior segment of PDR eyes. Understanding the mechanisms of neolymphovascularization may provide new approaches to suppressing the ischemia-driven

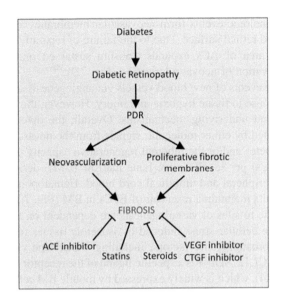

Diagram illustrating the development of retinal fibrosis in diabetic retinopathy and potential inhibitory strategies for the prevention of proliferative fibrotic membranes associated with PDR.

Modified from Roy et al.[88]

angiogenic process in PDR. (6) Cell proliferation, extracellular matrix remodeling, epithelial–mesenchymal transition, and neovascularization are key events in the progression of PDR. These events are secondary to hypoxic and inflammatory insults, and they promote the formation of fibrotic tissue in the interface between posterior hyaloid and retinal surface in PDR.[87] Therefore, anti-fibrosis therapy is an important approach to inhibit DR progression and prevent vision loss in PDR. The currently tested strategies for anti-fibrosis are illustrated in Fig. 7.8.[88]

Vasculogenesis deficit in PDR and endothelial progenitor cells—based therapy

Clinically progressive capillary nonperfusion and ACs formation in the diabetic retina induce hypoxia-related structural and functional abnormalities of microvessels. Starting from the severe stage of NPDR, persistent vasoregression indicates a failure of vessel repair for the area that lost blood supply. Such acellular retinal vessels may be repairable in early disease by de novo vasculogenesis. With the progression of retinopathy, EC replicative capacity is exhausted, reaching the so-called Hayflick limit,[89] meaning that the retinal vasculature in patients with diabetes gradually loses its regenerative capacity. The impaired de novo vasculogenesis and pathologically stimulated sprouting angiogenesis cannot revascularize ischemic retina.

Instead, these pathologic events form neovascular membranes at the interface between vitreous and retinal surface. Due to the failure of reparative functions in diabetic retina, the area of ACs expands, causing sustained retinal ischemia and consequent aggravation of neovascularization (Fig. 7.9).[90]

The reparative events of new blood vessels via angiogenesis and vasculogenesis can occur in response to tissue hypoxia and injury. However, they differ in the molecular triggers and underlying mechanisms. Overall, the outcome of reparative events is determined by either molecular signals from the devascularized microenvironment in diabetes and/or the inherent regenerative capacity of endothelial progenitor cells (EPCs) per se. EPCs are bone marrow (BM)—derived cells that can be found in the peripheral and umbilical cord blood. Hematopoietic BM cells provide EPCs.[91] Adults maintain a reservoir of EPCs in BM (Fig. 7.10). EPCs homing from the BM niche to sites of vasculogenesis are dependent on a cytokine/chemokine gradient. The cellular stress induced by ischemic tissues leads to the release of a number of proangiogenic factors, including VEGF and chemokine SDF-1, also known as CXCL12. SDF-1 is a specific ligand of the receptor C-X-C chemokine receptor 4 (CXCR4), which is widely expressed by mobile BM cells. It plays a major role in the recruitment and retention of $CXCR4^+$ BM cells to the proangiogenic niches, supporting revascularization of ischemic tissue.[92,93] The underlying mechanisms by which SDF-1 activates EPCs have recently been described.[94] Circulating SDF-1 is translocated from the plasma to the BM. After SDF-1 enters the BM microenvironment, it induces the activation of matrix metalloproteinase-9 (MMP-9) and the release of soluble kit-ligand (s-KitL). Subsequently, s-KitL induces the release of more SDF-1, enhancing mobilization of the $CXCR4^+$ and $s\text{-}Kit^+$ cells to the circulation.[95] Once established in the circulation, $CXCR4^+$ BM cells preferably incorporate into ischemic microenvironments via specific adhesion molecules.[96] SDF-1 expressed and presented by EPCs, at the site of injury, probably has an important role in triggering EPCs arrest and resettlement into the neoangiogenic niches.[97]

Under hypoxic conditions, transcription factors like HIF-1 are activated leading to upregulation of VEGF. VEGF contributes regulatory functions in both angiogenesis and vasculogenesis. In the latter, VEGF modulates EPCs kinetics for postnatal neovascularization.[99] VEGF stimulation of stromal cells leads to an increase in eNOS, nitric oxide (NO) production, and MMP-9 secretion. MMP-9 then converts membrane-bound Kit Ligand (m-KitL) to s-KitL, aiding in the release of EPCs from BM stromal cells. The EPCs then migrate toward the angiogenic gradient via chemokine receptors including CXCR4 and VEGFR-2.[100]

Accumulating evidence supports the findings that both type 1 and type 2 diabetic patients have reduced numbers, and altered differentiation function, of circulating EPCs.[101–103] In a clinical study, poor glycemic control with high hemoglobin A_{1c} levels is associated with a reduction in numbers of circulating EPCs, whereas adequate glycemic control seems to increase their numbers.[104] Hu and Lei in our laboratory investigated the number and function of EPCs isolated from patients with different stages of DR. EPCs were reduced remarkably in number in NPDR compared with the control group, whereas the number of circulating EPCs

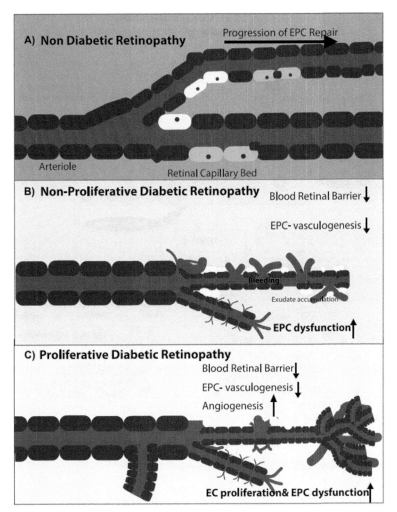

FIGURE 7.9

Vasculogenesis by reparative endothelial progenitor cells (EPCss) in different stages of diabetic retinopathy. (A) Functional EPCs can repair minor EC damage (*yellow*: unhealthy ECs, green: recovering ECs, *blue*: healthy ECs, *purple*: EPCs); (B) shows nonproliferative diabetic retinopathy, dysfunctional EPCs lose their reparative capacity, leading to vasoregression of ischemia retina; (C) shows proliferative diabetic retinopathy, pathological neovascularization following the progression of nonproliferative diabetic retinopathy, represents stimulated angiogenesis, and failed vasculogenesis to regenerate ischemic retina.

Modified from Shao et al.[90]

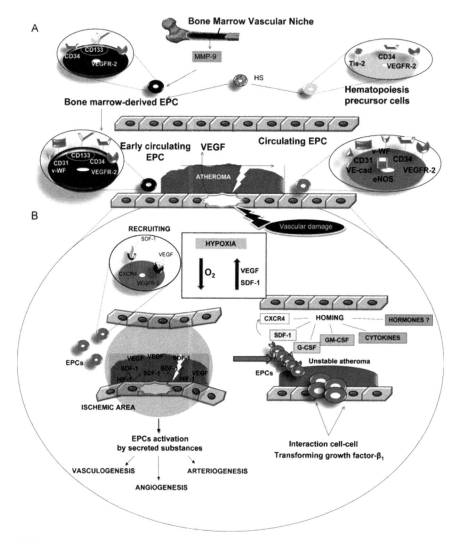

FIGURE 7.10

From bone marrow to blood circulation: differentiation and key role of endothelial progenitor cells (EPCs). (A) EPCs are BMCs that originate from vascular niche, a network of thin-walled and fenestrated sinusoidal vessels whose integrity is maintained and supported by surrounding hematopoietic cells. EPC recruitment is mediated by matrix metalloproteinase type 9 (MMP-9), in response to different stimuli. Two different populations of progenitor cells originate from a common precursor, the Hemangioblast (HS): EPCs and hematopoietic stem cells (HSCs). HSCs and EPCs share some common surface markers. During differentiation, EPC surface markers undergo changes, for example, the CD133 marker is lost. This marker is present on BM-derived EPCs and on early circulating EPCs; the adult circulating EPCs do not express this marker and begin to rebounded in PDR groups to varying degrees. This finding suggests three aspects: (1) the reduced EPCs number observed in patients with NPDR correlates with vasore-gressive status; (2) the rebound in circulating EPCs number in PDR patients indi-cates a phenomenon of mobilized release of EPCs from BM as a compensatory function; (3) the reparative capacity of vascularization by mechanism of vasculogen-esis may not be exhausted even in PDR and might be restored by an EPCs-based therapy.[105]

Due to the decreased number and dysfunction of EPCs in patients with different stages of DR including PDR, treatment of vasculogenesis impairment by EPCs-based therapy is challenging. First, it is notable that in the evaluation of preclinical and clinical EPC-based therapy, the results have been variable.[100] It is likely that a heterogeneous mixture of cells has been used. If highly specific BM-derived EPCs are utilized, EPC-specific biomarkers need to be further defined. Second, efficacious EPCs that can be modulated by various endogenous factors in de novo vasculogen-esis are essential. For example, these EPCs should be capable of responding to the ischemia-driven HIF-1/VEGF/VEGFR system and stimulating MMP-9 and the release of s-KitL (Fig. 7.10).[106] EPCs are also responsive to other key proangiogenic factors, such as the Ang/Tie2 system, as well as to cytokines and chemokines in the impaired devascularized area. For example, NO is critical for maturation of ECs and neovascularization involving EPCs.[107] Therefore, EPCs with adequate NO bioavail-ability is essential (Fig. 7.10). Recent study revealed that the quantity and function changes of EPCs in DR are attributed to mitochondrial dysfunction because mito-chondria regulate energy balance and cell fate determination.[90] Third, a prerequisite of successful EPC-based therapy is adequate diabetic control of recipients. DR is an essentially ischemia-driven complication of diabetes. The ischemic insult creates detrimental conditions for endogenous EPCs. Uncontrolled hyperglycemia can induce a variety of disturbed mechanisms which may make EPCs unable to cover devascularized area (Fig. 7.10).[98,100] Therefore, the successful vasculogenesis re-quires EPCs with adequate quantity and angiogenic functions.

Finally, vitreoretinal surgery, specifically pars plana vitrectomy for the late com-plications of PDR, continues to be required even in some patients who have received optimal systemic medical treatment, laser treatment, and anti-VEGF therapy. The current status and future direction of vitrectomy for PDR are discussed in Chapters 1 and 9.

---

show new EC-similar surface markers. (B) The hypoxia of ischemic area induces ECs to produce HIF-1-mediated stromal cell—derived factor-1 (SDF-1) and VEGF in high concentration; these two signaling proteins bind their respective receptors C-X-C chemokine receptor 4 (CXCR4) and VEGFR-2 on EPCs recruiting them to ischemic area. The homing of EPCs to the site of vascular damage is mediated by various factors such as SDF-1. Once in the damaged area, EPCs form a patch, mediated by cell—cell interaction with mature EPCs and transforming growth factor-β1 that leads to vascular repair.

Modified from Napoli et al.[98]

References

1. Centers for Disease Control and Prevention. *National Diabetes Fact Sheet*. 2007.
2. Gross JG, Glassman AR, Liu D, et al. Five-year outcomes of panretinal photocoagulation vs intravitreous ranibizumab for proliferative diabetic retinopathy: a randomized clinical trial. *JAMA Ophthalmol*. 2018;136(10):1138. https://doi.org/10.1001/jamaophthalmol.2018.3255.
3. Díaz-Flores L, Gutiérrez R, Gayoso S, et al. Intussusceptive angiogenesis and its counterpart intussusceptive lymphangiogenesis. *Histol Histopathol*. 2020;35(10):1083−1103. https://doi.org/10.14670/HH-18-222.
4. Gerhardt H, Betsholtz C. How do endothelial cells orientate? *EXS*. 2005;(94):3−15. https://doi.org/10.1007/3-7643-7311-3_1.
5. Takahashi H, Shibuya M. The vascular endothelial growth factor (VEGF)/VEGF receptor system and its role under physiological and pathological conditions. *Clin Sci (Lond)*. 2005;109(3):227−241. https://doi.org/10.1042/CS20040370.
6. Majumder S, Advani A. VEGF and the diabetic kidney: more than too much of a good thing. *J Diabetes Complicat*. 2017;31(1):273−279. https://doi.org/10.1016/j.jdiacomp.2016.10.020.
7. Blanco R, Gerhardt H. VEGF and Notch in tip and stalk cell selection. *Cold Spring Harb Perspect Med*. 2013;3(1). https://doi.org/10.1101/cshperspect.a006569. a006569-a006569.
8. Shibuya M. Structure and dual function of vascular endothelial growth factor receptor-1 (Flt-1). *Int J Biochem Cell Biol*. 2001;33(4):409−420. https://doi.org/10.1016/S1357-2725(01)00026-7.
9. Ambati BK, Nozaki M, Singh N, et al. Corneal avascularity is due to soluble VEGF receptor-1. *Nature*. 2006;443(7114):993−997. https://doi.org/10.1038/nature05249.
10. Benedito R, Roca C, Sörensen I, et al. The Notch ligands Dll4 and Jagged1 have opposing effects on angiogenesis. *Cell*. 2009;137(6):1124−1135. https://doi.org/10.1016/j.cell.2009.03.025.
11. Suchting S, Eichmann A. Jagged gives endothelial tip cells an edge. *Cell*. 2009;137(6):988−990. https://doi.org/10.1016/j.cell.2009.05.024.
12. Wu Q, Xu WD, Huang AF. Role of angiopoietin-2 in inflammatory autoimmune diseases: a comprehensive review. *Int Immunopharm*. 2020;80:106223. https://doi.org/10.1016/j.intimp.2020.106223.
13. Augustin HG, Koh GY, Thurston G, Alitalo K. Control of vascular morphogenesis and homeostasis through the angiopoietin-Tie system. *Nat Rev Mol Cell Biol*. 2009;10(3):165−177. https://doi.org/10.1038/nrm2639.
14. Kim I, Kim JH, Moon SO, Kwak HJ, Kim NG, Koh GY. Angiopoietin-2 at high concentration can enhance endothelial cell survival through the phosphatidylinositol 3′-kinase/Akt signal transduction pathway. *Oncogene*. 2000;19(39):4549−4552. https://doi.org/10.1038/sj.onc.1203800.
15. Yu X, Seegar TCM, Dalton AC, et al. Structural basis for angiopoietin-1-mediated signaling initiation. *Proc Natl Acad Sci USA*. 2013;110(18):7205−7210. https://doi.org/10.1073/pnas.1216890110.
16. Regula JT, Lundh von Leithner P, Foxton R, et al. Targeting key angiogenic pathways with a bispecific Cross MA b optimized for neovascular eye diseases. *EMBO Mol Med*. 2016;8(11):1265−1288. https://doi.org/10.15252/emmm.201505889.

17. Cai J, Kehoe O, Smith GM, Hykin P, Boulton ME. The angiopoietin/tie-2 system regulates pericyte survival and recruitment in diabetic retinopathy. *Invest Ophthalmol Vis Sci.* 2008;49(5):2163. https://doi.org/10.1167/iovs.07-1206.

18. Campochiaro PA. Molecular pathogenesis of retinal and choroidal vascular diseases. *Prog Retin Eye Res.* 2015;49:67−81. https://doi.org/10.1016/j.preteyeres.2015.06.002.

19. Fachinger G, Deutsch U, Risau W. Functional interaction of vascular endothelial-protein-tyrosine phosphatase with the angiopoietin receptor Tie-2. *Oncogene.* 1999; 18(43):5948−5953. https://doi.org/10.1038/sj.onc.1202992.

20. Yacyshyn OK, Lai PFH, Forse K, Teichert-Kuliszewska K, Jurasz P, Stewart DJ. Tyrosine phosphatase beta regulates angiopoietin-Tie2 signaling in human endothelial cells. *Angiogenesis.* 2009;12(1):25−33. https://doi.org/10.1007/s10456-008-9126-0.

21. Hussain RM, Neiweem AE, Kansara V, Harris A, Ciulla TA. Tie-2/Angiopoietin pathway modulation as a therapeutic strategy for retinal disease. *Expet Opin Invest Drugs.* 2019;28(10):861−869. https://doi.org/10.1080/13543784.2019.1667333.

22. Hammes HP, Feng Y, Pfister F, Brownlee M. Diabetic retinopathy: targeting vasoregression. *Diabetes.* 2011;60(1):9−16. https://doi.org/10.2337/db10-0454.

23. Hammes HP, Lin J, Wagner P, et al. Angiopoietin-2 causes pericyte dropout in the normal retina: evidence for involvement in diabetic retinopathy. *Diabetes.* 2004; 53(4):1104−1110. https://doi.org/10.2337/diabetes.53.4.1104.

24. Yao D, Taguchi T, Matsumura T, et al. High glucose increases angiopoietin-2 transcription in microvascular endothelial cells through methylglyoxal modification of mSin3A. *J Biol Chem.* 2007;282(42):31038−31045. https://doi.org/10.1074/jbc.M704703200.

25. Park SW, Yun JH, Kim JH, Kim KW, Cho CH, Kim JH. Angiopoietin 2 induces pericyte apoptosis via α3β1 integrin signaling in diabetic retinopathy. *Diabetes.* 2014;63(9): 3057−3068. https://doi.org/10.2337/db13-1942.

26. Lee J, Kim KE, Choi DK, et al. Angiopoietin-1 guides directional angiogenesis through integrin αvβ5 signaling for recovery of ischemic retinopathy. *Sci Transl Med.* 2013; 5(203):203ra127. https://doi.org/10.1126/scitranslmed.3006666.

27. Niranjan G, Srinivasan AR, Srikanth K, et al. Evaluation of circulating plasma VEGF-A, ET-1 and magnesium levels as the predictive markers for proliferative diabetic retinopathy. *Indian J Clin Biochem.* 2019;34(3):352−356. https://doi.org/10.1007/s12291-018-0753-y.

28. Semenza GL. Hydroxylation of HIF-1: oxygen sensing at the molecular level. *Physiology (Bethesda).* 2004;19:176−182. https://doi.org/10.1152/physiol.00001.2004.

29. Campochiaro PA. Ocular neovascularization. *J Mol Med (Berl).* 2013;91(3):311−321. https://doi.org/10.1007/s00109-013-0993-5.

30. Sweeney MD, Ayyadurai S, Zlokovic BV. Pericytes of the neurovascular unit: key functions and signaling pathways. *Nat Neurosci.* 2016;19(6):771−783. https://doi.org/10.1038/nn.4288.

31. Ribatti D, Nico B, Crivellato E. The role of pericytes in angiogenesis. *Int J Dev Biol.* 2011;55(3):261−268. https://doi.org/10.1387/ijdb.103167dr.

32. Hill J, Rom S, Ramirez SH, Persidsky Y. Emerging roles of pericytes in the regulation of the neurovascular unit in health and disease. *J Neuroimmune Pharmacol.* 2014;9(5): 591−605. https://doi.org/10.1007/s11481-014-9557-x.

33. Hellström M, Phng LK, Hofmann JJ, et al. Dll4 signalling through Notch1 regulates formation of tip cells during angiogenesis. *Nature.* 2007;445(7129):776−780. https://doi.org/10.1038/nature05571.

34. Bentley K, Gerhardt H, Bates PA. Agent-based simulation of notch-mediated tip cell selection in angiogenic sprout initialisation. *J Theor Biol.* 2008;250(1):25−36. https://doi.org/10.1016/j.jtbi.2007.09.015.

35. Gerhardt H, Golding M, Fruttiger M, et al. VEGF guides angiogenic sprouting utilizing endothelial tip cell filopodia. *J Cell Biol.* 2003;161(6):1163−1177. https://doi.org/10.1083/jcb.200302047.

36. Pitulescu ME, Schmidt I, Giaimo BD, et al. Dll4 and Notch signalling couples sprouting angiogenesis and artery formation. *Nat Cell Biol.* 2017;19(8):915−927. https://doi.org/10.1038/ncb3555.

37. Rattner A, Williams J, Nathans J. Roles of HIFs and VEGF in angiogenesis in the retina and brain. *J Clin Invest.* 2019;129(9):3807−3820. https://doi.org/10.1172/JCI126655.

38. Duh EJ, Sun JK, Stitt AW. Diabetic retinopathy: current understanding, mechanisms, and treatment strategies. *JCI Insight.* 2017;2(14):93751. https://doi.org/10.1172/jci.insight.93751.

39. Patel JI. Angiopoietin concentrations in diabetic retinopathy. *Br J Ophthalmol.* 2005;89(4):480−483. https://doi.org/10.1136/bjo.2004.049940.

40. Praidou A, Papakonstantinou E, Androudi S, Georgiadis N, Karakiulakis G, Dimitrakos S. Vitreous and serum levels of vascular endothelial growth factor and platelet-derived growth factor and their correlation in patients with non-proliferative diabetic retinopathy and clinically significant macula oedema. *Acta Ophthalmol.* 2011;89(3):248−254. https://doi.org/10.1111/j.1755-3768.2009.01661.x.

41. Loukovaara S, Robciuc A, Holopainen JM, et al. Ang-2 upregulation correlates with increased levels of MMP-9, VEGF, EPO and TGFβ1 in diabetic eyes undergoing vitrectomy. *Acta Ophthalmol.* 2013;91(6):531−539. https://doi.org/10.1111/j.1755-3768.2012.02473.x.

42. Butler JM, Guthrie SM, Koc M, et al. SDF-1 is both necessary and sufficient to promote proliferative retinopathy. *J Clin Invest.* 2005;115(1):86−93. https://doi.org/10.1172/JCI22869.

43. Mitamura Y, Tashimo A, Nakamura Y, et al. Vitreous levels of placenta growth factor and vascular endothelial growth factor in patients with proliferative diabetic retinopathy. *Diabetes Care.* 2002;25(12). https://doi.org/10.2337/diacare.25.12.2352, 2352-2352.

44. Funatsu H, Yamashita H, Noma H, et al. Outcome of vitreous surgery and the balance between vascular endothelial growth factor and endostatin. *Invest Ophthalmol Vis Sci.* 2003;44(3):1042. https://doi.org/10.1167/iovs.02-0374.

45. Wang S. Modulation of thrombospondin 1 and pigment epithelium−derived factor levels in vitreous fluid of patients with diabetes. *Arch Ophthalmol.* 2009;127(4):507. https://doi.org/10.1001/archophthalmol.2009.53.

46. Boehm BO, Lang G, Volpert O, et al. Low content of the natural ocular anti-angiogenic agent pigment epithelium-derived factor (PEDF) in aqueous humor predicts progression of diabetic retinopathy. *Diabetologia.* 2003;46(3):394−400. https://doi.org/10.1007/s00125-003-1040-9.

47. Nawaz IM, Rezzola S, Cancarini A, et al. Human vitreous in proliferative diabetic retinopathy: characterization and translational implications. *Prog Retin Eye Res.* 2019;72:100756. https://doi.org/10.1016/j.preteyeres.2019.03.002.

48. Zhang W, Liu H, Al-Shabrawey M, Caldwell RW, Caldwell RB. Inflammation and diabetic retinal microvascular complications. *J Cardiovasc Dis Res.* 2011;2(2):96−103. https://doi.org/10.4103/0975-3583.83035.

49. Kuwano T, Nakao S, Yamamoto H, et al. Cyclooxygenase 2 is a key enzyme for inflammatory cytokine-induced angiogenesis. *FASEB J*. 2004;18(2):300−310. https://doi.org/10.1096/fj.03-0473com.

50. Capitão M, Soares R. Angiogenesis and inflammation crosstalk in diabetic retinopathy: vascularization in Dr. *J Cell Biochem*. 2016;117(11):2443−2453. https://doi.org/10.1002/jcb.25575.

51. Joussen AM, Poulaki V, Mitsiades N, et al. Nonsteroidal anti-inflammatory drugs prevent early diabetic retinopathy via TNF-alpha suppression. *FASEB J*. 2002;16(3):438−440. https://doi.org/10.1096/fj.01-0707fje.

52. Demircan N, Safran BG, Soylu M, Ozcan AA, Sizmaz S. Determination of vitreous interleukin-1 (IL-1) and tumour necrosis factor (TNF) levels in proliferative diabetic retinopathy. *Eye (Lond)*. 2006;20(12):1366−1369. https://doi.org/10.1038/sj.eye.6702138.

53. Vincent JA, Mohr S. Inhibition of caspase-1/interleukin-1beta signaling prevents degeneration of retinal capillaries in diabetes and galactosemia. *Diabetes*. 2007;56(1):224−230. https://doi.org/10.2337/db06-0427.

54. Kowluru RA, Odenbach S. Role of interleukin-1beta in the development of retinopathy in rats: effect of antioxidants. *Invest Ophthalmol Vis Sci*. 2004;45(11):4161−4166. https://doi.org/10.1167/iovs.04-0633.

55. Murugeswari P, Shukla D, Rajendran A, Kim R, Namperumalsamy P, Muthukkaruppan V. Proinflammatory cytokines and angiogenic and anti-angiogenic factors in vitreous of patients with proliferative diabetic retinopathy and eales' disease. *Retina*. 2008;28(6):817−824. https://doi.org/10.1097/IAE.0b013e31816576d5.

56. Maier R, Weger M, Haller-Schober EM, et al. Multiplex bead analysis of vitreous and serum concentrations of inflammatory and proangiogenic factors in diabetic patients. *Mol Vis*. 2008;14:637−643.

57. Meleth AD, Agrón E, Chan CC, et al. Serum inflammatory markers in diabetic retinopathy. *Invest Ophthalmol Vis Sci*. 2005;46(11):4295−4301. https://doi.org/10.1167/iovs.04-1057.

58. Mocan MC, Kadayifcilar S, Eldem B. Elevated intravitreal interleukin-6 levels in patients with proliferative diabetic retinopathy. *Can J Ophthalmol*. 2006;41(6):747−752. https://doi.org/10.3129/i06-070.

59. dell'Omo R, Semeraro F, Bamonte G, Cifariello F, Romano MR, Costagliola C. Vitreous mediators in retinal hypoxic diseases. *Mediat Inflamm*. 2013;2013:1−16. https://doi.org/10.1155/2013/935301.

60. Ali Z, Mukwaya A, Biesemeier A, et al. Intussusceptive vascular remodeling precedes pathological neovascularization. *ATVB*. 2019;39(7):1402−1418. https://doi.org/10.1161/ATVBAHA.118.312190.

61. Folkman J, D'Amore PA. Blood vessel formation: what is its molecular basis? *Cell*. 1996;87(7):1153−1155. https://doi.org/10.1016/s0092-8674(00)81810-3.

62. Hellström M, Kalén M, Lindahl P, Abramsson A, Betsholtz C. Role of PDGF-B and PDGFR-beta in recruitment of vascular smooth muscle cells and pericytes during embryonic blood vessel formation in the mouse. *Development*. 1999;126(14):3047−3055.

63. Shyy YJ, Hsieh HJ, Usami S, Chien S. Fluid shear stress induces a biphasic response of human monocyte chemotactic protein 1 gene expression in vascular endothelium. *Proc Natl Acad Sci U S A*. 1994;91(11):4678−4682. https://doi.org/10.1073/pnas.91.11.4678.

64. Gale NW, Baluk P, Pan L, et al. Ephrin-B2 selectively marks arterial vessels and neovascularization sites in the adult, with expression in both endothelial and smooth-muscle cells. *Dev Biol*. 2001;230(2):151−160. https://doi.org/10.1006/dbio.2000.0112.

65. Shin D, Garcia-Cardena G, Hayashi S, et al. Expression of ephrinB2 identifies a stable genetic difference between arterial and venous vascular smooth muscle as well as endothelial cells, and marks subsets of microvessels at sites of adult neovascularization. *Dev Biol*. 2001;230(2):139−150. https://doi.org/10.1006/dbio.2000.9957.

66. Burri PH, Djonov V. Intussusceptive angiogenesis—the alternative to capillary sprouting. *Mol Aspects Med*. 2002;23(6S):S1−27. https://doi.org/10.1016/s0098-2997(02)00096-1.

67. Thurston G, Suri C, Smith K, et al. Leakage-resistant blood vessels in mice transgenically overexpressing angiopoietin-1. *Science*. 1999;286(5449):2511−2514. https://doi.org/10.1126/science.286.5449.2511.

68. Crivellato E, Nico B, Vacca A, Djonov V, Presta M, Ribatti D. Recombinant human erythropoietin induces intussusceptive microvascular growth in vivo. *Leukemia*. 2004;18(2):331−336. https://doi.org/10.1038/sj.leu.2403246.

69. van Royen N, Piek JJ, Buschmann I, Hoefer I, Voskuil M, Schaper W. Stimulation of arteriogenesis; a new concept for the treatment of arterial occlusive disease. *Cardiovasc Res*. 2001;49(3):543−553. https://doi.org/10.1016/s0008-6363(00)00206-6.

70. Taylor AC, Seltz LM, Yates PA, Peirce SM. Chronic whole-body hypoxia induces intussusceptive angiogenesis and microvascular remodeling in the mouse retina. *Microvasc Res*. 2010;79(2):93−101. https://doi.org/10.1016/j.mvr.2010.01.006.

71. Mentzer SJ, Konerding MA. Intussusceptive angiogenesis: expansion and remodeling of microvascular networks. *Angiogenesis*. 2014;17(3):499−509. https://doi.org/10.1007/s10456-014-9428-3.

72. Wang W, Lo A. Diabetic retinopathy: pathophysiology and treatments. *Indian J Manag Sci*. 2018;19(6):1816. https://doi.org/10.3390/ijms19061816.

73. Lee SHS, Kim HJ, Shin OK, et al. Intravitreal injection of AAV expressing soluble VEGF receptor-1 variant induces anti-VEGF activity and suppresses choroidal neovascularization. *Invest Ophthalmol Vis Sci*. 2018;59(13):5398. https://doi.org/10.1167/iovs.18-24926.

74. Kurihara T, Westenskow PD, Bravo S, Aguilar E, Friedlander M. Targeted deletion of Vegfa in adult mice induces vision loss. *J Clin Invest*. 2012;122(11):4213−4217. https://doi.org/10.1172/JCI65157.

75. Hofmann JJ, Luisa Iruela-Arispe M. Notch expression patterns in the retina: an eye on receptor-ligand distribution during angiogenesis. *Gene Expr Patterns*. 2007;7(4):461−470. https://doi.org/10.1016/j.modgep.2006.11.002.

76. Sahni J, Patel SS, Dugel PU, et al. Simultaneous inhibition of angiopoietin-2 and vascular endothelial growth factor-A with Faricimab in diabetic macular edema: boulevard phase 2 randomized trial. *Ophthalmology*. 2019;126(8):1155−1170. https://doi.org/10.1016/j.ophtha.2019.03.023.

77. Khan M, Aziz AA, Shafi NA, Abbas T, Khanani AM. Targeting angiopoietin in retinal vascular diseases: a literature review and summary of clinical trials involving faricimab. *Cells*. 2020;9(8):E1869. https://doi.org/10.3390/cells9081869.

78. Gucciardo E, Loukovaara S, Salven P, Lehti K. Lymphatic vascular structures: a new aspect in proliferative diabetic retinopathy. *Indian J Manag Sci*. 2018;19(12):4034. https://doi.org/10.3390/ijms19124034.

79. Korhonen A, Gucciardo E, Lehti K, Loukovaara S. Proliferative diabetic retinopathy transcriptomes reveal angiogenesis, anti-angiogenic therapy escape mechanisms, fibrosis and lymphatic involvement. *Sci Rep*. 2021;11(1):18810. https://doi.org/10.1038/s41598-021-97970-5.

80. Yuan HT, Venkatesha S, Chan B, et al. Activation of the orphan endothelial receptor Tie1 modifies Tie2-mediated intracellular signaling and cell survival. *FASEB J*. 2007; 21(12):3171−3183. https://doi.org/10.1096/fj.07-8487com.

81. Ha JM, Jin SY, Lee HS, et al. Regulation of retinal angiogenesis by endothelial nitric oxide synthase signaling pathway. *Korean J Physiol Pharmacol*. 2016;20(5):533. https://doi.org/10.4196/kjpp.2016.20.5.533.

82. Jacot JL, Sherris D. Potential therapeutic roles for inhibition of the PI3K/Akt/mTOR pathway in the pathophysiology of diabetic retinopathy. *J Ophthalmol*. 2011;2011: 1−19. https://doi.org/10.1155/2011/589813.

83. Hawinkels LJ, Garcia de Vinuesa A, Ten Dijke P. Activin receptor-like kinase 1 as a target for anti-angiogenesis therapy. *Expert Opin Investig Drugs*. 2013;22(11): 1371−1383. https://doi.org/10.1517/13543784.2013.837884.

84. Cai W, Rook SL, Jiang ZY, Takahara N, Aiello LP. Mechanisms of hepatocyte growth factor-induced retinal endothelial cell migration and growth. *Invest Ophthalmol Vis Sci*. 2000;41(7):1885−1893.

85. Gucciardo E, Loukovaara S, Korhonen A, et al. The microenvironment of proliferative diabetic retinopathy supports lymphatic neovascularization: PDR microenvironment and neovasculature. *J Pathol*. 2018;245(2):172−185. https://doi.org/10.1002/path.5070.

86. Cioffi S, Martucciello S, Fulcoli FG, et al. Tbx1 regulates brain vascularization. *Hum Mol Genet*. 2014;23(1):78−89. https://doi.org/10.1093/hmg/ddt400.

87. Ban CR, Twigg SM. Fibrosis in diabetes complications: pathogenic mechanisms and circulating and urinary markers. *Vasc Health Risk Manag*. 2008;4(3):575−596. https://doi.org/10.2147/vhrm.s1991.

88. Roy S, Amin S, Roy S. Retinal fibrosis in diabetic retinopathy. *Exp Eye Res*. 2016;142: 71−75. https://doi.org/10.1016/j.exer.2015.04.004.

89. Linskens MH, Harley CB, West MD, Campisi J, Hayflick L. Replicative senescence and cell death. *Science*. 1995;267(5194):17. https://doi.org/10.1126/science.7848496.

90. Shao Y, Li X, Wood JW, Ma JX. Mitochondrial dysfunctions, endothelial progenitor cells and diabetic retinopathy. *J Diabet Complicat*. 2018;32(10):966−973. https:// doi.org/10.1016/j.jdiacomp.2018.06.015.

91. Grant MB, May WS, Caballero S, et al. Adult hematopoietic stem cells provide functional hemangioblast activity during retinal neovascularization. *Nat Med*. 2002;8(6): 607−612. https://doi.org/10.1038/nm0602-607.

92. Ceradini DJ, Kulkarni AR, Callaghan MJ, et al. Progenitor cell trafficking is regulated by hypoxic gradients through HIF-1 induction of SDF-1. *Nat Med*. 2004;10(8): 858−864. https://doi.org/10.1038/nm1075.

93. Petit I, Jin D, Rafii S. The SDF-1−CXCR4 signaling pathway: a molecular hub modulating neo-angiogenesis. *Trends Immunol*. 2007;28(7):299−307. https://doi.org/ 10.1016/j.it.2007.05.007.

94. Dar A, Goichberg P, Shinder V, et al. Chemokine receptor CXCR4−dependent internalization and resecretion of functional chemokine SDF-1 by bone marrow endothelial and stromal cells. *Nat Immunol*. 2005;6(10):1038−1046. https://doi.org/10.1038/ni1251.

95. Heissig B, Hattori K, Dias S, et al. Recruitment of stem and progenitor cells from the bone marrow niche requires MMP-9 mediated release of kit-ligand. *Cell*. 2002;109(5): 625−637. https://doi.org/10.1016/S0092-8674(02)00754-7.

96. Vajkoczy P, Blum S, Lamparter M, et al. Multistep nature of microvascular recruitment of ex vivo−expanded embryonic endothelial progenitor cells during tumor

angiogenesis. *J Exp Med*. 2003;197(12):1755−1765. https://doi.org/10.1084/jem.20021659.

97. Yao L, Salvucci O, Cardones AR, et al. Selective expression of stromal-derived factor-1 in the capillary vascular endothelium plays a role in Kaposi sarcoma pathogenesis. *Blood*. 2003;102(12):3900−3905. https://doi.org/10.1182/blood-2003-02-0641.

98. Napoli C, Hayashi T, Cacciatore F, et al. Endothelial progenitor cells as therapeutic agents in the microcirculation: an update. *Atherosclerosis*. 2011;215(1):9−22. https://doi.org/10.1016/j.atherosclerosis.2010.10.039.

99. Asahara T, Takahashi T, Masuda H, et al. VEGF contributes to postnatal neovascularization by mobilizing bone marrow-derived endothelial progenitor cells. *EMBO J*. 1999;18(14):3964−3972. https://doi.org/10.1093/emboj/18.14.3964.

100. George AL, Bangalore-Prakash P, Rajoria S, et al. Endothelial progenitor cell biology in disease and tissue regeneration. *J Hematol Oncol*. 2011;4:24. https://doi.org/10.1186/1756-8722-4-24.

101. Lois N, McCarter RV, O'Neill C, Medina RJ, Stitt AW. Endothelial progenitor cells in diabetic retinopathy. *Front Endocrinol*. 2014;5. https://doi.org/10.3389/fendo.2014.00044.

102. van Ark J, Moser J, Lexis CPH, et al. Type 2 diabetes mellitus is associated with an imbalance in circulating endothelial and smooth muscle progenitor cell numbers. *Diabetologia*. 2012;55(9):2501−2512. https://doi.org/10.1007/s00125-012-2590-5.

103. Loomans CJM, de Koning EJP, Staal FJT, et al. Endothelial progenitor cell dysfunction: a novel concept in the pathogenesis of vascular complications of type 1 diabetes. *Diabetes*. 2004;53(1):195−199. https://doi.org/10.2337/diabetes.53.1.195.

104. Kusuyama T, Omura T, Nishiya D, et al. Effects of treatment for diabetes mellitus on circulating vascular progenitor cells. *J Pharmacol Sci*. 2006;102(1):96−102. https://doi.org/10.1254/jphs.fp0060256.

105. Hu L, mei, Lei X, Ma B, et al. Erythropoietin receptor positive circulating progenitor cells and endothelial progenitor cells in patients with different stages of diabetic retinopathy. *Chin Med Sci J*. 2011;26(2):69−76. https://doi.org/10.1016/S1001-9294(11)60023-0.

106. Déry MAC, Michaud MD, Richard DE. Hypoxia-inducible factor 1: regulation by hypoxic and non-hypoxic activators. *Int J Biochem Cell Biol*. 2005;37(3):535−540. https://doi.org/10.1016/j.biocel.2004.08.012.

107. Duda DG, Fukumura D, Jain RK. Role of eNOS in neovascularization: NO for endothelial progenitor cells. *Trends Mol Med*. 2004;10(4):143−145. https://doi.org/10.1016/j.molmed.2004.02.001.

Pathogenesis of diabetic macular edema

Overview of diabetic macular edema

Diabetic macular edema (DME) is the leading cause of vision loss in diabetic patients, increasing along with the growing prevalence of type 2 diabetic mellitus worldwide.[1] DME refers to abnormal increase of fluid in the macula under diabetic condition. Depending upon the anatomic, functional, and mechanistic features of the fluid accumulation, DME can be defined as different types. Among multiple, intricate mechanisms, the two major underlying mechanisms of DME consist of breakdown of blood–retinal barrier (BRB), including inner BRB and outer BRB, leading to the increased fluid influx into retina from retinal and choroidal vasculatures, and decrease in drainage functions by Müller glia and retinal pigment epithelium (RPE), causing reduced fluid efflux out of retina. As a result, DME develops.[2,3] When fluid is extravasated from retinal vessels, that is, inner BRB and leakage of outer BRB, it accumulates as intraretinal fluid (IRF) or subretinal fluid (SRF) (Fig. 8.1). According to the Starling equation, in normal retina, the balance of influx and efflux of the fluid in retina is maintained by the integrity of BRB and the normal functions of Müller glial cells and RPE.[1,4] DME results from an imbalance between fluid entry, fluid exit, and retinal hydraulic conductivity, leading to IRF or SRF accumulation (Fig. 8.1).[1] An intact BRB and the active drainage function of both Müller glia and RPE maintain the retina in a relatively dehydrated status.[1]

The pathophysiology of DME starts with decreased retinal oxygen tension, which leads to retinal capillary hyperpermeability and increased intravascular pressure due to dysfunction of vascular autoregulation. The capillary hyperpermeability is attributed to hypoxia-induced upregulation of vascular endothelial growth factor (VEGF). VEGF is known to play a major role in the development of DME. The favorable outcome by anti-VEGF agents has established the guideline of DME treatment, in which intravitreal anti-VEGF injection is the first-line therapy. The clinical benefits of anti-VEGF therapy consist of improved visual acuity, decreased macular thickness, and delayed or even reversed progression of diabetic retinopathy (DR). The current anti-VEGF therapies for DME patients mainly focus on maintaining the integrity of BRB by antagonizing VEGF-A and/or placental growth factor (PlGF) to reduce retinal edema. However, it remains largely unknown whether or not these anti-VEGF agents can restore the drainage functions of Müller glia and

Therapeutic Targets for Diabetic Retinopathy. https://doi.org/10.1016/B978-0-323-93064-2.00003-2

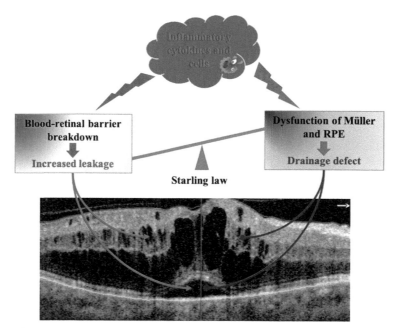

FIGURE 8.1

A simplified illustration of pathogenesis of extracellular diabetic macular edema (DME). According to Starling's law, DME results from increased leakage of fluid due to the breakdown of the blood—retinal barrier (BRB) and the decreased drainage function of Müller glia and retinal pigment epithelium (RPE). In addition, inflammatory cytokines and inflammatory cells also participate in the formation of DME, exacerbating both the breakdown of BRB and dysfunction of the drainage cells.

Data from Zhang and Li.

RPE to facilitate the absorbance of excess fluid in retina. In addition to the VEGF pathway, DME formation is attributed to other factors including leakage of microaneurysms, tractional effects by epiretinal membranes or posterior vitreous cortex, and inflammatory cells as well as the inflammatory factors from both retina and vitreous pool.[1,5,6]

New DME classification based on anatomic features of fovea

In diabetic retina, when fluid accumulates in the macular area, it leads to increased central retinal thickness. Based on optical coherence tomography (OCT) findings, the location of the thickened central retina relative to the fovea is a determinant for the diagnosis and treatment of DME. The classification of DME has been updated as center-involved DME (CI-DME) or non-center-involved DME (non-CI-DME) (see Chapter 1). Furthermore, due to anatomical and functional features of the central retina, the macula is the region most predisposed to the development of edema. The various predisposing factors include a high rate of fluid production due to the high cell count in this region along with the high metabolic activity, a low rate of extracellular fluid resorption due to the presence of a central avascular zone, and the peculiar arrangement of the Henle's fiber layer (HFL). HFL contains bundles of unmyelinated cone and rod photoreceptor axons terminating in the pedicles that synapse in the retinal outer plexiform layer (OPL). These fibers are intermingled with Müller cell processes and are obliquely oriented as a result of foveal pit development where photoreceptors migrate inward and ganglion cells migrate outward. Given the large number of central foveal photoreceptor nuclei and this marked displacement, HFL constitutes a significant fraction of the thickness of retinal layers within the macula. Therefore, the change of HFL thickness may significantly impact the central subfield thickness (CST). However, the exact roles of these anatomic features of the fovea in water accumulation into and drainage from the fovea remain to be determined.

Based on swept-source OCT measurable pathology, including fluid accumulation and disruption of various retinal layers, a new classification of DME has been proposed.[7] In this new DME classification, the retina is divided into: anterior portion, mainly comprising the inner nuclear layer and OPL, including HFL; and posterior portion, mainly comprising the outer nuclear layer. Fujiwara et al. reported that eyes with diffuse fluid at the posterior portion showed significantly poorer visual acuity, higher ellipsoid zone (EZ) disruption rates, and greater CST than did those without fluid at the posterior portion. These results not only indicate the importance of the localization and extent of the fluid for visual outcome in DME[7] but also suggest that the use of CST as the key biomarker measuring the outcome of DME in previous major clinical trials may need to be reconsidered.

In addition to the importance of the anatomic location of macular fluid accumulation, the fluid accumulation within the intracellular space is defined as cytotoxic edema or intracellular swelling, while fluid accumulation in the extracellular space is defined as vasogenic edema.[5] Most importantly, intracellular and extracellular retinal swelling may result from different pathophysiologic mechanisms in DME formation.

Intracellular/cytotoxic edema

Diabetic cytotoxic edema can result from intracellular accumulation of sorbitol, lactate, and phosphates secondary to hyperglycemia-induced metabolic abnormalities.[5] Under physiologic conditions, Müller cells remove the fluid from the retinal interstitial tissue to the blood vessels or vitreous, while RPE cells remove excess fluid from the retina to the choroid by active transport.[8,9] Müller cells are the most important glial cells in retina, spanning the whole retina from the inner limiting membrane (ILM) to the external limiting membrane (ELM). The extensions of Müller cells contact all types of retinal cells, with their processes wrapping the blood vessels. Müller cells facilitate contact among retinal cells and different ocular compartments such as vitreous, retinal vessels, and the subretinal space. Müller cells have many aquaporins, ion channels, transmembrane proteins, and enzymes. An important characteristic of Müller cells is their great conductance for potassium. The numerous functions of Müller cells include drainage of extracellular fluid into the retinal vessels or vitreous body, regulation of retinal blood flow, maintenance of retinal pH by ionic homeostasis, glutamate recycling due to neuronal transmission, and maintenance of glucose metabolism. In DR, the metabolism of Müller cells is disturbed, which compromises the drainage function of Müller cells leading to intracellular accumulation of fluid and inadequate discharge of the fluid into blood vessels or vitreous. Consequently, the intracellular swelling or cytotoxic edema of Müller cells leads to rupture of cell membranes as well as increased liquid in the extracellular space, presenting intraretinal cystoid abnormal spaces visible by OCT.

In normal retina, excess SRF that accumulates under the neurosensory retina is usually absorbed and transported by the RPE cells. The active transport of RPE cells along with choroidal osmotic pressure keeps the subretinal space relatively dry to maintain retinal attachment.[10,11] In experimental DR, the degeneration of RPE and the breakdown of outer BRB were observed.[12,13] In both 2- and 4-week diabetic rats, the major leakage of fluorescein isothiocyanate-dextran is detected in the outer nuclear layer indicating the dysfunction of RPE. Furthermore, the protein levels of zonula occludens-1 (ZO-1) and occludin in the RPE–Bruch's membrane–choriocapillaris complex are significantly decreased, whereas hypoxia-inducible factor 1α and c-Jun N-terminal kinase pathways are activated.[13] However, direct evidence showing intracellular edema of RPE cells per se still needs to be validated both experimentally and clinically.

Intracellular edema in the form of DME as a consequence of metabolic disturbances[14,15] appears to localize within RPE cells, Müller cells, and retinal neurons. With the development of DME, the intracellular edema of the involved cells results in neuronal toxicity, contributing to vision loss and extracellular fluid volume increase.[1]

Cytotoxic edema and dysfunction of Müller cells

Retinal Müller glia, macroglial cells unique to the retina, are responsible for the transport and removal of excess fluid from retinal parenchyma into the vitreous and retinal vessels.[1,16,17] Based on our clinical observation, in a cohort study of DME (CST > 275 μm), there is a strong correlation between the thickness of the inner nuclear layer, where somas of Müller cells are located, and the CST, suggesting that intracellular edema, especially Müller intracellular edema, contributes to DME development.[18] The intracellular edema of Müller cells is also observed in patients with DR when examined with OCT angiography (OCTA), as indicated by the hyporeflective cystoid edema spaces in the deep capillary network in both b-scan and en face of OCTA.[1]

Müller cells regulate the homeostasis of ion and water in the retina mainly through inward rectifying potassium channel 4.1 (Kir4.1) and aquaporin 4 (AQP4).[1,8,19] The polarized distribution of Kir4.1 enables the potassium efflux away from the neural retina.[18] While the water, accompanied with potassium and powered by osmotic pressure, is transported through AQP4, a selective water transport protein colocalized with Kir4.1. Both Kir4.1 and AQP4 are anchored by Dystrophin 71 (Dp71) on the membranes of Müller cells.[20,21] Studies showed that the swelling of Müller cells is caused by the downregulation or redistribution of Kir4.1, AQP4, and Dp71 in many retinal disease models, such as retinal vein occlusion, ischemia-reperfusion injury, and DR.[22−24]

In 3-month rat experimental DR, Kir4.1 was absent in the ILM and perivascular areas.[25] The altered distribution of Kir4.1 was also detected in 6-month diabetic rat retinas, with a global decrease in the ELM and perivascular region.[16] In our previous study using 3-month diabetic rat retinas, Kir4.1 and AQP4 were decreased significantly. The immunofluorescence of Kir4.1 was greatly decreased, especially at the end feet of Müller cells.[24] The decreased expression and the altered distribution of Kir4.1 and AQP4 may be a molecular marker of the dysfunction of Müller cells. The dysfunction of water and ion transport out of the retina may cause intracellular edema of Müller cells. To further confirm the contributing role of Kir4.1 and AQP4 in the drainage function of Müller cells, a partial lens surgery was performed in C57BL6/J mice to establish an experimental model of intracellular edema, in which inner BRB breakdown and swollen Müller cells are accompanied with the downregulation of Kir4.1, AQP4, and Dp71, as well as delocalization of Kir4.1. Upregulation of Kir4.1 and AQP4 by dexamethasone in Müller cells could protect the retina from swelling.[26] These data support the roles Kir4.1 and AQP4 in regulation of the drainage function of Müller cells. The downregulation or redistribution of Kir4.1 and AQP4 plays a detrimental role in the formation of intracellular edema in Müller cells.

Drainage dysfunction of RPE cells

Under physiologic conditions, intraocular pressure (IOP) establishes the power to push the movement of water from the vitreous body into the neural retina, the subretinal space, and the choroid, allowing the constant removal of water from the inner retina to the choriocapillaris.[27] Tight junctions among the RPE cells create a barrier between the subretinal space and the choriocapillaris.[9,28] Evidence exists that the paracellular resistance is 10 times higher than transcellular resistance, specifying RPE as a tight epithelium forming outer BRB.[29,30] With this barrier, water transport occurs mainly by transcellular pathways which are facilitated by aquaporin 1 (AQP1).[31,32] The RPE transports ions and water from the subretinal space or apical side of RPE to the choroid or basolateral side of RPE.[33] The Na^+-K^+-ATPase, which is located in the apical membrane, provides the energy for transepithelial transport.[34] There is a large amount of water produced in the retina, mainly as a consequence of the large metabolic turnover in retinal neurons. Constant elimination of water from the subretinal space produces an adhesive force between the neural retina and the RPE. This function is lost when Na^+-K^+-ATPase is inhibited with ouabain or furosemide experimentally.[35] The study on changes of tight junctional proteins in RPE under hyperglycemia produced some controversial results. In diabetic rat retinas, the protein expression of tight junction proteins, that is, ZO-1 and occludin are significantly decreased, implying the pro-breakdown of outer BRB and dysfunction of RPE cells.[13] In contrast, an in vitro study showed no significant difference for mRNA and protein levels of occludin and ZO-1 in ARPE-19 cells under different concentrations of glucose (5.5 and 25 mM).[36] However, evidence exists that high glucose could induce overexpression of claudin-1, another component of tight junction in ARPE-19 cell line.[36] Nevertheless, high glucose concentrations increase transepithelial but decrease apical-basolateral permeability of ARPE-19 cells, while the permeability changes of the RPE induced by high glucose seems not directly related to tight junction expression.[36] In cultured bovine RPE cells, it has been demonstrated that hyperglycemia induces a loss of Na^+-K^+-ATPase function, which can be restored by treatment with an aldose reductase inhibitor.[37] Therefore, it appears that hyperglycemia impairs the transport of water from subretinal space to the choriocapillaris, contributing to DME development.

In a light-evoked model of diabetic chick retina, RPE cells are responsible for modifying subretinal space hydration via apical membrane Na—K—Cl cotransporters and the conductive efflux of K^+ across the apical membrane and Cl^- across the basal membrane. In other words, the hydration status of subretinal space is dependent on RPE functions.[38] Morphologically, electron microscopic studies on RPE of retinas in diabetic animal models further demonstrated shrunken nuclei, reduced endoplasmic reticulum, infolding of cell membranes, altered melanosomes, and reduced number of RPE cells.[39] OCT characteristics of outer retina in DME have proven that EZ disruption occurs subsequent to the disruption of the ELM.[40] Since the ELM, apical microvilli of Müller cells, functions like a third retinal barrier, ELM disruption may result in photoreceptor and RPE damage. In fact, decreased RPE thickness was observed in DME patients with NPDR or PDR.[41] Nevertheless, these OCT biomarkers may be useful in assessing the drainage function of outer retinal layers, especially the RPE layer in eyes with DME.

Extracellular/vasogenic edema

The BRB protects retinal neuronal functions by maintaining an adequate microenvironment. The tight and restrictive BRB regulate ion, protein, and water flux into and out of the retina. The BRB is composed of both inner BRB and outer BRB. Abnormal fluid accumulation secondary to DME is mainly attributed to the breakdown of BRB.

Inner and outer BRB breakdown

DME is the result of an accumulation of fluid in the retinal layers around the fovea. The increase in water content of the retinal tissue initially occurs in the form of cytotoxic or intracellular edema, resulting from an alteration of the cellular ionic distribution as described above. In the second phase of DME, the extracellular accumulation of fluid is directly associated with breakdown of the inner and outer BRB. In this phase, the protective function of the BRB is lost and Starling law applies. Following breakdown of the BRB, the loss of equilibrium between hydrostatic and oncotic pressure gradients across the BRB leads to further progression of the macular edema (Fig. 8.1).[42] The amount of accumulated extracellular fluid is determined by the difference between the osmotic and hydrostatic pressure in the retinal veins and arterioles.[43] The result of vasogenic edema is an accumulation of fluid in retinal parenchyma that is called IRF, mainly in the extracellular spaces of the OPL and the inner and outer nuclear retinal layers. In diabetic patients, the accumulation of fluid underneath the neurosensory retina is called SRF. The loss of protective function of BRB is attributed to the impairment of cells comprising the BRB and cell—cell junctions. Three BRB pathologies in DR are critical in the development of DME, that is, pericyte loss, impaired cell—cell junctions, and capillary basement membrane thickening.[44] In DR, loss of cell—cell junctions in the endothelium results in the leakage of red blood cells, plasma, and lipid.[45,46] This leakage manifests clinically as intraretinal hemorrhages, edema, and hard exudates.

The predominant mechanisms leading to BRB breakdown and subsequent vasogenic DME comprise activated VEGF downstream pathways and inflammation leading to the release of cytokines and growth factors.[47,48] Since there is substantial overlapping of the pathogenic role of the VEGF pathway in both DME formation and DR progression, it has been discussed in detail in Chapters 5 and 6 and need not be replicated here. On the other hand, various other growth factors and cytokines play a causative role in BRB breakdown through multiple signaling pathways.[47] For instance, tumor necrosis factor α (TNF-α) promotes leukostasis in early DR and increases intercellular adhesion molecule 1 (ICAM-1). TNF-α is essential for progressive BRB breakdown, and its inhibition might provide a therapeutic target for the prevention of the progressive BRB breakdown, retinal leukostasis, and apoptosis associated with DR.[47,49] Interleukin-1β (IL-1β) stimulates the production of reactive oxygen species (ROS) and can accelerate apoptosis of retinal capillary endothelial cells through the activation of the nuclear factor kappa B pathway, a process exacerbated in high glucose conditions.[50,51] Hyperglycemia-induced oxidative stress upregulates multiple cytokines, chemokines, and enzymes such as angiopoietins, interleukins, cyclooxygenase-2 (COX-2), inducible nitric oxide synthase (iNOS), and matric metalloproteinases, which potentiate BRB breakdown.[44,52] Apart from these, the activated kallikrein—kinin system in diabetic retina also contributes to neovascularization and retinal hemorrhage through bradykinin B1 and B2 receptor activation, promoting vasodilation, vascular permeability, inflammation, and leukostasis.[53] B2 receptor specifically stimulates endothelial nitric oxide synthase and phospholipase

A2, leading to vasodilation by increasing the production of nitric oxide and prosta-cyclin.[54] B2 receptor also activates the Src kinases, thereby promoting vascular endothelial (VE)-cadherin phosphorylation, which contributes to the plasma leakage through reversible opening of the endothelial cell junctions.[55] Concomitant activation of iNOS by B1 receptor can also cause peroxynitrite formation contributing to oxidative stress and leukostasis in the inflammatory diabetic retina.[54,55]

Inflammation and vasogenic DME

There is an accumulating body of evidence that immunological and inflammatory mechanisms play a prominent role in the pathogenesis of DR and DME.[1,6] In DR, a low-grade inflammation is maintained by the production of cytokines such as IL-6, IL-8, and monocyte chemoattractant protein-1 (MCP-1).[6,56] IL-6 alters the function of the astrocytes that give structural support to the capillaries in the retina, leading to disruption of the inner BRB causing leakage of retinal capillaries. The inflammatory factors, such as IL-8 and MCP-1 act on neutrophils and monocytes, promoting infiltration of these cells into the retina. Besides inflammation-related factors, inflammatory cells, such as leukocytes and microglia, also play pivotal roles in DME.

Inflammation and vasogenic edema

Leukostasis is the early inflammatory response in DME. The upregulation of ICAM-1 on endothelial cells leads to increased leukostasis, resulting in retinal vascular leakage.[57] Neutrophils from diabetic animals exhibit higher levels of surface integrin expression such as CD18, and integrin-mediated adhesion, whereas antibodies against CD-18 or ICAM-1, or genetic knockout of these genes in animals can inhibit the leukostasis and decreased BRB breakdown.[58] In DR, chronic hyperglycemia increases expression of chemokines, including the C-C motif chemokine ligand-2 (CCL2), also known as MCP-1 that increase leukostasis, diapedesis, and influx of monocytes into the retina and extravascular space.[59] Leukocytes migrate through the endothelium into the extravascular space where they differentiate into activated macrophages and secrete various cytokines and inflammation-related factors, including VEGF, IL-6, TNF-α, and angiopoietin-2 (Ang-2).[44] These mediators disrupt the cell—cell junctions, resulting in BRB breakdown. The disruption of the BRB in diabetes involves numerous factors and signal cascades within the vascular lumen and in the retinal parenchyma. A prominent factor contributing to BRB breakdown in DME is VEGF. However, there are many other factors involved in the pathogenesis of DME, particularly inflammatory cytokines, chemokines, and growth factors such as TNF-α, IL-1β, hepatocyte growth factor, insulin-like growth factor-1, ICAM-1, IL-6, MCP-1, and histamine.[57] VEGF, IL-1α, IL-1β, IL-6, IL-8, IL-10, ICAM-1, MCP-1, TNF-α, PlGF, and complement factors were detected and reported in the vitreous or aqueous humor of diabetic patients with DME,[6] indicating the heavy contribution of inflammation in the pathogenesis of vasogenic DME.

Activated inflammatory cells in DME

In addition to inflammatory cytokines and leukostasis, microglia activation is involved in the inflammatory reactions of DME and DR.[60] In retina, resident microglia can be regarded as the immunological watchdogs. Microglial cells are the active sensors of retinal microenvironment and rapidly respond to various insults with a morphological and functional transformation into reactive phagocytes.[61,62] In diabetic retina, activated microglial cells, releasing the inflammatory factors and phagocytosing the apoptotic neurons, contribute to the anatomical and functional abnormalities in retina.[63] Activated microglial cells acquire a more ameboid phenotype with increased motility, and they migrate from inner retina to the subretinal space (see Chapter 5). In eyes with DR, microglia are markedly increased in number and are hypertrophic. These cells are clustered around the retinal vasculature, especially the dilated veins, microaneurysms, intraretinal hemorrhages, cotton wool spots, as well as the optic nerve, and sites of retinal and vitreous neovascularization.[64] In some retinas with cystoid macular edema, microglia infiltrate the outer retina and subretinal space.[64] In addition, microglial cells synthesize cytokines, proteases, nitrous oxide, and ROS in the extracellular medium, accompanying with neuronal death.[61,63] The subretinal space is an immune-privileged space that can be altered by the presence of microglial cells and the production of cytokines. A previous study showed that porous holes are present between the RPE layer and the choroid, which facilitate the passage of cells between both layers.[1] In the same study, Graeber et al. [65] observed, in a murine diabetic model, that, in the case of diabetes, the number of holes in the RPE layer is increased to permit the migration of more inflammatory cells into the choroid. They also observed an increase in ICAM-1 and Caveolin-1 (CAV-1), both of which are implicated in leukostasis, with the number of holes diminishing after one year. Microglia participate in the inflammatory response by increasing their number around the vessels and are activated by CCL2/MCP-1 that also induces the recruitment of macrophages to the retina.[59,66]

Advanced OCT techniques have revealed fluid accumulation at various macular layers, which is direct evidence of DME caused by vasogenic edema. Recently, hyperreflective foci (HRF) viewed with OCT or OCTA in the diabetic retina have been considered as a biomarker of active inflammatory cells, especially microglia and macrophages. HRF were first described by Coscas et al. as hyperreflective dots by spectral-domain OCT in patients with age-related macular degeneration.[67] Subsequently, HRF have been reported in many retinal diseases, including DR and DME (Fig. 8.2), retinal vein occlusion, choroideremia, and other retinal degenerative diseases.[68-70] One previous study demonstrated a positive correlation between soluble CD14, a cytokine released by microglia and macrophages in the aqueous humor, and the increased number of HRF in patients with DME, indicating that inflammatory cells, such as microglia, participate in the pathogenesis of DME.[60]

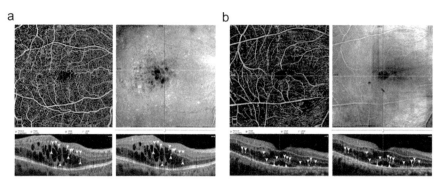

FIGURE 8.2

Hyperreflective foci (HRF) in patients with diabetic macular edema (DME). (A) One female patient with DME in her right eye demonstrating cystoid edema with HRF around the cysts. (B) One male patient with DME demonstrating the subretinal fluid accumulation with many HRF around the subretinal space. The HRF are indicated by *yellow arrowhead*.

Data from Zhang and Li.

Anti-inflammation for DME treatment

Based on the inflammatory theory of DME formation, ongoing translational research targeting inflammatory cells and factors is shedding new light on the management of DME beyond anti-VEGF therapy. Anti-inflammation treatment can be roughly classified into two categories, that is, regulation/inhibition of inflammatory cells (by minocycline, dextromethorphan) and targeting inflammatory mediators (by dexamethasone, TAK-779, TNF-α inhibitor). Several proof-of-concept studies have shown that anti-inflammation is an effective mechanism of drug action for DME. Minocycline, besides its antimicrobial activity, is reported to have anti-inflammatory, antioxidant, anti-apoptotic, neuroprotective, and immunomodulatory effects.[71] In a pilot study, oral minocycline was tested in DME patient for the safety and efficacy in a single-center, prospective, open-label phase I/II clinical trial (ClinicalTrials.gov number, NCT01120899).[72] In this study, minocycline treatment improved visual function and decreased central macular edema and vascular leakage. Thus, microglial inhibition with oral minocycline might be a promising therapeutic strategy targeting the inflammatory etiology of DME. Dextromethorphan, a drug capable of inhibiting microglial activation, was effective in decreasing vascular leakage in 5 DME patients in a single-center, prospective, open-label phase I/II clinical trial with oral dextromethorphan 60 mg twice daily for 6 months as monotherapy.[73]

Evidence exists that both intravitreal injection of anti-VEGF drugs and dexamethasone treatment decrease the number of HRF in patients with DME.[68,74,75] A retrospective, observational, single-center study showed the number of HRF to be decreased significantly for refractory DME patients after switching to an intravitreal dexamethasone implant following bevacizumab treatment.[76] A recent study showed that a chemokine receptor (CCR2/CCR5) inhibitor, TAK-779 (a dual CCR2/CCR5 inhibitor), significantly decreased retinal vascular permeability in diabetic mice.[77] TAK-779 also decreased infiltration of macrophage/microglia, reduced the levels of stromal cell—derived factor 1 (SDF-1) and ICAM-1, and restored cell junction molecules (ZO-1) in the retina of diabetic mice.[77] Targeting the chemokine pathway may be a novel therapeutic strategy for DME management. Anti-inflammatory treatments for DR and DME have also been discussed in detail in Chapter 5.

Therapeutic strategy for DME

Targeting various pathways implicated in the pathogenesis of DME is a fundamental strategy for treating this complication.[78] According to evidence-based medicine, current DME treatments can be summarized as follows. First, primary prevention is the systemic management of diabetes, such as control of hyperglycemia, hyperlipidemia, and high blood pressure. Second, the newer generation focal laser therapy is promising (see Chapter 10); the efficacy and safety of focal laser for treating DME were validated by the Early Treatment of Diabetic Retinopathy Study in 1980s.[79] Today, the focal/grid laser is an alternative in eyes with DME, being reserved mostly for non-CI-DME. Third, the upregulated VEGF causes BRB breakdown in DME. The DRCR.net Protocol T recommended anti-VEGF therapy as the mainstay of DME treatment. Anti-VEGF therapy has become the first-line treatment for CI-DME.[78] However, suboptimal responses to anti-VEGF for DME have prompted researchers to develop novel approaches. New generation anti-VEGF agents and multiple therapeutic routes are under development (see Chapters 9 and 10). Fourth, corticosteroids that effectively suppress inflammation can inhibit VEGF and decrease fluid extravasation from leaking retinal vessels. Thus, intravitreal preservative-free triamcinolone, the extended-release dexamethasone implant (Ozurdex), and the fluocinolone acetonide implant (Iluvein) are Food and Drug Administration (FDA)—approved for treating DME. However, due to concerns regarding IOP elevation and cataract formation, corticosteroids are used as the second-line therapy for DME. Fifth, diabetic vitrectomy for patients with DME and its clinical indications are discussed in Chapters 1 and 10. Sixth, anti-inflammation drugs combined with or without anti-VEGF drugs are promising for the management of DME.

Based on these underlying mechanisms, the future direction of DME treatment should be focused on the following aspects. First, newer anti-VEGF agents are required. For instance, brolucizumab has demonstrated robust visual gains and anatomical improvements with a favorable benefit/risk profile in patients with DME.[80] Second, the recently FDA-approved bispecific antibody faricimab that binds both Ang-2 and VEGF-A produces favorable outcomes in treating DME[81] (see Chapters 9 and 10). Third, for protecting BRB in diabetic retina, inhibitors of VE-protein tyrosine phosphatase that activates Tie-2 receptors have achieved primary goal of decreased retinal vascular permeability (see Chapter 9).[82] Fourth, in order to enhance anti-inflammatory efficacy of corticosteroids in DME treatment, the suprachoroidal route has been explored. While an unconventional route of drug delivery, suprachoroidal delivery of corticosteroids using microneedles has the potential to increase drug concentrations at the posterior retina, thereby reducing cataract formation and IOP elevation by minimizing exposure to anterior segment structures.[83] Fifth, anti-inflammatory effects on diabetic retina also have been achieved by using integrin antagonists. For instance, risuteganib downregulates oxidative stress by inhibiting the $\alpha v\beta 3$, $\alpha v\beta 5$, and $\alpha 5\beta 1$ integrin receptors and has met the primary end point in a phase II trial for DME.[84] Sixth, for maintaining the integrity of inner and outer BRB, cell-specific treatments need to be developed. For example, recently a key enzyme that initiates the pericyte "dropout" and loss of endothelial barrier function has been identified as soluble epoxide hydrolase (sEH). In this reaction, a diol is generated from docosahexaenoic acid. Overexpression of sEH and elevated levels of the precursor of the diol have been found in human diabetic retinas. The diol is able to alter the localization of cholesterol-binding proteins and disturb pericyte-endothelial cell, as well as inter-endothelial cell junctions.[85] Therefore, inhibition of sEH, which can prevent the pericyte loss and vascular hyperpermeability, may be translated into a cell-specific strategy for treating DR and DME. The growing achievements of translational research will lead to future treatments for DME with better efficacy, longer duration, and greater cost-effectiveness (see Chapters 9 and 10).

References

1. Daruich A, Matet A, Moulin A, et al. Mechanisms of macular edema: beyond the surface. *Prog Retin Eye Res*. 2018;63:20−68. https://doi.org/10.1016/j.preteyeres.2017.10.006.
2. Reichenbach A, Bringmann A. New functions of Müller cells. *Glia*. 2013;61(5): 651−678. https://doi.org/10.1002/glia.22477.
3. Caplan MJ. Membrane polarity in epithelial cells: protein sorting and establishment of polarized domains. *Am J Physiol*. 1997;272(4 Pt 2):F425−F429. https://doi.org/10.1152/ajprenal.1997.272.4.F425.
4. Bringmann A, Reichenbach A, Wiedemann P. Pathomechanisms of cystoid macular edema. *Ophthalmic Res*. 2004;36(5):241−249. https://doi.org/10.1159/000081203.
5. Romero-Aroca P, Baget-Bernaldiz M, Pareja-Rios A, Lopez-Galvez M, Navarro-Gil R, Verges R. Diabetic macular edema pathophysiology: vasogenic versus inflammatory. *J Diabetes Res*. 2016;2016:2156273. https://doi.org/10.1155/2016/2156273.
6. Rübsam A, Parikh S, Fort PE. Role of inflammation in diabetic retinopathy. *Int J Mol Sci*. 2018;19(4):E942. https://doi.org/10.3390/ijms19040942.
7. Fujiwara A, Kanzaki Y, Kimura S, et al. En face image-based classification of diabetic macular edema using swept source optical coherence tomography. *Sci Rep*. 2021; 11(1):7665. https://doi.org/10.1038/s41598-021-87440-3.
8. Reichenbach A, Wurm A, Pannicke T, Iandiev I, Wiedemann P, Bringmann A. Müller cells as players in retinal degeneration and edema. *Graefes Arch Clin Exp Ophthalmol*

Albrecht Von Graefes Arch Klin Exp Ophthalmol. 2007;245(5):627–636. https://doi.org/10.1007/s00417-006-0516-y.

9. Simó R, Villarroel M, Corraliza L, Hernández C, Garcia-Ramírez M. The retinal pigment epithelium: something more than a constituent of the blood–retinal barrier-implications for the pathogenesis of diabetic retinopathy. *J Biomed Biotechnol.* 2010;2010:190724. https://doi.org/10.1155/2010/190724.

10. Fields MA, Del Priore LV, Adelman RA, Rizzolo LJ. Interactions of the choroid, Bruch's membrane, retinal pigment epithelium, and neurosensory retina collaborate to form the outer blood–retinal-barrier. *Prog Retin Eye Res.* 2020;76:100803. https://doi.org/10.1016/j.preteyeres.2019.100803.

11. Yang S, Zhou J, Li D. Functions and diseases of the retinal pigment epithelium. *Front Pharmacol.* 2021;12:727870. https://doi.org/10.3389/fphar.2021.727870.

12. Zhang J, Wu Y, Jin Y, et al. Intravitreal injection of erythropoietin protects both retinal vascular and neuronal cells in early diabetes. *Invest Ophthalmol Vis Sci.* 2008;49(2):732–742. https://doi.org/10.1167/iovs.07-0721.

13. Zhang C, Xie H, Yang Q, et al. Erythropoietin protects outer blood–retinal barrier in experimental diabetic retinopathy by up-regulating ZO-1 and occludin. *Clin Exp Ophthalmol.* 2019;47(9):1182–1197. https://doi.org/10.1111/ceo.13619.

14. Kohno T, Ishibashi T, Inomata H, Ikui H, Taniguchi Y. Experimental macular edema of commotio retinae: preliminary report. *Jpn J Ophthalmol.* 1983;27(1):149–156.

15. Yanoff M, Fine BS, Brucker AJ, Eagle RC. Pathology of human cystoid macular edema. *Surv Ophthalmol.* 1984;28(suppl):505–511. https://doi.org/10.1016/0039-6257(84)90233-9.

16. Bringmann A, Pannicke T, Grosche J, et al. Müller cells in the healthy and diseased retina. *Prog Retin Eye Res.* 2006;25(4):397–424. https://doi.org/10.1016/j.preteyeres.2006.05.003.

17. Spaide RF. Retinal vascular cystoid macular edema: review and new theory. *Retina Phila Pa.* 2016;36(10):1823–1842. https://doi.org/10.1097/IAE.0000000000001158.

18. Lange J, Hadziahmetovic M, Zhang J, Li W. Region-specific ischemia, neovascularization and macular oedema in treatment-naïve proliferative diabetic retinopathy. *Clin Exp Ophthalmol.* 2018;46(7):757–766. https://doi.org/10.1111/ceo.13168.

19. Kofuji P, Biedermann B, Siddharthan V, et al. Kir potassium channel subunit expression in retinal glial cells: implications for spatial potassium buffering. *Glia.* 2002;39(3):292–303. https://doi.org/10.1002/glia.10112.

20. Fort PE, Sene A, Pannicke T, et al. Kir4.1 and AQP4 associate with Dp71- and utrophin-DAPs complexes in specific and defined microdomains of Müller retinal glial cell membrane. *Glia.* 2008;56(6):597–610. https://doi.org/10.1002/glia.20633.

21. Sene A, Tadayoni R, Pannicke T, et al. Functional implication of Dp71 in osmoregulation and vascular permeability of the retina. *PLoS One.* 2009;4(10):e7329. https://doi.org/10.1371/journal.pone.0007329.

22. Pannicke T, Iandiev I, Uckermann O, et al. A potassium channel-linked mechanism of glial cell swelling in the postischemic retina. *Mol Cell Neurosci.* 2004;26(4):493–502. https://doi.org/10.1016/j.mcn.2004.04.005.

23. Rehak M, Hollborn M, Iandiev I, et al. Retinal gene expression and Müller cell responses after branch retinal vein occlusion in the rat. *Invest Ophthalmol Vis Sci.* 2009;50(5):2359–2367. https://doi.org/10.1167/iovs.08-2332.

24. Wang T, Zhang C, Xie H, et al. Anti-VEGF therapy prevents Müller intracellular edema by decreasing VEGF-A in diabetic retinopathy. *Eye Vis Lond Engl*. 2021;8(1):13. https://doi.org/10.1186/s40662-021-00237-3.

25. McDowell RE, Barabas P, Augustine J, et al. Müller glial dysfunction during diabetic retinopathy in rats is reduced by the acrolein-scavenging drug, 2-hydrazino-4,6-dimethylpyrimidine. *Diabetologia*. 2018;61(12):2654−2667. https://doi.org/10.1007/s00125-018-4707-y.

26. Siqueiros-Marquez L, Bénard R, Vacca O, et al. Protection of glial Müller cells by dexamethasone in a Mouse model of Surgically induced blood−retinal barrier breakdown. *Invest Ophthalmol Vis Sci*. 2017;58(2):876−886. https://doi.org/10.1167/iovs.16-20617.

27. Hamann S. Molecular mechanisms of water transport in the eye. *Int Rev Cytol*. 2002;215:395−431. https://doi.org/10.1016/s0074-7696(02)15016-9.

28. Erickson KK, Sundstrom JM, Antonetti DA. Vascular permeability in ocular disease and the role of tight junctions. *Angiogenesis*. 2007;10(2):103−117. https://doi.org/10.1007/s10456-007-9067-z.

29. Miller SS, Steinberg RH. Active transport of ions across frog retinal pigment epithelium. *Exp Eye Res*. 1977;25(3):235−248. https://doi.org/10.1016/0014-4835(77)90090-2.

30. Miller SS, Steinberg RH. Passive ionic properties of frog retinal pigment epithelium. *J Membr Biol*. 1977;36(4):337−372. https://doi.org/10.1007/BF01868158.

31. Verkman AS, Ruiz-Ederra J, Levin MH. Functions of aquaporins in the eye. *Prog Retin Eye Res*. 2008;27(4):420−433. https://doi.org/10.1016/j.preteyeres.2008.04.001.

32. Stamer WD, Bok D, Hu J, Jaffe GJ, McKay BS. Aquaporin-1 channels in human retinal pigment epithelium: role in transepithelial water movement. *Invest Ophthalmol Vis Sci*. 2003;44(6):2803−2808. https://doi.org/10.1167/iovs.03-0001.

33. Strauss O. The retinal pigment epithelium in visual function. *Physiol Rev*. 2005;85(3):845−881. https://doi.org/10.1152/physrev.00021.2004.

34. Rizzolo LJ. Polarization of the Na^+, K^+-ATPase in epithelia derived from the neuroepithelium. *Int Rev Cytol*. 1999;185:195−235. https://doi.org/10.1016/s0074-7696(08)60152-7.

35. Frambach DA, Roy CE, Valentine JL, Weiter JJ. Precocious retinal adhesion is affected by furosemide and ouabain. *Curr Eye Res*. 1989;8(6):553−556. https://doi.org/10.3109/02713688908995753.

36. Villarroel M, García-Ramírez M, Corraliza L, Hernández C, Simó R. Effects of high glucose concentration on the barrier function and the expression of tight junction proteins in human retinal pigment epithelial cells. *Exp Eye Res*. 2009;89(6):913−920. https://doi.org/10.1016/j.exer.2009.07.017.

37. Crider JY, Yorio T, Sharif NA, Griffin BW. The effects of elevated glucose on Na^+/K^+-ATPase of cultured bovine retinal pigment epithelial cells measured by a new nonradioactive rubidium uptake assay. *J Ocul Pharmacol Ther*. 1997;13(4):337−352. https://doi.org/10.1089/jop.1997.13.337.

38. Li JD, Gallemore RP, Dmitriev A, Steinberg RH. Light-dependent hydration of the space surrounding photoreceptors in chick retina. *Invest Ophthalmol Vis Sci*. 1994;35(6):2700−2711.

39. Xia T, Rizzolo LJ. Effects of diabetic retinopathy on the barrier functions of the retinal pigment epithelium. *Vision Res*. 2017;139:72−81. https://doi.org/10.1016/j.visres.2017.02.006.

40. Saxena S, Ruia S, Prasad S, et al. Increased serum levels of urea and creatinine are surrogate markers for disruption of retinal photoreceptor external limiting membrane and

inner segment ellipsoid zone in type 2 diabetes mellitus. *Retina Phila Pa.* 2017;37(2): 344−349. https://doi.org/10.1097/IAE.0000000000001163.

41. Tălu Ş, Nicoara SD. Malfunction of outer retinal barrier and choroid in the occurrence and progression of diabetic macular edema. *World J Diabetes.* 2021;12(4):437−452. https://doi.org/10.4239/wjd.v12.i4.437.

42. Cunha-Vaz J, Bernardes R, Lobo C. Blood−retinal barrier. *Eur J Ophthalmol.* 2011; 21(6_suppl):3−9. https://doi.org/10.5301/EJO.2010.6049.

43. Cunha-Vaz J. Diabetic macular edema. *Eur J Ophthalmol.* 1998;8(3):127−130.

44. Urias EA, Urias GA, Monickaraj F, McGuire P, Das A. Novel therapeutic targets in diabetic macular edema: beyond VEGF. *Vision Res.* 2017;139:221−227. https://doi.org/10.1016/j.visres.2017.06.015.

45. Antonetti DA, Klein R, Gardner TW. Diabetic retinopathy. *N Engl J Med.* 2012;366(13): 1227−1239. https://doi.org/10.1056/NEJMra1005073.

46. Frank RN. Diabetic retinopathy. *N Engl J Med.* 2004;350(1):48−58. https://doi.org/10.1056/NEJMra021678.

47. Rudraraju M, Narayanan SP, Somanath PR. Regulation of blood−retinal barrier cell-junctions in diabetic retinopathy. *Pharmacol Res.* 2020;161:105115. https://doi.org/10.1016/j.phrs.2020.105115.

48. Peach CJ, Mignone VW, Arruda MA, et al. Molecular pharmacology of VEGF-A isoforms: binding and signalling at VEGFR2. *Int J Mol Sci.* 2018;19(4):E1264. https://doi.org/10.3390/ijms19041264.

49. Huang H, Gandhi JK, Zhong X, et al. TNFα is required for late BRB breakdown in diabetic retinopathy, and its inhibition prevents leukostasis and protects vessels and neurons from apoptosis. *Invest Ophthalmol Vis Sci.* 2011;52(3):1336−1344. https://doi.org/10.1167/iovs.10-5768.

50. Mittal M, Siddiqui MR, Tran K, Reddy SP, Malik AB. Reactive oxygen species in inflammation and tissue injury. *Antioxid Redox Signal.* 2014;20(7):1126−1167. https://doi.org/10.1089/ars.2012.5149.

51. Liu Y, Biarnés Costa M, Gerhardinger C. IL-1β is upregulated in the diabetic retina and retinal vessels: cell-specific effect of high glucose and IL-1β autostimulation. *PLoS One.* 2012;7(5):e36949. https://doi.org/10.1371/journal.pone.0036949.

52. Kowluru RA, Chan PS. Oxidative stress and diabetic retinopathy. *Exp Diabetes Res.* 2007;2007:43603. https://doi.org/10.1155/2007/43603.

53. Liu J, Feener EP. Plasma kallikrein-kinin system and diabetic retinopathy. *Biol Chem.* 2013;394(3):319−328. https://doi.org/10.1515/hsz-2012-0316.

54. Kuhr F, Lowry J, Zhang Y, Brovkovych V, Skidgel RA. Differential regulation of inducible and endothelial nitric oxide synthase by kinin B1 and B2 receptors. *Neuropeptides.* 2010;44(2):145−154. https://doi.org/10.1016/j.npep.2009.12.004.

55. Bhat M, Pouliot M, Couture R, Vaucher E. The kallikrein-kinin system in diabetic retinopathy. *Prog Drug Res Fortschritte Arzneimittelforschung Progres Rech Pharm.* 2014;69:111−143. https://doi.org/10.1007/978-3-319-06683-7_5.

56. Ambrosini E, Aloisi F. Chemokines and glial cells: a complex network in the central nervous system. *Neurochem Res.* 2004;29(5):1017−1038. https://doi.org/10.1023/b:nere.0000021246.96864.89.

57. Adamis AP, Berman AJ. Immunological mechanisms in the pathogenesis of diabetic retinopathy. *Semin Immunopathol.* 2008;30(2):65−84. https://doi.org/10.1007/s00281-008-0111-x.

58. Joussen AM, Poulaki V, Le ML, et al. A central role for inflammation in the pathogenesis of diabetic retinopathy. *FASEB J.* 2004;18(12):1450−1452. https://doi.org/10.1096/fj.03-1476fje.

59. Rangasamy S, McGuire PG, Franco Nitta C, Monickaraj F, Oruganti SR, Das A. Chemokine mediated monocyte trafficking into the retina: role of inflammation in alteration of the blood−retinal barrier in diabetic retinopathy. *PLoS One.* 2014;9(10):e108508. https://doi.org/10.1371/journal.pone.0108508.

60. Lee H, Jang H, Choi YA, Kim HC, Chung H. Association between soluble CD14 in the aqueous humor and hyperreflective foci on optical coherence tomography in patients with diabetic macular edema. *Invest Ophthalmol Vis Sci.* 2018;59(2):715−721. https://doi.org/10.1167/iovs.17-23042.

61. Karlstetter M, Scholz R, Rutar M, Wong WT, Provis JM, Langmann T. Retinal microglia: just bystander or target for therapy? *Prog Retin Eye Res.* 2015;45:30−57. https://doi.org/10.1016/j.preteyeres.2014.11.004.

62. Kettenmann H, Hanisch UK, Noda M, Verkhratsky A. Physiology of microglia. *Physiol Rev.* 2011;91(2):461−553. https://doi.org/10.1152/physrev.00011.2010.

63. Saijo K, Glass CK. Microglial cell origin and phenotypes in health and disease. *Nat Rev Immunol.* 2011;11(11):775−787. https://doi.org/10.1038/nri3086.

64. Zeng H yang, Green WR, Tso MOM. Microglial activation in human diabetic retinopathy. *Arch Ophthalmol Chic Ill 1960.* 2008;126(2):227−232. https://doi.org/10.1001/archophthalmol.2007.65.

65. Graeber MB, Li W, Rodriguez ML. Role of microglia in CNS inflammation. *FEBS Lett.* 2011;585(23):3798−3805. https://doi.org/10.1016/j.febslet.2011.08.033.

66. Taghavi Y, Hassanshahi G, Kounis NG, Koniari I, Khorramdelazad H. Monocyte chemoattractant protein-1 (MCP-1/CCL2) in diabetic retinopathy: latest evidence and clinical considerations. *J Cell Commun Signal.* 2019;13(4):451−462. https://doi.org/10.1007/s12079-018-00500-8.

67. Coscas G, De Benedetto U, Coscas F, et al. Hyperreflective dots: a new spectral-domain optical coherence tomography entity for follow-up and prognosis in exudative age-related macular degeneration. *Ophthalmol J Int Ophtalmol Int J Ophthalmol Z Augenheilkd.* 2013;229(1):32−37. https://doi.org/10.1159/000342159.

68. Vujosevic S, Torresin T, Bini S, et al. Imaging retinal inflammatory biomarkers after intravitreal steroid and anti-VEGF treatment in diabetic macular oedema. *Acta Ophthalmol.* 2017;95(5):464−471. https://doi.org/10.1111/aos.13294.

69. Romano F, Arrigo A, MacLaren RE, et al. Hyperreflective FOCI as a pathogenetic biomarker in choroideremia. *Retina Phila Pa.* 2020;40(8):1634−1640. https://doi.org/10.1097/IAE.0000000000002645.

70. Frizziero L, Midena G, Longhin E, et al. Early retinal changes by OCT angiography and multifocal electroretinography in diabetes. *J Clin Med.* 2020;9(11):E3514. https://doi.org/10.3390/jcm9113514.

71. Singh S, Khanna D, Kalra S. Minocycline and doxycycline: more than antibiotics. *Curr Mol Pharmacol.* 2021;14(6):1046−1065. https://doi.org/10.2174/1874467214666621021012628.

72. Cukras CA, Petrou P, Chew EY, Meyerle CB, Wong WT. Oral minocycline for the treatment of diabetic macular edema (DME): results of a phase I/II clinical study. *Invest Ophthalmol Vis Sci.* 2012;53(7):3865−3874. https://doi.org/10.1167/iovs.11-9413.

73. Valent DJ, Wong WT, Chew EY, Cukras CA. Oral dextromethorphan for the treatment of diabetic macular edema: results from a phase I/II clinical study. *Transl Vis Sci Technol.* 2018;7(6):24. https://doi.org/10.1167/tvst.7.6.24.

74. Qin S, Zhang C, Qin H, et al. Hyperreflective foci and subretinal fluid are potential imaging biomarkers to evaluate anti-VEGF effect in diabetic macular edema. *Front Physiol.* 2021;12:791442. https://doi.org/10.3389/fphys.2021.791442.

75. Huang CH, Yang CH, Hsieh YT, Yang CM, Ho TC, Lai TT. Hyperreflective foci in predicting the treatment outcomes of diabetic macular oedema after anti-vascular endothelial growth factor therapy. *Sci Rep.* 2021;11(1):5103. https://doi.org/10.1038/s41598-021-84553-7.

76. Kim KT, Kim DY, Chae JB. Association between hyperreflective foci on spectral-domain optical coherence tomography and early recurrence of diabetic macular edema after intravitreal dexamethasone Implantation. *J Ophthalmol.* 2019;2019:3459164. https://doi.org/10.1155/2019/3459164.

77. Monickaraj F, Oruganti SR, McGuire P, Das A. A potential novel therapeutic target in diabetic retinopathy: a chemokine receptor (CCR2/CCR5) inhibitor reduces retinal vascular leakage in an animal model. *Graefes Arch Clin Exp Ophthalmol Albrecht Von Graefes Arch Klin Exp Ophthalmol.* 2021;259(1):93−100. https://doi.org/10.1007/s00417-020-04884-5.

78. Kim EJ, Lin WV, Rodriguez SM, Chen A, Loya A, Weng CY. Treatment of diabetic macular edema. *Curr Diabetes Rep.* 2019;19(9):68. https://doi.org/10.1007/s11892-019-1188-4.

79. Early treatment diabetic retinopathy study research group. Photocoagulation for diabetic macular edema. Early treatment diabetic retinopathy study report number 1. *Arch Ophthalmol Chic Ill 1960.* 1985;103(12):1796−1806.

80. Brown DM, Emanuelli A, Bandello F, et al. KESTREL and KITE: 52-week results from two Phase III pivotal trials of brolucizumab for diabetic macular edema. *Am J Ophthalmol.* January 13, 2022. https://doi.org/10.1016/j.ajo.2022.01.004. S0002-9394(22) 00006-X.

81. Sahni J, Patel SS, Dugel PU, et al. Simultaneous inhibition of angiopoietin-2 and vascular endothelial growth factor-A with faricimab in diabetic macular edema: BOULEVARD phase 2 Randomized trial. *Ophthalmology.* 2019;126(8):1155−1170. https://doi.org/10.1016/j.ophtha.2019.03.023.

82. Campochiaro PA, Sophie R, Tolentino M, et al. Treatment of diabetic macular edema with an inhibitor of vascular endothelial-protein tyrosine phosphatase that activates Tie2. *Ophthalmology.* 2015;122(3):545−554. https://doi.org/10.1016/j.ophtha.2014.09.023.

83. Willoughby AS, Vuong VS, Cunefare D, et al. Choroidal changes after suprachoroidal injection of triamcinolone acetonide in eyes with macular edema secondary to retinal vein occlusion. *Am J Ophthalmol.* 2018;186:144−151. https://doi.org/10.1016/j.ajo.2017.11.020.

84. Shaw LT, Mackin A, Shah R, et al. Risuteganib-a novel integrin inhibitor for the treatment of non-exudative (dry) age-related macular degeneration and diabetic macular edema. *Expert Opin Investig Drugs.* 2020;29(6):547−554. https://doi.org/10.1080/13543784.2020.1763953.

85. Hu J, Dziumbla S, Lin J, et al. Inhibition of soluble epoxide hydrolase prevents diabetic retinopathy. *Nature.* 2017;552(7684):248−252. https://doi.org/10.1038/nature25013.

Treatments for diabetic retinopathy and diabetic macular edema in pipeline

Impact of the protocols by DRCR.net on treatment of diabetic retinopathy and diabetic macular edema

The Diabetic Retinopathy Clinical Research (DRCR) Retina Network is funded by the National Eye Institute. The mission of the DRCR Retina Network is to conduct high-quality, collaborative clinical research that improves vision and quality of life for people with retinal diseases. The DRCR network was established in September 2002. In 2018, the Network expanded its scope beyond diabetic retinopathy (DR) to consider research on other retinal disorders. Thus, the name was changed to the DRCR Retina Network in April of 2019. The Network currently includes over 160 participating sites with over 500 physicians throughout the United States and Canada. The DRCR Retina Network supports the identification, design, and implementation of multicenter clinical research initiatives for retinal disorders.

The clinical studies carried out by DRCR Retina Network are available online;[1] those studies related to DR and diabetic macular edema (DME) are listed in Table 9.1. These clinical trials comprise different treatments for DR and DME, including anti-vascular endothelial growth factor (anti-VEGF) agents, triamcinolone acetonide, sustainable release of dexamethasone, photocoagulation, pars plana vitrectomy (PPV), etc. Current pharmacologic treatments for DR and DME have been introduced in Chapter 1. Herein, only the treatment guidelines that are established by DRCR Retina Network are reemphasized.

Currently, intravitreal injection of anti-VEGF agents is the first-line therapy and standard of care in the treatment of DME. Protocol I showed that intravitreal ranibizumab with prompt or deferred laser is more effective through at least one year compared with prompt laser alone for the treatment of center-involved DME (CI-DME).[2] The expanded two-year results are similar, reinforcing that ranibizumab should be considered for patients with CI-DME.[3] Five-year results suggest focal/grid laser treatment at the initiation of intravitreal ranibizumab is no better than deferring laser treatment for more than 24 weeks in eyes with CI-DME with vision impairment. Most eyes treated with ranibizumab and either prompt or deferred laser maintain vision gains obtained by the first year through 5 years with little additional treatment after 3 years.[4] The five-year follow-up provided valuable information that

Therapeutic Targets for Diabetic Retinopathy. https://doi.org/10.1016/B978-0-323-93064-2.00011-1

Table 9.1 The clinical trials for DR and DME by DRCR Retina Network.[1]

Protocol	Protocol description	Start date	End date	Clinical trial ID
A	A Pilot Study of Laser Photocoagulation for Diabetic Macular Edema	06/07/2003	01/31/2008	NCT00071773
B	A Randomized Trial Comparing Intravitreal Triamcinolone Acetonide and Laser Photocoagulation for Diabetic Macular Edema	07/01/2004	10/03/2008	NCT00367133
D	Evaluation of Vitrectomy for Diabetic Macular Edema Study	08/09/2004	02/26/2009	NCT00709319
E	A Pilot Study of Peribulbar Triamcinolone Acetonide for Diabetic Macular Edema	08/31/2004	11/01/2007	NCT00369486
C	Temporal Variation in Optical Coherence Tomography Measurements of Retinal Thickening in Diabetic Macular Edema	10/01/2004	05/20/2005	
H	A Phase 2 Evaluation of Anti-VEGF Therapy for Diabetic Macular Edema: Bevacizumab (Avastin)	05/01/2005	02/29/2008	NCT00336323
F	An Observational Study of the Development of Diabetic Macular Edema Following Scatter Laser Photocoagulation	09/29/2005	01/31/2008	NCT00687154
G	Subclinical Diabetic Macular Edema Study	11/28/2005	04/22/2009	
K	The Course of Response to Focal Photocoagulation for Diabetic Macular Edema	11/17/2006	06/19/2008	NCT00442156
I	Intravitreal Ranibizumab or Triamcinolone Acetonide in Combination with Laser Photocoagulation for Diabetic Macular Edema	03/20/2007	12/31/2013	NCT00444600
J	Intravitreal Ranibizumab or Triamcinolone Acetonide as Adjunctive Treatment to Panretinal Photocoagulation for Proliferative Diabetic Retinopathy	03/20/2007	07/07/2010	NCT00445003
L	Evaluation of Visual Acuity Measurements in Eyes with Diabetic Macular Edema	06/01/2007	11/06/2010	
O	Comparison of Time Domain OCT and Spectral Domain OCT Retinal Thickness Measurement in Diabetic Macular Edema	05/14/2009	01/31/2013	
P	A Pilot Study in Individuals with Center-Involved DME Undergoing Cataract Surgery	06/01/2009	11/12/2010	
Q	An Observational Study in Individuals with Diabetic Retinopathy without Center-Involved DME Undergoing Cataract Surgery	07/01/2009	05/19/2011	
N	An Evaluation of Intravitreal Ranibizumab for Vitreous Hemorrhage Due to Proliferative Diabetic Retinopathy	06/14/2010	12/21/2012	NCT00996437
M	Effect of Diabetes Education during Retinal Ophthalmology Visits on Diabetes Control	04/04/2011	12/31/2014	NCT01323348
R	A Phase II Evaluation of Topical NSAIDs in Eyes with Non-central Involved DME	05/19/2011	12/18/2013	NCT01331005

Table 9.1 The clinical trials for DR and DME by DRCR Retina Network.[1]—cont'd

Protocol	Protocol description	Start date	End date	Clinical trial ID
S	Prompt Panretinal Photocoagulation versus Intravitreal Ranibizumab with Deferred Panretinal Photocoagulation for Proliferative Diabetic Retinopathy	02/27/2012	02/05/2018	NCT01489189
GEN	Genes in Diabetic Retinopathy Project	03/02/2012		
T	A Comparative Effectiveness Study of Intravitreal Aflibercept, Bevacizumab and Ranibizumab for Diabetic Macular Edema	08/21/2012	10/18/2018	NCT01627249
V	Treatment for Central-Involved Diabetic Macular Edema in Eyes with Very Good Visual Acuity	11/01/2013	09/11/2018	NCT01909791
U	Short-term Evaluation of Combination Corticosteroid + Anti-VEGF Treatment for Persistent Central-Involved Diabetic Macular Edema Following Anti-VEGF Therapy	02/19/2014	06/01/2017	NCT01945866
AA	Peripheral Diabetic Retinopathy (DR) Lesions on Ultrawide-field Fundus Images and Risk of DR Worsening Over Time	01/01/2015		NA
W	Intravitreous Anti-VEGF Treatment for Prevention of Vision Threatening Diabetic Retinopathy in Eyes at High Risk	01/04/2016	01/04/2022	NCT02634333
AB	Intravitreous Anti-VEGF vs. Prompt Vitrectomy for Vitreous Hemorrhage from Proliferative Diabetic Retinopathy	11/14/2016	01/09/2020	NCT02858076
TX	A Comparative Effectiveness Study of Intravitreal Aflibercept, Bevacizumab and Ranibizumab for Diabetic Macular Edema—Follow-up Extension Study	06/01/2017	04/18/2019	
AC	Randomized Trial of Intravitreous Aflibercept versus Intravitreous Bevacizumab + Deferred Aflibercept for Treatment of Central-Involved Diabetic Macular Edema	12/01/2017		NCT03321513
AD	PROMINENT-Eye Ancillary Study: Diabetic Retinopathy Outcomes in a Randomized Trial of Pemafibrate versus Placebo	12/15/2017	12/31/2018	NCT03345901
AE	A Pilot Study Evaluating Photobiomodulation Therapy for Diabetic Macular Edema	04/09/2019		NCT03866473
AF	A Randomized Trial Evaluating Fenofibrate for Prevention of Diabetic Retinopathy Worsening	03/01/2021		NCT04661358
AK	Home OCT Monitoring System: Feasibility Study	07/13/2021		

Abbreviations: Anti-VEGF, anti-vascular endothelial growth factor; DME, diabetic macular edema; DR, diabetic retinopathy; NSAIDs, nonsteroid antiinflammatory drugs; OCT, optical coherence tomography.

eyes receiving initial ranibizumab therapy for CI-DME were having better long-term vision improvements than eyes managed with laser or triamcinolone plus laser followed by deferred ranibizumab, in terms of persistent thickening and vision impairment.[5]

Protocol T compared the effectiveness of three anti-VEGF reagents including aflibercept, bevacizumab and ranibizumab, for the treatment of CI-DME in a two-year clinical trial. The results showed that within one year of intravitreal anti-VEGF treatment, all three anti-VEGF reagents improved vision in eyes with CI-DME, but the relative effect depended on baseline visual acuity.[6] When the initial visual acuity loss was mild, there were no apparent differences among study groups. At worse levels of baseline visual acuity (20/50 or worse), aflibercept was more effective at improving vision.[6] Two years observation demonstrated all three anti-VEGF groups had visual acuity improvement at 2 years with a decreased number of injections in the second year. Among eyes with worse baseline visual acuity, aflibercept, on average, had superior two-year visual acuity outcomes compared with bevacizumab, but the superiority of aflibercept over ranibizumab, noted at one year, was no longer evident.[7] The cardiovascular thrombotic end point of this study was measured by Anti-platelet Trialists' Collaboration (APTC) event. A higher APTC event rates with ranibizumab over 2 years warrants continued evaluation in future trials.[7] As an extension study of Protocol T, Protocol TX showed 5 years observation for anti-VEGF treatments for DME.[8] The two-thirds of eligible Protocol T participants completed a five-year visit. The mean visual acuity improved from baseline to 5 years without protocol-defined treatment.[8] Although mean retinal thickness was similar at 2 and 5 years, the mean visual acuity worsened during this period. Additional strategies improving long-term outcomes of anti-VEGF therapy in eyes with DME are warranted to maintain better visual acuity.[8]

Protocol S compared the effectiveness of panretinal photocoagulation (PRP) with ranibizumab + PRP in the treatment of proliferative diabetic retinopathy (PDR). The two-year results showed that treatment with ranibizumab resulted in visual acuity that was not inferior to PRP treatment at two years.[9] Although longer-term follow-up is needed, ranibizumab may be a reasonable treatment alternative for patients with PDR.[10] Five-year follow-up in Protocol S showed that although loss to follow-up was relatively high, visual acuity in most study eyes that completed follow-up was very good at 5 years and was similar in both groups.[11] Severe vision loss or serious PDR complications were uncommon with PRP or ranibizumab; however, the ranibizumab group had lower rates of developing vision-impairing DME and less visual field loss. Patient-specific factors, including anticipated visit compliance, cost, and frequency of visits, should be considered when choosing treatment for patients with PDR. These findings support either anti-VEGF therapy or PRP as viable treatments for patients with PDR.[11]

As for vitreous hemorrhage from PDR, Protocol AB showed, there was no statistically significant difference in the primary outcome of mean visual acuity letter score over 24 weeks following initial treatment with intravitreal aflibercept versus vitrectomy with PRP.[12] Both initial aflibercept and vitrectomy with PRP are viable approaches for PDR-related vitreous hemorrhage. However, the study may have been underpowered, considering the range of the 95% confidence interval (CI), to detect a clinically important benefit in favor of initial vitrectomy with PRP. Further analysis demonstrated that eyes receiving initial vitrectomy with PRP had faster recovery of vision over 24 weeks when baseline visual acuity was worse than 20/800 and faster vitreous hemorrhage clearance.[13] Approximately one-third of the eyes in each group received the alternative treatment (aflibercept or vitrectomy with PRP).

Protocol V compared the changes of vision at 2 years among eyes with CI-DME and good visual acuity, which were managed with aflibercept, laser photocoagulation, or observation.[14] The results showed that among eyes with CI-DME and good visual acuity, there was no significant difference in vision loss at 2 years whether eyes were initially managed with aflibercept or with laser photocoagulation or observation and given aflibercept only if visual acuity worsened.[14] Thus, for patients with relatively good vision, observation without treatment unless visual acuity worsens may be a reasonable strategy for CI-DME.

Protocol U studied the effect of adding dexamethasone to continued ranibizumab treatment in patients with persistent DME. The data showed that the addition of intravitreal dexamethasone to continued ranibizumab therapy (combo-therapy) does not improve visual acuity at 24 weeks relative to continued ranibizumab therapy alone among eyes with persistent DME following anti-VEGF therapy. However, the addition of dexamethasone is more likely to reduce retinal thickness in persistent DME treated with several anti-VEGF injections.[15] The clinical trials of an anti-VEGF drug in combination with dexamethasone for treatment-naïve DME or refractory DME were conducted to determine whether the combo-therapy as a primary treatment or a sequential therapy can provide additional benefit to treatment with anti-VEGF agents alone.

Protocol W determined the efficacy of intravitreal aflibercept injections compared with sham treatment in preventing potentially vision-threatening complications in eyes with moderate to severe nonproliferative diabetic retinopathy (NPDR).[16] In this randomized clinical trial, among eyes with moderate to severe NPDR, the proportion of eyes that developed PDR or vision-reducing CI-DME was lower with periodic aflibercept compared with sham treatment. However, through 2 years, preventive treatment did not confer visual acuity benefit compared with observation plus treatment with aflibercept only after the development of PDR or vision-reducing CI-DME.[16]

Protocol AE studied the photobiomodulation (PBM) therapy for CI-DME with good visual acuity and found PBM therapy was safe and well tolerated but was not found to be effective in further improving visual acuity.[17]

Targeting VEGF family

VEGF plays a causal role in inducing blood–retinal barrier (BRB) breakdown, macular edema, and angiogenesis.[18] The identification of VEGF as a key mediator in the pathogenesis of DR and DME has revolutionized the management of this sight-threatening disease. Because of superior anatomic and functional outcomes, anti-VEGF agents have rapidly replaced macular laser photocoagulation as the first-line therapy in the treatment of CI-DME and have become a crucial alternative therapy for vision-threatening DR. Current anti-VEGF treatment comprises intravitreal aflibercept, ranibizumab, conbercept, and off-label use of bevacizumab as introduced in Chapter 1.[8,19–23]

Development of anti-VEGF treatment

Anti-VEGF therapy has created a paradigm shift for treating various retinochoroidal disorders.[24] The commercially available anti-VEGF drugs differ in molecular structure, molecular weight, receptor binding affinity, VEGF isoforms being targeted, production methods, etc (see Table 9.2 and Chapter 1). There are several clinical limitations to current anti-VEGF treatment, including (1) most patients need repeated injections; (2) for patients with persistent DME, 31.6%−65.6% edema still exists even after regular monthly intravitreal injection for at least four injections within 24 weeks;[25] (3) some patients respond incompletely or are unresponsive to anti-VEGF treatment (nonresponders); and (4) the high cost of multiple anti-VEGF treatments. These limitations demand the development of other treatment strategies, such as increasing doses of each anti-VEGF treatment, improving treatment durability, developing biosimilars to reduce cost of current anti-VEGF drugs, and exploring other novel treatments and new delivery routes.

The current trend for anti-VEGF development is toward either smaller molecular weight targeting VEGF-A (e.g., Beovu and abicipar), fusion proteins targeting VEGF-A in combination with other factors (e.g., faricimab), or targeting other VEGF family members such as VEGF-C and VEGF-D. The following are new agents under development:

OPT-302 (Opthea; Victoria, Australia) is a soluble form of VEGF receptor 3 (VEGFR-3) comprising the extracellular domains 1−3 of human VEGFR-3 and the Fc fragment of human IgG1. OPT-302 is being explored as an adjuvant intravitreal injection for patients undergoing standard anti-VEGF therapies. OPT-302 blocks the activity of the proteins VEGF-C and VEGF-D, which cause blood vessels to grow and leak and contribute to the pathophysiology of retinal diseases.[26] OPT-302 may serve a complementary therapeutic role in VEGF-mediated DR pathogenesis and overcome some limitations of therapies that only target VEGF-A in neovascular eye diseases. Intravitreal OPT-302 inhibition of VEGF-C and -D was well tolerated, and OPT-302 combination therapy may overcome an escape mechanism to VEGF-A suppression in the management of neovascular age-related macular degeneration (nAMD).[26] A multicenter phase 1b/2a trial has evaluated OPT-302 in combination with aflibercept for refractory DME.[27]

Combo-therapy targeting all the VEGF family members might be beneficial to patients with fundus vascular diseases. In mammals, the VEGF family has five members, that is, VEGF-A, VEGF-B, VEGF-C, VEGF-D, and placental growth factor

Table 9.2 Anti-VEGF biosimilars.

Anti-VEGF biosimilars		Manufacturer	Status
Biosimilar to ranibizumab	Razumab	Intas Pharmaceuticals Ltd., India	Approved by DGCI in 2015
	Ranizurel/R-TPR-024	Reliance Life Sciences, India	Approved by DGCI in 2020
	SB11 Byooviz	Samsung Bioepis, South Korea	US FDA (2021), EMA (2021)
	FYB201	Formycon AG/Bioeq	BLA review accepted by FDA
	Xlucane	Xbrane Biopharma, Sweden	Phase 3 trial active
	SJP-0133/ GBS-007	Senju Pharmaceutical, Japan	Phase 3 trial completed; results awaited
	LUBT010	Lupin Ltd., India	Phase 3 trial active; recruitment completed
	CKD-701	Chong Kun Dang, South Korea	Phase 3 trial completed
	PF582	Pfenex, USA	Phase 1/2 trial completed; on hold
	BCD100	BIOCND, South Korea; Qilu Pharmaceuticals, China	Phase 3 clinical trial active; recruiting
Biosimilar to aflibercept	MYL-1701P	Momenta Pharmaceuticals and Mylan NV, USA	Phase 3 trial completed
	ABP-938	Amgen, USA	Phase 3 trial active; recruitment stage
	FYB203	Formycon AG/Bioeq, Germany	Phase 3 trial active; recruitment stage
	SB-15	Samsung Bioepis Co. Ltd, South Korea	Phase 3 trial active; recruitment stage
	SOK583A19	Sandoz, Switzerland	Phase 3 trial active; recruitment stage
	CT-P42	Celltrion, South Korea	Phase 3 trial active; recruitment stage
	ALT-L9	Alteogen, South Korea	Phase 1 trial begun; not yet recruiting
	OT-702	Ocumension Therapeutics/ Shandong Boan Biological Technology, China	Phase 3 trial active

DGCI, *Directorate General Commercial Intelligence;* EMA, *European Medicines Agency;* FDA, *Food and Drug Administration.*

(PlGF). Both aflibercept and conbercept can bind VEGF-A, -B and PlGF, while OPT-302 binds VEGF-C and -D. Thus, the strategy of combo-therapy using aflibercept or conbercept with OPT-302 is worth trying.

KSI-301 (KODIAK sciences, Palo Alto, CA) is an investigational anti-VEGF therapy, built on Kodiak's Antibody Biopolymer Conjugate Platform. It is designed to maintain potent and effective drug levels in ocular tissues.[28,29] It has two components comprising a specific anti-VEGF IgG1 antibody and an inert immune effector. These two components are covalently and stably linked to a high molecular weight phosphorycholine biopolymer (950 kDa). Increasing the molecular weight of intravitreal drugs is one of the approaches to increase injection interval, since larger molecules are known to enhance intraocular stability. The prolonged intravitreal half-life, due to slow diffusion in the vitreous cavity and decreased elimination by both anterior and posterior routes,[30,31] could create a high intraocular durability of intravitreal KSI-301. It is designed to have a duration of approximately 6 months. Clinical trials called GLEAM study and GLIMMER study are underway. Phase-3 of multicenter, randomized studies aim to evaluate the safety, efficacy, and durability of KSI-301 in treatment-naïve patients with DME. In each of these studies, patients are randomized to receive either intravitreal KSI-301 or aflibercept. Patients will be administered KSI-301 every 8—24 weeks after three loading doses and aflibercept every 8 weeks after five loading doses.[32] However, a randomized, double-masked, active comparator-controlled Phase 2b/3 clinical trial of KSI-301 in patients with nAMD did not meet the primary endpoint.[33] The results show that, although KSI-301 demonstrated strong durability and was safe and well tolerated, it did not meet the primary efficacy endpoint of showing visual acuity gains for subjects dosed on extended regimens compared to aflibercept given every 8 weeks.

Abicipar pegol (AGN-150998, Allergan plc/Molecular Partners) belongs to a family of the designed ankyrin repeat proteins (DARPin) which are composed of several ankyrin repeats bound to a 20 kDa polyethylene glycol (PEG) tail. Abicipar pegol specifically binds with high affinity to all soluble isoforms of VEGF-A.[34] It has improved pharmacokinetic properties compared with ranibizumab as it has a lower molecular weight (34 vs. 48 kDa), higher target binding affinity (2 vs. 46 pM) and longer ocular half-life ($\geq$13 vs. 7 days in the aqueous humor).[35–37] In phase I/II, open-label, multicenter dose-escalation trial for DME, a single intraocular injection of abicipar pegol (0.4 mg) resulted in levels higher than the half-maximal inhibitory concentration of VEGF in aqueous humor for 8—12 weeks.[36] Although there was prolonged edema reduction and visual improvement in several patients, ocular inflammation was a major concern.[36] In the phase II REACH study (NCT01397409), abicipar pegol showed a favorite profile in terms of the improvement of visual acuity and central retinal thickness up to 20 weeks when intravitreally injected at baseline and 4 and 8 month time points, compared to monthly ranibizumab intravitreal injections in nAMD.[35,38] Phase III clinical trials, SEQUOIA (NCT02462486) and CEDAR (NCT02462928), evaluating abicipar pegol given every 2—3 months in nAMD patients demonstrated non-inferior in improving visual acuity compared with monthly treatment of ranibizumab.[38,39] However, it failed to gain the Food and Drug Administration (FDA) approval in 2020 due to significant intraocular inflammation (8.9%−15.4%) and an unfavorable risk−benefit ratio.[39,40] Abicipar pegol, as the smaller, longer lasting anti-VEGF biologics, might offer an exciting opportunity to increase the timeframe between intravitreal injections, and the two-year results from two multicenter, randomized, phase 3 clinical trials with identical protocols (CEDAR and SEQUOIA) showed efficacy of abicipar pegol in the treatment of nAMD given every 8 or 12 weeks.[40] The extended duration of effect of abicipar allows for quarterly dosing and reduced treatment burden.[40] Further knowledge of the efficacy and safety of abicipar pegol is needed before its approval for the treatment of DR.[41]

Anti-VEGF biosimilars

The recombinant anti-VEGF drugs, including Lucentis (Ranibizumab), Eylea (Aflibercept), Lumitin (Conbercept), Beovu (Brolucizumab), and off-label Avastin (Bevacizumab) are used worldwide because the anti-VEGF therapy can significantly improve visual outcomes in patients with nAMD and DME. These anti-VEGF medications have been available for more than a decade, and their patent expiration dates are coming. In fact, bevacizumab's patent expired in July 2019 in the United States (2022 in the European Union), ranibizumab's patent expired in June 2020 in the United States (2022 in the European Union), and aflibercept's patent will expire in 2023 in the United States (2025 in the European Union). 42 With the expiry of these patents, biosimilars can be used as a suitable and cheaper alternative. The transition to biosimilars can have a substantial impact all over the world because of the favorable cost-effectiveness.[43]

According to the World Health Organization (WHO), biosimilars are defined as biotechnological products that[44] are highly similar to a biological product already approved by the FDA (reference product) and have no clinically meaningful differences in terms of safety, purity, and potency (i.e., safety and effectiveness), in addition to meeting other criteria specified by law.[45] Thus, anti-VEGF biosimilars should demonstrate similarities in pharmacokinetics, pharmacodynamics, safety, and efficacy that resemble approved reference biologics (anti-VEGF drugs).[46] Biosimilars are increasing competition among biologics. Patients and physicians can expect the same safety and effectiveness from the biosimilar over the course of treatment as from the reference product. Biosimilars hold the potential to reduce the financial burden of the highly efficacious biologic therapy in retinal pathologies.[47] As more and more patents of anti-VEGF agents are expiring, the production of biosimilars is bound to increase in the future.

Many bevacizumab biosimilars have already been approved for the treatment of various cancers. However, due to the better cost-effectiveness of bevacizumab than ranibizumab, its off-label use in ophthalmology is still increasing.[43]

Currently, there are several anti-VEGF biosimilars to ranibizumab and aflibercept in the development stage or acquiring approval (Table 9.2).[43] Razumab (Intas Pharmaceutical Ltd, Ahmedabad, GJ, India) is the first biosimilar to ranibizumab that has been approved for ophthalmic use; it is approved for use in India by the drug controller general of India for nAMD, myopic choroidal neovascularization (CNV), DME, and retinal vein occlusion-macular edema (RVO-ME).[43,46,48,49] In 2021, the US FDA approved Byooviz (ranibizumab-nuna) as the first biosimilar to Lucentis (ranibizumab injection) for the treatment of several eye diseases, including nAMD, RVO-ME, and CNV. Byooviz (SB11), from Samsung Bioepis, South Korea, has been approved by the US FDA and European Medicines Agency (EMA).[50] Other biosimilars to ranibizumab (FYB201, Germany; R TPR 024 and Lupin's ranibizumab, India; Xlucane, Sweden; SB11, and SJP-0133, Japan) are in the advanced stages of clinical trials.[51] As for aflibercept biosimilars, ABP-938 (Amgen, USA) is under phase 3 trial, and the study is scheduled to be completed by July 2023 (NCT04270747). A randomized multicentric trial with 566 patients of nAMD is included. These patients will receive either injections of ABP-938 or aflibercept (randomized 1:1) every 8 weeks. The subjects receiving aflibercept will again be randomized 1:1 at 16 weeks, with 50% of patients being switched to ABP-938 injection. The patients will receive injections every 8 weeks for 48 weeks with follow up until 52 weeks. Other biosimilars to aflibercept (MYL-1710P, ABP-938, and CHS-2020, USA; FYB203, Germany; SB15, South Korea) are also in advanced stages of clinical trials.[51]

Targeting HIF-1α

Hypoxia-inducible factors (HIFs) are the key regulators of oxygen homeostasis in response to hypoxia. In the course of diabetes, the retina is hypoxic, but adaptive responses to hypoxia are impaired due to insufficient activation of HIF signaling. This impaired adaptive response to hypoxia contributes to diabetic pathology, including DR.[52]

In fact, HIF-1α expression was found to be significantly higher in the vitreous of patients with PDR compared with the patients with NPDR.[53,54] Furthermore, the expression of HIF-1α and VEGF was demonstrated to be higher in active PDR than in quiescent PDR.[54,55] These findings suggest that HIF-1α is a key regulator in the development of retinal neovascularization during hypoxia; therefore, strategies designed to target HIF-1α may lead to more effective treatments for pathologic angiogenesis of PDR. Most importantly, the HIF-1α/VEGF mechanistic pathways leading to DR progression share incredible similarity with pathogenic events of cancer. The cancer research has prompted us to study the feasibility of anti-HIF-1α for treating neovascular events of DR.[56,57] HIF-1α inhibition can be achieved by several mechanisms: (1) inhibition of HIF-1α mRNA expression;[58–60] (2) inhibition of HIF-1α protein expression;[61] (3) promotion of HIF-1α protein degradation;[62–64] (4) inhibition of HIF-1α and HIF-1β dimerization;[65] and (5) inhibition of HIF-1α DNA-binding activity.[66–68]

Inhibition of HIF-1α mRNA by RNA interference significantly reduced retinal neovascularization in C57BL/6J mice with ischemic retinopathy.[58] A reagent such as EZN-2968, an antisense oligonucleotide inhibitor of HIF-1α, demonstrated a reduction of HIF-1α mRNA and protein expression in a pilot trial for patients with refractory solid tumors.[60]

Cardiac glycosides, such as Digoxin and Cedilanid, are effective inhibitors of HIF-1α transcriptional activity and can inhibit tumor metastasis by inhibiting HIF-1α.[61] In mouse models with ischemic retinopathy, intraocular or intraperitoneal injection of Digoxin markedly reduced retinal levels of HIF-1α protein and mRNAs and resulted in the suppression of retinal and CNV.[69] In the C57BL/6 mouse model of oxygen-induced retinopathy (OIR), retinal neovascular areas and obliterative areas were significantly reduced after injection with Cedilanid compared with control mice.[70]

β-Lapachone, a quinone-containing compound, is a substrate of NAD(P)H: quinone oxidoreductase (NQO1) that can inhibit retinal neovascularization by promoting HIF-1α protein degradation. In the OIR mice model, intraocular administration of β-lapachone results in significant reduction in hypoxia-induced retinal neovascularization without retinal toxicity or perturbation of developmental retinal angiogenesis.[64]

Scutellarin, a flavone glycoside, was reported to reduce VEGF expression by promoting HIF-1α protein degradation.[62] Unlike β-lapachone, scutellarin not only enhances HIF-1α protein degradation but also interrupts the interaction between HIF-1α and P300, a coactivator, thus, reducing the transcriptional activity of HIF-1α and exerting antiangiogenic effects.[62]

Acriflavine, a mixture of trypaflavin (3,6-diamino-10-methylacridinium chloride) and proflavine (3,6-diaminoacridine), was found to inhibit tumor growth and angiogenesis by binding to HIF-1α and preventing HIF-1α dimerization with HIF-1β in a xenograft tumor model.[71] In the OIR mouse model, intraocular injection of acriflavine prevented the dimerization of HIF-1α and HIF-1β. Blocking the transcriptional activation of HIF-1α and reducing the expression of multiple HIF-1α-mediated genes including angiopoietin-2 (Ang-2), platelet-derived growth factor-B (PDGF-B), and VEGF-A, resulted in reduced angiogenesis in the OIR mice.[65]

Since HIF-1α upregulation plays a pivotal role in the pathogenesis of DR, targeting of HIF-1α or blocking the HIF-1α pathway may lead to more effective treatment for DR. It should be concerned about off-target effects of HIF-1α inhibition to treat DR. Since HIF-1α is an upstream transcription factor affecting many key genes, its inhibition might cause unwanted effects. The efficacy and safety of HIF-1α inhibitors require more work before moving from bench to bedside.

Targeting VEGFRs

VEGFRs (VEGFR1 and VEGFR2) mediate the signaling transduction of VEGF-A, -B and PlGF. Inhibition of VEGFRs is one of the promising strategies for the treatment of VEGF-driven neovascular diseases.[72–76] Targeting VEGFRs has been extensively studied in clinical oncology. There are several approaches to inhibiting VEGFR signaling, that is, VEGFR antibodies, VEGFR allosteric inhibitors, and inhibition of the intracellular tyrosine kinase of VEGFR by small molecules (tyrosine kinase inhibitors, TKIs).

VEGFR antibody

Tanibirumab (TTAC-0001), a humanized monoclonal antibody, specifically binds VEGFR-2 and is currently being developed in preclinical stage by PharmAbcine (Daejon, Korea).[73] The preclinical pharmacokinetics, interspecies scaling, and pharmacokinetics of a phase 1 clinical trial of TTAC-0001 were reported and designed for first-in-human studies.[77]

Ramucirumab (Cyramza), a fully humanized anti-VEGFR2 monoclonal antibody, has been approved for the treatment of cancer, such as advanced or metastatic gastric cancer or gastroesophageal junction adenocarcinoma in patients who experience disease progression on or after fluoropyrimidine- or platinum-containing chemotherapy.[74] It deserves to try its ophthalmic use for retinal vascular diseases.

VEGFR allosteric inhibitor

The VEGF-A/VEGFR2 complex is the major signaling pathway involved in angiogenesis. The inhibition of their downstream events causes reduced vessel sprouting, retarding tumor growth, and progression of inflammatory disorders. VEGF-A/VEGFR2 signaling requires receptor dimerization and a well-defined orientation of monomers in the active dimer. The extracellular portion of the receptor is composed of seven Ig-like domains, among which domain 2 (D2) and D3 are the ligand-binding domains, while D4 and D7 establish homotypic contacts. The extracellular portions of the receptor allosterically regulate receptor activity. The allosteric targeting of D4 and D7 of VEGFR2 represents a promising alternative treatment for neovascular disorders without direct binding to VEGF.[75,78]

Tyrosine kinase inhibitors for VEGFRs

The activation of VEGFRs upon binding VEGF is involved in the pathogenesis of retinal vascular diseases and microinflammation.[79,80] Binding of VEGF to its receptors, VEGFR1/2, induces dimerization and activation of the tyrosine kinase domain of the VEGF receptor, resulting in autophosphorylation of tyrosine residues. The phosphorylated tyrosine residues are used as docking sites for signaling proteins that relay the transduction signals for cell proliferation, migration, tube formation, and increased permeability of vascular endothelial cells. Thus, inhibition of VEGF receptor activation using TKIs might provide an alternative approach for treating retinal vascular diseases, including DME and nAMD.[76]

GB-102 (GrayBug Vision; Redwood City, CA) is sunitinib maleate, a TKI with activity against both VEGF-A and PDGF. The drug is encapsulated within bioerodible polymer nanoparticles that degrade slowly over time.[81] After injection, it forms a depot in the inferior vitreous, which gradually biodegrades over time and functions as a durable method of antiangiogenesis. GB-102 treatment can last up to 6 months with comparable visual acuity and central subfield thickness (CST) outcomes before another dose is required.[29,82] Phase 1/2a study (ADAGIO) results reported that 88% of the nAMD patients at 3 months and 68% of the patients at

6 months were maintained on a single dose of GB-102.[83] Some patients maintained positive outcomes as far as 8 months.[83] Of the emerging therapies, GB-102 has by far the longest duration between treatments, which would have a significant impact on the patient's life with less frequent follow-up and less expenditure.[83]

X-82 (Tyrogenex) is an oral anti-PDGF and VEGF-A inhibitor. In a Phase 1 dose-escalation study (NCT02348359) for nAMD, 10 of 35 patients (29%) did not complete the 24-week endpoint, with six (17%) withdrawing due to adverse events, including diarrhea, nausea, fatigue, and transaminase elevation.[84] Phase 2 APEX study (NCT02348359) comparing X-82 (Tyrogenex) with as-needed aflibercept injections to aflibercept monotherapy is underway.

PAN-90806 (PanOptica; Mount Arlington, NJ), a TKI eyedrop, has been shown to produce anti-VEGF-A biological signaling with topical once daily dosing, according to a phase 1/2 study (NCT03479372). PAN-90806 shows potential as a monotherapy treatment for nAMD and for prophylaxis or chronic maintenance. This topical anti-VEGF eyedrop has demonstrated safety and biological response as monotherapy. However, it may be only appropriate for certain patients, as seen in the results of the masked review and further studies are needed to confirm these findings.[29]

Pazopanib (GlaxoSmithKline) is a topical VEGF-A TKI, inhibiting both VEGF-A and PDGF. Phase 2b trial results were released in 2015. At the 52-week endpoint in a 510-patient study for nAMD, pazopanib QID (4 times daily) combined with as-needed ranibizumab was found to be noninferior to ranibizumab dosed as-needed or monthly; however, the addition of pazopanib did not decrease the number of as-needed ranibizumab injections by >50% (the prespecified minimum criterion of efficacy). There was no significant difference in retinal thickness and size of lesion between the pazopanib group, with allowance for as-needed ranibizumab injections, and the monthly ranibizumab treatment groups.[85]

Targeting VEGF coreceptor or auxiliary proteins
Targeting neuropilin1/2

Vesencumab is a human IgG1 monoclonal antibody against neuropilin-1 (NRP1), with potential anti-angiogenic and anti-neoplastic activities. NRP1 is a membrane-bound coreceptor normally expressed by endothelial cells and plays a role in angiogenesis, cell survival, migration, and invasion (see Fig. 7.1 of Chapter 7). Vesencumab specifically targets and binds to NRP1; the antibody-NRP1 complex prevents the subsequent coupling of NRP1 to VEGFR2, thereby potentially inhibiting VEGF-mediated signaling and preventing angiogenesis. In combination with other anti-VEGF therapies, vesencumab may enhance their anti-angiogenic effect.[86] Vesencumab is currently undergoing clinical study for cancer patients.[87]

Targeting integrin

Integrins, members of a family of heterodimeric, noncovalently bound cell adhesion proteins, are transmembrane receptors consisting of a larger α subunit and a smaller β subunit. Integrins serve as physical and biochemical bridges between cells and regulate cellular interaction through signal transduction pathways with surrounding cells and with the extracellular matrix.[88] Physiologically, they play important roles in cell adhesion, proliferation, shape, and motility. They are involved in a variety of biological processes and are also central to the etiology and pathology of many diseases. Some integrins are closely associated with vitreolysis, choroidal and retinal angiogenesis, as well as ocular surface diseases.[89] For example, integrins αvβ3, αvβ5, and α5β1 are closely associated with CNV in nAMD,[90,91] and increased levels of αvβ3, αvβ5, and α5 integrins have been reported in fibrovascular membranes (FVMs) of individuals with PDR.[90] Leukocytes adhesion and leukostasis are the early pathologic features of DR,[92] in which integrins play a critical role. In experimental DR models, integrin-mediated adherence of leukocytes to the retinal vasculature was observed.[93,94] Anti-intercellular adhesion molecule 1 (anti-ICAM-1) or anti-β2-integrin decreased leukocyte adhesion, endothelial cell death, and BRB breakdown.[92–94] Therefore, targeting integrins, independent of anti-VEGF therapies has the potential to halt vision loss (see Chapter 10). Many anti-integrin treatments have undergone clinical trials for DME (Table 9.3) and preclinical studies for other retinal vascular diseases (Table 9.4).

Risuteganib (RSG; also known as Luminate, ALG-1001, Allegro Ophthalmics, LLC, San Juan Capistrano, CA) is an engineered arginyl-glycyl-aspartic acid (RGD) class synthetic peptide that modulates integrin receptors. RGD peptide

Table 9.3 Summary of major clinical trials of integrin inhibitors for diabetic macular edema.

Drug/ Company	Target integrin receptors	Trial stage	Key findings
Risuteganib/ Allegro Ophthalmics	αvβ3, αvβ5, α5β1, and α5β3	Ph 2	Intravitreal risuteganib was well-tolerated with no drug toxicity or intraocular inflammation and showed 12-week durability after the completion of three loading doses.[95]
THR-687/ Oxurion	αvβ3, αvβ5, and α5β1	Ph 1	THR-687 was found to be safe and well-tolerated with no dose-limiting toxicities or serious adverse events.[96,97]
SF-0166/ SciFluor Life Sci.	αvβ3, αvβ6, and αvβ8	Ph 1/2	Treatment with SF-0166 was associated with a reduction in retinal thickness of 53% of patients with improvement in visual acuity.[98]

Table 9.4 Summary of preclinical investigational integrin inhibitors.

Drug/ Company	Target integrin receptors	Preclinical animal models	Key findings
SB-267268/ GlaxoSmithKline	αvβ3 and αvβ5	ROP mouse model	Reduced pathologic angiogenesis and lowered VEGF and VEGFR2 mRNA levels[99]
AXT-107/ AsclepiX Therapeutics	αvβ3 and α5β1	Ang-2-transgenic mouse model and LPS-induced inflammation model	Inhibited vascular leakage and inflammation[100]
JNJ-26076713/ Johnson & Johnson Pharmaceutical	αvβ3 and αvβ5	ROP mouse model and diabetic rats	Inhibited retinal neovascularization and retinal vascular permeability[101]
Cilengitide/ Merck-Serono	αvβ3	Tenascin-C knockout and tenascin-C silenced mouse model	Inhibited CNV formation[102]
Lebecetin/SATT Lutech	αvβ1, and αv-containing integrins	Mouse CNV and ROP mouse model	Inhibited choroidal and retinal neovascularization[103]

Abbreviations: Ang-2, *angiopoietin-2;* CNV, *choroidal neovascularization;* LPS, *lipopolysaccharide;* ROP, *retinopathy of prematurity;* VEGF, *vascular endothelial growth factor;* VEGFR2, *vascular endothelial growth factor receptor 2.*

treatment suppresses retinal neovascularization and facilitates the release of cellular adhesion between the vitreous and the retina, inducing posterior vitreous detachment (PVD).[104,105] Risuteganib has potential as a therapy for DR and DME.[89,106]

SB-267268 (GlaxoSmithKline) is a small molecule antagonist of αvβ3 and αvβ5 integrins.[99] In *in vitro* studies, SB-267268 is found to be 1,000-fold selective in binding to αvβ3 and αvβ5 receptors compared to other integrins αIIbβ3, α5β1, and α3β1. In an animal model of retinopathy of prematurity (ROP), SB-267268 reduced pathologic angiogenesis by 50%, along with a decrease in VEGF and VEGFR2 messenger RNA.[99] The clinical trials of integrin inhibitors for DME are summarized in Table 9.3.

Targeting Ang-2/tyrosine kinase with immunoglobulin-like and EGF-like domains 2 (Tie2) system

The angiopoietin (Ang)/Tie2 pathway is a therapeutic target for the treatment of retinal vascular diseases (see Chapters 7 and 10). Angiopoietin-1 (Ang-1) and Ang-2 ligands compete for the Tie2 receptor. Tie2 is a tyrosine kinase receptor located predominantly on vascular endothelial cells that plays a central role in vascular stability. Activated Tie2 increases endothelial cell survival, adhesion, and cell junction integrity, thereby stabilizing the vasculature, while Ang-2 interferes with the Ang-1/Tie2 axis, resulting in vascular leakage. Vascular endothelial-protein tyrosine phosphatase (VE-PTP), an endothelial cell-specific phosphatase forms a complex with Tie2, dephosphorylates Tie2, and thus, like Ang-2, acts to oppose the actions of Ang-1.[107] Ang-1 stimulates Tie2 phosphorylation in endothelial cells, but unlike VEGF, it does not promote endothelial cell proliferation or tube formation. Ang-2 and VE-PTP are negative regulators increased by hypoxia. They inactivate Tie2, destabilizing the vasculature and increasing responsiveness to VEGF and other inflammatory cytokines that stimulate vascular leakage and neovascularization.

In DR, there is an increased production of Ang-2, competing with Ang-1 for binding Tie2 and reducing phosphorylation of Tie2, whereas VE-PTP directly reduces phosphorylation of Tie2. Inactivation of Tie2 destabilizes the vasculature, resulting in pericyte dropout, reduction of endothelial cell viability, endothelial cell adherence to extracellular matrix, cell junction integrity, and increased responsiveness to VEGF and other proangiogenic/permeability factors. Thus, activating the Tie2 signaling pathway, by inhibiting Ang-2 or VE-PTP, should be a therapeutic strategy for retinal vascular diseases, such as DME, PDR, and nAMD.

Targeting Ang-2

Nesvacumab (Regeneron, Tarrytown, NY, USA) is a fully human IgG1 monoclonal antibody that selectively binds Ang-2 with high affinity and specifically blocks Ang-2 binding to the Tie2 receptor. Nesvacumab was coformulated with aflibercept with goal of increasing the duration of aflibercept's antipermeability effect but failed to show benefit over aflibercept monotherapy in achieving visual gains in phase 2 studies of nAMD and DME.[108]

AXT107 (Asclepix Therapeutics, Baltimore, MD, USA) is a peptide derived from the noncollagenous domain of collagen IV.[108] AXT107 promotes conversion of Ang-2 into a Tie2 agonist and blocks signaling through VEGFR2 and other receptor tyrosine kinases.[108] AXT107 modifies Ang-2 to act more like Ang-1 by enabling Tie2 activation instead of blocking its activity. In the presence of Ang-2 and AXT107, $\alpha5\beta1$ integrin is disrupted, which promotes clustering of Tie2 at junctions and converts Ang-2 into a strong agonist, similar to responses observed when Ang-1 levels greatly exceed those of Ang-2.[100] Currently, AXT107 is in the preclinical phase of study.[108]

Targeting VE-PTP

ARP-1536 (Aerpio Therapeutics, Cincinnati, OH, USA) is a novel monoclonal antibody that activates the Tie2 receptor by targeting VE-PTP. ARP-1536 is intravitreally administered, currently undergoing preclinical studies.[81]

AKB-9778 (Aerpio Therapeutics, Cincinnati, OH, USA) is a small molecule antagonist of VE-PTP, which increases phosphorylation of Tie2 even in the presence of high Ang-2 levels. AKB-9778 differs from ARP-1536 in that it is administered by subcutaneous injection. In preclinical studies, AKB-9778 reduced VEGF-induced leakage and ocular neovascularization and showed additive benefit when combined with VEGF suppression.[109] AKB-9778, when combined with monthly ranibizumab, reduced DME more effectively than ranibizumab monotherapy in a phase 2 study.[110]

Bispecific drug

Faricimab, previously known as RG7716 (Roche, Basel, Switzerland and Genentech, South San Francisco, CA, USA), is a bispecific antibody that simultaneously binds both VEGF-A and Ang-2. Phase 3 trials for DME (YOSEMITE NCT03622580 and RHINE NCT03622593) showed robust vision gains and anatomical improvements in patients treated with faricimab, and the personalized treatment interval was extended to 16 weeks, demonstrating the potential for faricimab to extend the duration of the treatment regimen for patients with DME.[111] Faricimab was approved by the US FDA in February 2022 (see Chapters 7 and 10).

Other targets

ICON-1, a product of Iconic Therapeutics (South San Francisco, CA), is a recombinant modified factor VIIIa protein linked with the Fc portion of a human immunoglobulin G1. ICON-1 binds to tissue factor (also called coagulation factor III) that is overexpressed in CNV in nAMD but does not interfere with normal blood coagulation. The Fc portion of this molecule can bind to the Fc receptor of cells like natural killer cells and prompt antibody-dependent cellular toxicity to suppress CNV. There is potential for ICON-1 to be combined with existing anti-VEGF medication. Currently, an antitissue factor monoclonal antibody ICON-4 is being evaluated as a potential therapy for nAMD with clinical trials that started in 2020.[29]

AKST4290 (formerly ALK4290) is an oral treatment that targets eotaxin, an immunomodulatory chemokine that is highly expressed in CNV, choroidal endothelial cells, and in the circulation in nAMD. The increased eotaxin and C—C chemokine receptor type 3 (CCR3) lead to increase in membrane permeability and degradation, and immune cell recruitment. The agent is an inhibitor against CCR3, which is the natural receptor for eotaxin. CCR3 and its ligand C—C motif chemokine ligand 11 (CCL11, also known as eotaxin-1) are expressed in neovascular lesions, and CCL11 levels are increased in choroidal endothelial cells and systemic circulations in patients with nAMD.[29] AKST4290 ameliorates inflammatory cytokines in preclinical models.

DE-122 (Carotuximab), from Santen (Osaka, Japan) and TRACON Pharmaceuticals (San Diego, CA), is an antibody to endoglin, a protein that plays a critical role in angiogenesis. Endoglin is a growth factor that is expressed in the endothelium.[112]

Endoglin has been shown to release angiogenic factors from inflammatory cells in vivo. Endoglin is elevated in endothelial cells of choroidal neovascular membranes. DE-122 is undergoing clinical evaluation.

Targeting inflammation

Corticosteroids

Difluprednate (difluprednisolone butyrate acetate, DFBA) is an anti-inflammatory steroid, which is effective in the treatment of anterior uveitis, postoperative ocular inflammation, and pain.[113,114] Difluprednate ophthalmic emulsion 0.05% (Durezol (TM), Sirion Therapeutics Inc., USA) effectively reduces refractory DME postvitrectomy[115] and diffuses DME without surgical intervention.[116] In another clinical study, 20 patients with persistent DME who were treated with difluprednate ophthalmic emulsion (0.05%) achieved improved visual acuity and decreased retinal thickness.[117]

Topical dexamethasone-cyclodextrin eye drops are well tolerated and decrease central macular thickness (CMT), and improve visual acuity in DME.[118] In a randomized, controlled trial, topical 1.5% dexamethasone γ-cyclodextrin nanoparticle eye drops significantly improved visual acuity and decreased macular thickness in patients with DME.[119] However, the potential side effect of increased intraocular pressure limits the use of steroids, thus, it is considered only as an adjunct therapy for DME.[117]

Nonsteroid anti-inflammatory drugs

Nonsteroid anti-inflammatory drugs (NSAIDs) were reported effective in DME with various and heterogeneous results. NSAIDs inhibit the cyclooxygenase (COX) enzyme system, that is, an essential mediator of ocular inflammation through the regulation of prostaglandin-dependent pathways.[120]

Bromfenac acts primarily on COX-2[121] and nepafenac, a prodrug through its active metabolite amfenac, inhibits the activity of COX-1 and COX-2.[122] In a pilot study, topical bromfenac significantly reduced CMT in patients with DME, however, without obvious effect on visual acuity.[123] The safety and efficacy of topical nepafenac 0.1% were tested in six eyes of five patients for the treatment of DME. The results showed that topical nepafenac treatment improved vision and decreased retinal thickness.[124] Topical nepafenac was reported to have a significant effect on narrowing retinal arteriolar diameter and on reducing CMT in eyes with mild DR during six-week follow-up.[125] Topical nepafenac adjunctive to phacoemulsification in diabetic patients was shown to be effective for prophylaxis of macular edema.[126] In a prospective study, diabetic patients with visually significant cataract and no DME, undergoing uncomplicated phacoemulsification and intraocular lens implantation, were randomly assigned to receive postoperative topical nepafenac, intraoperative intravitreal ranibizumab, or no prophylactic treatment (control group). At 3 months postoperative follow-up, there was a significant improvement in vision and reduction in CMT in the topical nepafenac group relative to controls, with no significant difference between the nepafenac and ranibizumab-treated groups. The data indicated that postoperative topical nepafenac could be an effective adjunctive therapy to phacoemulsification in diabetic patients for prophylaxis of macular edema.[126]

Further investigations on whether topical NSAIDs could serve as a treatment alternative or an adjunctive to intravitreal anti-VEGF therapy are required.

Vascular adhesion protein-1 inhibitor

Vascular adhesion protein-1 (VAP-1), also known as amine oxidase copper-containing 3 (AOC3) and semicarbazide-sensitive amine oxidase, is a membrane-bound adhesion protein that facilitates the binding of leukocytes to endothelial cells and their subsequent transmigration to sites of inflammation.[127] VAP-1 is a bifunctional protein. It can catalyze the deamination of primary amines and is also involved in the production of hydrogen peroxide, aldehydes, and advanced glycation end products (AGEs).[128] Previous studies showed that soluble VAP-1 levels were higher in the vitreous fluid of PDR patients than in those of nondiabetic patients,[129] mediating inflammation and oxidative stress in PDR.[129] VAP-1 is stored in intracellular vesicles and rapidly translocates to the luminal surface of endothelial cells during inflammation.[130]

VAP-1 on the retinal endothelial cells mediates rolling, adhesion, transmigration of leukocytes, and leukostasis.[127,131] VAP-1 is involved in leukocyte recruitment, which is a predominant feature of experimental DR.[127] In streptozotocin-induced diabetic rats, leukocyte transmigration rate was reduced by the specific inhibitor of VAP-1, known as UV-002, indicating that VAP-1 inhibition might have therapeutic potential for DR.[127] Overexpression of VAP-1 exacerbates oxidative stress and modulates a variety of inflammatory mediators.[128] In the laser-induced CNV model, VAP-1 inhibition significantly suppressed CNV formation and reduced macrophage infiltration into CNV lesions.[132] Furthermore, VAP-1 inhibition decreases the expression of ICAM-1 and monocyte chemoattractant protein-1 (MCP-1).[132] In mice after retinal laser photocoagulation, RTU-1096, a VAP-1 inhibitor, reduced intraocular leukocyte recruitment and expression of ICAM-1, resulting in reduced levels of hydrogen peroxide.[133] Thus, VAP-1 inhibition may be a potential therapeutic strategy for the prevention of macular edema secondary to scatter laser photocoagulation in patients with DR. In diabetic animals, the beneficial effect of VAP-1 inhibition on retinal function and structure was evidenced by electroretinogram and histopathological studies.[134] Thus, VAP-1 inhibition could be an adjuvant therapy for the treatment of DR.[128]

The preclinical and clinical findings of VAP-1 inhibitor in DR and DME are listed in Table 9.5. A phase 2, double-masked, randomized, active-controlled study

Table 9.5 The preclinical and clinical findings of VAP-1 inhibitor in DR and DME.

Agent	Preclinical findings	Clinical findings
ASP8232	Inhibited plasma VAP-1 activity and improved retinal hyperpermeability and plasma total antioxidant status in diabetic rat model. More effective in reducing ocular hyperpermeability when combined with intravitreal antirat VEGF antibody than either agent alone.[135]	VIDI study phase 2a CI-DME. Failed to reduce CST alone, no additional benefit in combination with ranibizumab.[135]
RTU-1096	Abrogated outer nuclear layer thickening and reduced upregulation of ICAM-1 in mice after retinal laser photocoagulation.[133]	Phase 1-healthy volunteers. Well tolerated at all tested doses.[136]
BI 1467335 (formerly PXS-4728A)	Inhibited neutrophil tethering and rolling, reduced inflammation in mouse models.[137,138]	ROBIN (NCT03238963) phase 2a NPDR. Primary safety endpoint met, unable to demonstrate a clear efficacy signal (development discontinued due to risk of drug—drug interaction).[139,140]

Abbreviations: CI-DME, center-involved diabetic macular edema; CST, central subfield thickness; DME, diabetic macular edema; DR, diabetic retinopathy; ICAM-1, intercellular adhesion molecule 1; NPDR, nonproliferative diabetic retinopathy; VAP-1, vascular adhesion protein-1; VEGF, vascular endothelial growth factor; VIDI, VAP-1 inhibition in DME.

(VIDI study, NCT02302079) tested the effect of ASP8232, a potent and specific small molecule VAP-1 inhibitor, on CI-DME.[135] The primary data showed that near complete inhibition of plasma VAP-1 activity with ASP8232 had no effect on CST in patients with CI-DME. Furthermore, combination therapy with ranibizumab did not provide additional benefit for DME. Thus, the clinical application of VAP-1 inhibition requires further study.

Interleukin-6/IL-6 receptor inhibitor

Interleukin-6 (IL-6) is produced by a variety of cells. IL-6 signals intensify local pathological processes that are associated with chronic inflammation. A metaanalysis showed that an increased level of IL-6 is generally detected in vitreous and/or serum of diabetic patients and correlates with the severity of DR.[141] In DR, IL-6 is one of the major mediators of retinal vascular inflammation.[142–146] IL-6 plays a significant role in initiating BRB breakdown in DR,[147,148] because IL-6 signaling disturbs barrier function in retinal endothelial cells and increases vascular leakage through downregulation of tight junction proteins.[149] IL-6 signaling through its membrane-bound IL-6 receptor (IL-6R) is known as "classical signaling."

Importantly, IL-6 signaling is also observed in cells that do not express the membrane-bound IL-6R through a soluble IL-6R (sIL-6R), known as "trans-signaling".[150,151] The downstream consequences of IL-6 trans-signaling result in oxidative stress, inflammation, and endothelial barrier disruption in human retinal endothelial cells.[148] Inhibition of IL-6 trans-signaling significantly reduced diabetes-induced oxidative damage at the systemic and local retinal level in a mouse model of early DR.[152] There is increasing evidence that IL-6 classical signaling is anti-inflammatory, whereas trans-signaling induces the proinflammatory effects of IL-6.[153–155] Therefore, inhibition of IL-6 trans-signaling is able to prevent inflammation and endothelial barrier disruption in retinal endothelial cells.[148]

Recent advances have led to the development of several therapeutic interventions targeting IL-6 signaling pathways,[156] including anti-IL-6 antibodies: siltuximab, sirukumab, olokizumab, and clazakizumab; anti-IL-6R antibodies: tocilizumab, sarilumab, satralizumab, and vobarilizumab; and selective inhibitors of IL-6 trans-signaling: sgp130Fc (olamkicept). Anti-IL-6 and anti-IL-6R strategies globally block IL-6 signaling, essentially targeting both classical and trans-signaling pathways. Tocilizumab, an IL-6R-inhibiting monoclonal antibody, is useful in the treatment of various autoimmune and inflammatory conditions, notably rheumatoid arthritis.[157] Thus, blocking IL-6 and IL-6R may be potential approaches for treating DR. In fact, a clinical study quantifying vitreous concentrations of cytokines including IL-6 in patients with DR may provide evidence for targeting specific inflammatory factors.[158]

Tumor necrosis factor-α inhibitor

Tumor necrosis factor-α (TNF-α), a pleiotropic cytokine, induces proinflammatory and proangiogenic changes in inflammatory diseases such as rheumatoid arthritis, inflammatory bowel diseases, DR, and nAMD.[159–163] TNF-α is an inflammatory cytokine that promotes the upregulation of adhesion molecule expression, leukocyte recruitment, and monocyte attraction. TNF-α was found to be increased in the aqueous and vitreous of diabetic patients compared to control subjects.[146,164,165] A meta-analysis showed that serum TNF-α was increased in diabetic patients compared to healthy individuals. The elevated serum TNF-α was correlated with the presence and severity of DR.[166] Targeting TNF-α might provide an option to treat DR and DME. In clinical settings, three monoclonal anti-TNF-α full IgG1 antibodies, that is, infliximab, adalimumab, and golimumab, as well as PEGylated Fab' fragment of anti-TNF-α antibody certolizumab pegol and extracellular domain of TNF receptor 2/IgG1-Fc fusion protein etanercept, are almost equally effective for rheumatoid arthritis.[159]

In fact, a clinical study with infliximab that achieved anatomical and functional improvement in a cohort of DME patients is a proof-of-concept study, highlighting the pathogenic role of TNF-α in DR.[167]

Minocycline

Minocycline is a second-generation, semisynthetic tetracycline that exerts anti-inflammatory effects independent from its anti-microbial actions. Minocycline is effective in a number of animal models of neurodegeneration in which microglia and inflammation have been implicated. Minocycline dramatically reduces inflammation and protects against excitotoxic neuronal death after cerebral ischemia[168] and light-induced photoreceptor degeneration.[169,170] Minocycline exerts its neuroprotection in part by inhibiting the proliferation and activation of microglia.[171] Minocycline reduces the expression of inflammatory mediators, microglial activation, and caspase-3 activation in experimental DR.[172] Minocycline also has been shown to exert antiapoptotic effects by inhibiting caspases-1 and -3 in a transgenic mouse model of Huntington disease[173] and by inhibiting cytochrome c release from mitochondria in the spinal cord injury model.[174] Oral minocycline was used to treat patients with DME in a single-center perspective phase I/II clinical trial. In this study, the minocycline treatment improved visual function, central macular edema, and vascular leakage. Therefore, the preliminary clinical data suggest that microglial inhibition with oral minocycline is a therapeutic strategy for the inflammatory etiology of DME.[175]

Neuroprotection

Erythropoietin

Besides hematopoietic action, the anti-inflammatory, anti-apoptotic, anti-oxidative, and cytoprotective functions of erythropoietin (EPO) have been demonstrated in experimental DR.[176–178] Carbamylated EPO, an EPO derivative, has anti-apoptotic effects similar to EPO on experimental DR.[179,180] The protective mechanisms of EPO via its receptor on diabetic retina are complex. To date, the EPO protective mechanisms that have been investigated comprise anti-apoptosis and neuroprotection via activating the ERK and AKT pathways,[176,181] neurotrophic effect and anti-reactive gliosis,[182] anti-VEGF via inhibition of HIF-1α,[183] anti-inflammatory effect by decreasing inflammatory factors from Müller glia,[184] increase in the expression of zinc transporter 8 (ZnT8),[185] downregulation of glutamate,[186] and maintenance of the expression of VE-cadherin by inhibiting its phosphorylation and internalization through VEGF/VEGFR2/Src pathway. In addition, EPO is able to improve the integrity of the inner BRB[187] and maintains outer BRB integrity through downregulation of HIF-1α and c-Jun N-terminal kinase signaling, and upregulation of ZO-1 and occludin expressions in retinal pigment epithelial (RPE) cells.[188] Recently, we found that EPO protects the inner BRB by inhibiting microglia phagocytosis via Src/Akt/cofilin signaling in experimental DR.[189]

A clinical cohort study showed that intravitreal injection of EPO could improve the visual acuity and reduce macular edema in refractory DME patients.[190] It has been proposed that application of EPO for DR may be stage-specific. The detailed working mechanism and clinical application of EPO for DR are further discussed in Chapter 10.

ARA290

Cibinetide, also known as ARA 290 and helix B surface peptide, is a synthetic 11 amino acid peptide, derived from the structure of the B helix of EPO, with marked anti-apoptotic, anti-inflammatory, and anti-permeability effects, but without erythropoietic function.[191–193] In an experimental DR model, cibinetide administered systemically inhibited vascular leakage and edema and protected retinal blood vessels against neuroglial degeneration.[192] Furthermore, cibinetide participates in metabolic control of diabetes in both preclinical and clinical studies.[194,195] Thus, the potential of ARA290 application for DR treatment merits further study.

Somatostatin and brimonidine

Somatostatin and brimonidine are two other drugs with potential neuroprotective function. In diabetic rats, topical administration of somatostatin prevented retinal neurodegeneration and minimized electroretinography abnormalities, glial activation, apoptosis, and the misbalance between proapoptotic and survival signaling.[196] An experimental study also demonstrated that brimonidine is a potential neuroprotective agent.[197] Both somatostatin and brimonidine were tested in diabetic patients; however, no neuroprotective effect was found for either when the primary end point was evaluated.[198] However, the topical administration of somatostatin and brimonidine appears to be useful in preventing the worsening of preexisting retinal neurodysfunction.[198] Topical treatment with either somatostatin or brimonidine was observed to cause retinal arteriolar and venous dilation in patients with type 2 diabetes and early DR.[199] Future studies should go into detail of these findings in arresting early DR.

Drug delivery and durability

The clinical indications for anti-VEGF intravitreal injection in retinal and choroidal diseases are expanding.[200] However, since intravitreal anti-VEGF drugs require repeated injections to achieve optimal efficacy, other routes of drug delivery targeting the posterior segment of the eye have been extensively investigated, such as topical, subtenon, subretinal, and suprachoroidal.[30] To lengthen drug durability, a variety of options are presently under preclinical and clinical investigation. These include dose escalation, prolonged vitreous half-life, and decreasing elimination by increasing molecular weight, use of intravitreal implants and nanoparticle formulation hydrogels, the port delivery system (PDS), and multiple combined systems.[30,200] Each type of administration carries its own advantages and disadvantages. Topical administration is the least invasive but is often ineffective due to poor penetrance and low therapeutic levels at the posterior segment structures.[201] Subretinal injections are targeted, yet require an invasive surgical procedure that carries significant risks.[30] Intravitreal injection is easy to administer and can be performed in an office setting; however, it does not target a specific area and can have adverse effects, including endophthalmitis as well as a relatively high treatment burden.[202]

Port delivery system with ranibizumab

Currently, the delivery of anti-VEGF drugs is largely dependent on repeated intravitreal injections. The newly developed PDS is a state-of-the-art nondegradable, refillable implant that is surgically placed in the sclera via pars plana. This novel drug delivery device allows continuous release of anti-VEGF agents such as ranibizumab and minimizes the need for frequent intravitreal injections while maintaining therapeutic intraocular drug levels controlling disease activity.[203] Passive diffusion results in movement of drugs from the port to the vitreous cavity, with sustained and controlled release achieved by the porous metal element.[204] Recently, Campochiaro et al. conducted a phase 2, multicenter, randomized, active treatment-controlled clinical trial of a ranibizumab-loaded PDS (LADDER; NCT02510794) to determine the efficacy and safety of the drug system in nAMD.[204] Participants were administered ranibizumab at 10 mg/mL, 40 mg/mL, 100 mg/mL, or monthly intravitreal ranibizumab 0.5 mg injections. After 9 months, visual outcomes were similar for patients administered the ranibizumab-loaded port 100 mg/mL and those receiving monthly intravitreal injections. Because the median time to initial refill was 15 months in the 100 mg/mL group, a significant reduction in treatment burden was achieved with the PDS compared to intravitreal injections. ARCHWAY (NCT03677934) randomized phase 3 trial of PDS with ranibizumab showed that PDS with ranibizumab met its primary objective, demonstrating equivalent efficacy to monthly ranibizumab, with 98.4% of PDS-treated patients not requiring supplemental treatment in the first 24-week interval.[205] Phase 3 clinical trials for DR (PAVILION; NCT04503551), and DME (PAGODA; NCT04108156) are currently in progress. The fully enrolled phase 3 PAGODA trial of DME patients compares the PDS (with refill exchanges at 6-month intervals) with monthly 0.5 mg ranibizumab.

Suprachoroidal injection

The suprachoroidal space (SCS) between the sclera and choroid is becoming an applicable route to deliver therapeutics to the back of the eye via suprachoroidal injection.[200] Suprachoroidal administration is minimally invasive. After the drug is delivered to the SCS, it can directly target both the retina and the choroid due to the posterior pole fluid flow, thereby avoiding multiple ocular tissue barriers and accomplishing drug efficacy at low doses.[30,206] In addition, sustained release could be achieved due to drug accumulation and distribution in SCS.[207] However, the risks of hemorrhage and choroidal detachment cannot be neglected. The Phase 1/2 HULK Study enrolled 20 eyes with DME, including 10 previously treated eyes and 10 treatment-naïve eyes.[208] The treatment-naïve eyes were treated with one-time intravitreal injection of aflibercept (2 mg/0.05 mL) and SCS injection of triamcinolone acetonide (TA) (CLS-TA, 4 mg/100 μL; Clearside Biomedical, Alpharetta, GA, USA), while the 10 previously treated eyes were treated with CLS-TA (4 mg/ 100 μL) monotherapy. The reported results were a mean BCVA change of +8.5 and +1.1 EDTRS letters and mean CST decrease of 91 and 128 μm in the treatment-naïve and previously treated groups, respectively. The study demonstrated a greater benefit for treatment-naïve eyes with SCS injection of CLS-TA. Although all eyes demonstrated anatomic improvement after CLS-TA injection, mean visual improvements were minimal among previously treated patients.[209] The phase 2 TYBEE clinical trial enrolled 71 eyes with treatment-naïve DME.[210] A total of 36 eyes were the active group and received CLS-TA (4 mg/100 μL) and aflibercept (2 mg/0.05 mL) at baseline and week 12. The control group consisted of 35 eyes which were treated with aflibercept (2 mg/0.05 mL) at baseline, week 4, week 8, and week 12. At 24 weeks from baseline, the mean BCVA improvement was 11.8 and 13.8 EDTRS letters ($P = .288$), there was a mean CST decrease of 212.1 and 178.6 μm ($P = .089$), and the mean number of treatments was 2.6 and 3.6 in the active and control groups, respectively. The visual benefit was similar between the arms, with modest anatomic benefit and potential to reduce treatment burden in the active group.[210] The benefit of SCS application is discussed in Chapter 10.

Topical eye drops

Topical administration is very efficient for the treatment of anterior segment diseases. However, because of multiple ocular barriers, such as tear drainage, cornea, conjunctiva, and blood—aqueous barrier, it is considered inefficient for posterior segment diseases. Nevertheless, because eye drops so convenient to administer, researchers have focused on developing topical formulations to treat retinal diseases. One topical agent developed by PanOptica (Mount Arlington, NJ), PAN-90806, is a TKI of VEGF-A and PDGF. A phase 1/2 clinical trial (NCT03479372) was performed with treatment-naïve nAMD patients who were administered eye drops (2, 6, and 10 mg/mL) daily for 12 weeks. Based on the study findings, no rescue injections were required for 51% of the participants, and improved visual outcomes were observed in 88% of patients in the no rescue group.[211]

Oral route

Vorolanib (X-82), an oral anti-VEGFR/platelet-derived growth factor receptor/ colony-stimulating factor 1 receptor targeting multiple tyrosine kinases, has a short half-life and limited tissue accumulation.[212] Phase 1 study of vorolanib with everolimus (mTOR inhibitor, 10 mg daily) in patients with solid tumors showed that vorolanib can safely be combined with everolimus (NCT01784861). Oral vorolanib might have potential usage in treating fundus vascular diseases, like DME and nAMD.

Subcutaneous injection

AKB-9778 is a novel small molecule inhibitor of VE-PTP.[213] In two clinical trials for DME patients, subcutaneous injections of AKB-9778 monotherapy were safe and provided added benefit to VEGF suppression.[109,214] In an open-label phase 1B clinical trial, patients with DME self-administered subcutaneous injections of AKB-9778 with four different doses (5, 15, 22.5, or 30 mg) bid for 4 weeks.[214] The results showed that visual acuity was mildly improved from 1.8 to 6.7 letters and that swelling was reduced in some, but not all patients with DME.[214] In phase II, randomized, double-masked clinical trials, the activation of Tie2 by subcutaneous injections of AKB-9778 in combination with ranibizumab caused a significantly greater reduction in macular edema than that seen with ranibizumab alone, indicating enhanced benefit in DME due to Tie2 activation by AKB-9778 in combination with VEGF suppression.[109,110]

High-dose aflibercept

Intravitreal injection of high-dose anti-VEGF agents might prolong the intravitreal injection intervals and improve drug efficacy. In a preclinical animal study, Kim et al. administered a 10-fold dose of ranibizumab in rabbit eyes that resulted in a twofold increase in retinal half-life and long-lasting effective concentration in the retinal compartment, without any adverse local or systemic effects.[215] The READ-3 study that enrolled DME patients found that increasing the conventional 0.5 mg dose of ranibizumab to 2 mg did not further improve vision at 24 months.[216] Currently, randomized, double-masked, phase 3 clinical trials are being conducted with high-dose aflibercept every 12 or 16 weeks after a loading phase in participants with DR (PHOTON; NCT04429503) and nAMD (PULSAR; NCT04423718).

Sustained/controlled release

Several intravitreal implants, including Ozurdex (Allergan Inc., Irvine, CA, USA), Retisert (Bausch & Lomb, Rochester, NY, USA), and Illuvien (Alimera Sciences Inc., Alpharetta, GA, USA), have been approved by the FDA for DME, RVO-ME, and posterior noninfectious uveitis.[30] Ozurdex (dexamethasone) and Retisert/Illuvien (fluocinolone acetonide) intravitreal implants target the retinal layer, with higher drug dose and longer drug concentration in the intraocular space.[217–219]

Ozurdex is a representative biodegradable intravitreal dexamethasone implant with poly(lactic-co-glycolic acid) conjugation. Biodegradable implants exhibit drug efficacy for 3–6 months due to the exponential decrease in drug concentration caused by three-dimensional drug release and gradual degradation of scaffolds in the vitreous cavity. MEAD Study evaluated the safety and efficacy of Ozurdex (0.7 and 0.35 mg) in the treatment of patients with DME and showed that both doses of dexamethasone in the implant met the primary efficacy endpoint for improvement in visual acuity with acceptable safety profile.[220]

Retisert and Illuvien are both nonbiodegradable polymer-conjugated formulations. As nonbiodegradable implants last for 2−3 years, sustained drug release is achieved by the steady linear decrease in drug concentration in the confined diffusion area. However, the devices remain in the vitreous cavity without decaying. FAME study evaluated long-term efficacy and safety of intravitreal inserts releasing 0.2 μg/d (low dose) or 0.5 μg/d (high dose) fluocinolone acetonide (Iluvien, Alimera Sciences, Alpharetta, GA, USA) in patients with DME and showed that fluocinolone acetonide inserts provide substantial visual benefit for up to 3 years for patients with DME and also provided an option for patients who do not respond to other therapy, such as anti-VEGF treatment.[221,222]

Gene therapy to deliver anti-VEGF agents

Given the burden of repeated anti-VEGF treatments, gene therapy holds the promise for long-term suppression of VEGF in retinal vascular diseases. Gene therapy has several advantages over current intravitreal anti-VEGF injections, including long-term therapeutic effects without repeated treatments, and the capacity for cell-targeted delivery using cell-specific promotors. In 2017, the US FDA approved the first gene therapy drug, Luxturna (voretigene neparvovec-rzyl, Spark Therapeutics),[223] which is delivered into the subretinal space for treating patients with Leber congenital amaurosis type-2 (LCA-2) due to *RPE65* mutation.[224] As for gene therapy to target VEGF in retinal vascular diseases, several gene therapy drugs, including RGX-314, ADVM-022, and rAAV-sFlt1, are currently under clinical evaluation.

RGX-314 is an adeno-associated virus 8 (AAV8) vector carrying an anti-VEGF monoclonal antibody fragment (Fab) that selectively binds to human VEGF-A. Preclinical studies with a transgenic mouse model expressing human VEGF in retina (rho/VEGF mice), a model of type 3 CNV showed that subretinal injection of RGX-314 resulted in significant reduction of neovascularization.[225] Besides subretinal delivery, suprachoroidal injection of the same dose of RGX-314 resulted in similar expression of anti-VEGF Fab and similar suppression of VEGF-induced vascular leakage in the rat.[226] A phase I/IIa clinical trial delivering RGX-314 by subretinal injections into patients with nAMD is currently ongoing (NCT03066258), and the interim assessment found that RGX-314 was well tolerated and continued to produce anti-VEGF Fab for 2 years.[227] The Phase II ALTITUDE trial is looking at patients with DR without DME who are treated with a single dose of RGX-314, delivered in SCS.[228] Positive three-month interim data from cohort 1, treated with a single injection at a dose level of 2.5×10^{11} genomic copies per eye, showed that treatment is well tolerated and 33% of patients had a $\geq$2-step improvement from baseline on the ETDRS-DRSS score compared with 0% of patients in the control arm.

ADVM-022, an AAV2-7m8 vector encoding aflibercept, has been optimized for intravitreal delivery and strong protein expression. To overcome the difficulties of subretinal injections, ADVM-022 employs the AAV2-7m8 vector to encode aflibercept to be given as an intravitreal injection. Long-term expression and efficacy of ADVM-022-derived aflibercept were evaluated in a laser-induced CNV model in nonhuman primates.[229] This preclinical study found ADVM-022 effective at maintaining high aflibercept levels in the vitreous for 3−9 months with no serious adverse effects, and preventing laser-induced CNV at levels comparable to a single intravitreal aflibercept at the time of CNV induction. In addition, ADVM-022 administration 13 months before laser-induced CNV prevented the occurrence of CNV lesions, to the same degree as a bolus of aflibercept delivered at the time of laser. These results demonstrate that a single intravitreal administration of ADVM-022 may provide a safe and effective long-term treatment option for neovascular AMD and DME and may ultimately improve patients' visual outcomes.[230] Clinical trials for nAMD (NCT04645212; NCT03748784) and DME (NCT04418427) are currently underway, evaluating safety and efficacy following a single intravitreal injection of ADVM-022.

rAAV-sFlt1, recombinant AAV2 vector expressing soluble VEGF receptor 1, works as a decoy receptor binding VEGF. Preclinical study using nonhuman primates showed that a single subretinal injection of rAAV-sFlt1 was safe and well tolerated.[231] Although phase I study (NCT01494805) in nAMD patients demonstrated the safety,[232] phase IIa randomized clinical trial (NCT01494805) with 32 patients showed no clear benefit in visual acuity or anatomy compared with baseline and control eyes.[233] The potential effect of rAAV-sFlt1 on DME deserves further study.[234]

Subthreshold micropulse laser for DME

Anti-VEGF therapy is the first-line treatment for DME, but its clinical outcomes are often suboptimal.[25] Subthreshold micropulse laser is a safe, nonscarring alternative procedure as evidenced by imaging modalities and microperimetry analyses.[235−238] Subthreshold micropulse laser therapy is known to improve RPE function, modulating the activation of heat-shock proteins and normalizing cytokine expression.[239] Subthreshold micropulse laser treatment seems to result in a long-term normalization of specific retinal neuroinflammatory metabolic pathways.[240] Subthreshold micropulse laser has been accepted as a viable and promising therapy in selected cases for DME treatment.[241] The infrared subthreshold micropulse laser (810-nm wavelength) is currently proven effective for the treatment of DME.[242] However, yellow subthreshold micropulse laser (577-nm wavelength) has also shown good success and safety[243] due to its intrinsic physiobiological characteristics, namely better penetration through media opacities, null absorbance by macular xanthophyll pigments, and an excellent combined absorbance by melanin and oxyhemoglobin.[239] In a prospective, randomized, single institution, comparative six-month pilot study, the retinal and choroidal morphologic changes and macular function were evaluated and compared in patients with CI-DME treated with yellow (577-nm) or infrared (810-nm) subthreshold micropulse laser.[244] The data showed that both treatments with the lowest duty cycle (5%) and fixed power parameters are safe from the morphologic and visual function points of view in mild CI-DME.[244] In a retrospective study analyzing 56 eyes from 36 patients with CI-DME treated with subthreshold micropulse laser monotherapy (EasyRet photocoagulator) with 577-nm wavelength, the DME patients with subretinal fluid (SRF) responded well, demonstrating the absorbance of SRF, while those with intraretinal edema responded poorly to laser monotherapy.[241]

In a retrospective, comparative study, the relative efficacy of fixed and variable treatment regimens using subthreshold yellow micropulse laser for treatment of DME was studied.[245] The study included 24 eyes receiving a fixed regimen of subthreshold micropulse laser treatment and 15 eyes receiving a variable treatment regimen of subthreshold micropulse laser. When followed up for 12 months, the results showed that both treatment regimens were effective for the treatment of mild CI-DME. The fixed treatment regimen appears more suitable by minimizing treatment time and reducing possible titration errors.[245]

Subthreshold micropulse laser in combination with intravitreal injections of bevacizumab has been proven to be effective and safe in the treatment of DME. Since the number and frequency of intravitreal injections of bevacizumab are markedly reduced,[246] it is a promising novel combination therapy for DME.[247]

Improvement of pars plana vitrectomy for PDR

Due to the rising frequency of obesity, increasing life span, the prevalence of DR is continuously increasing worldwide. PDR and other complications develop after 30 years in up to 20% of persons with diabetes.[248] Following this trajectory, PDR will continue to be a major cause of blindness in the future. Since the discovery of pars plana vitrectomy (PPV) 50 years ago, the experience of PPV practice suggests that PPV is the last defense for PDR patients with severe consequences. PPV is expected to stop vision loss or even to restore lost vision. As the continuation of the current diabetic vitrectomy described in Chapter 1, a recent retrospective cohort study showed more complex outcomes. In patients who underwent primary PPV for PDR, about a quarter of all patients required revitrectomy after 10 years. More than half of the patients needed a vitrectomy of the fellow eyes.[249] Therefore, improvement of PPV efficacy and long-term outcome for severe PDR is imperative in future. In order to achieve this goal, two major tasks must be completed.

On the one hand, better understanding of the pathological contributions of the vitreoretinal interface with its neighboring structures is required because this understanding could be translated into surgical skill during PDR vitrectomy.[250] For instance, there are two patterns of new retinal vessels growing at the vitreoretinal interface. First, new retinal vessels grow away from the retinal surface, penetrating into the vitreous cortex and interacting with vitreous microfibrils.[251] Second, the new vessels can also breach the internal limiting membrane along the retinal surface, forming abortive clumps of new vessels in PVD areas. These two patterns of new blood vessel growth reflect the derangement of the vitreoretinal interface in PDR. The derangement of vitreoretinal interface is landmark for heralding iatrogenic breaks, persistent vitreoretinal traction, and vitreous hemorrhage during PPV surgery, which is also an important cause of revitrectomy. Therefore, pre- and intraoperative imaging studies on the vitreoretinal interface are critical for improved visualization during vitrectomy for PDR. Another vitreoretinal interface derangement in PDR eyes relates to the status of PVD. It is known that PVD may protect against PDR progression, but partial PVD is more frequently encountered than complete PVD.[252] Partial PVD generates multiple stagnant pockets of liquid within the vitreoschisis cavity, especially around the macula. Therefore, achieving a complete PVD in vitrectomy is critical to eliminating accumulated angiogenic factors and improving oxygenation of retina, leading to a restoration of retinal structure and function.[252] The vitreoretinal interface interacts with neighboring fibrocytes/myofibroblasts and bioactive factors of the vitreous body. These cellular and molecular components are often associated with tractional retinal detachment and vitreous hemorrhage in PDR. Clinical acumen tells us that delamination of FVM is technically challenging.[253] Understanding the necessity of preoperative deactivation of fibrovascular tissue by anti-VEGF treatment and intraoperative bimanual dissection of vitreoretinal interface/adhesion with optimal visualization is the key for successful PDR vitrectomy.

On the other hand, with understanding of the challenges of PDR vitrectomy, improving vitrectomy instrumentation/equipment is essential in the future. The advance of PPV has been following the trend toward smaller and thinner microsurgical equipment. Many vitrectomy procedures can now be performed with self-sealing, sutureless (no-stitch) incisions. Although it has some limitations, small-gauge vitrectomy surgery is generally considered more comfortable for patients than surgery with larger instruments and offers faster visual recovery in many cases. PPV is continuously evolving. More advanced fluidics, high-speed vitrectors, a wider variety of instruments and perioperative agents, the preoperative and intraoperative imaging systems such as optical coherence tomography (OCT), and surgeon–artificial intelligence (AI) interaction robotics systems will optimize vitrectomy for the complex cases in patients with PDR and DME.[254]

In future PDR vitrectomy, the faster vitrectomy probe, so-called vitreous cutter, is needed. However, the mechanical speed of vitreous cutter has reached its limit. It is now thought that using an ultrasonic vitreous cutter can produce a "cut rate" of more than 1,000 K cycles per minute with 100% duty cycle. At this point, the port is always open.[255] Rizzo and Faraldi reported another possible technique called electrochemical viscosity modification. This technique is able to use a high-intensity electric field with a very high-frequency variation of charge between two or more electrodes mounted at the end of a vitrectomy probe and can also modify the nature of the vitreous, making vitreolysis and allowing smooth suction.[256] In the "medical vitreolysis" era, enzymatic vitreolysis is used as a preoperative adjunct to enhance complete detachment of the posterior hyaloid and reduce iatrogenic retinal breaks.[257] To meet the demand of vitreoretinal microsurgical technique, enzymatic, pneumatic, and combined vitreolysis are in developmental stage for routine use. How to improve precision, perception, and manipulation dexterity is the main challenge to vitreoretinal surgeons performing PPV for complicated cases of PDR. For instance, the visualization of the precise anatomy is limited through a dilated pupil, especially under complex intraocular lighting conditions. The retinal anatomy sometimes presents semitransparent features, which are difficult to see (e.g., retinal membrane). Because excessive reaction force applied to the retina can damage delicate anatomy, surgeons need assist devices to overcome the deficiency in tactile perception. Additionally, physiological tremors that are an intrinsic limitation of human surgeons need to be minimized by special devices. In vitreoretinal surgery, the instrument inserted through trocars with rigid shafts has limited distal tip dexterity. Fortunately, the advent of intraoperative OCT systems and the development of robotic surgical devices provide potential solutions to overcome these problems because these issues are usually beyond the natural capability of humans. Intraoperative OCT permits real-time retinal visualization during surgery offering additional operative information to surgeons. In a pilot study, intraoperative OCT-aided PPV for complex retinal detachment surgery showed superiority over the conventional PPV in terms of higher primary success rate and better final visual outcome.[258] A future prospective randomized study is needed to assess intraoperative OCT utility with a variety of designs. An excellent review of robotic systems for vitreoretinal surgery by Ahronovich et al. is the must-read material in the reference list.[254]

References

1. https://public.jaeb.org/drcrnet/view/home.
2. Diabetic Retinopathy Clinical Research Network, Elman MJ, Aiello LP, et al. Randomized trial evaluating ranibizumab plus prompt or deferred laser or triamcinolone plus prompt laser for diabetic macular edema. *Ophthalmology*. 2010;117(6). https://doi.org/10.1016/j.ophtha.2010.02.031, 1064-1077.e35.
3. Elman MJ, Bressler NM, Qin H, et al. Expanded 2-year follow-up of ranibizumab plus prompt or deferred laser or triamcinolone plus prompt laser for diabetic macular edema. *Ophthalmology*. 2011;118(4):609−614. https://doi.org/10.1016/j.ophtha.2010.12.033.
4. Elman MJ, Ayala A, Bressler NM, et al. Intravitreal ranibizumab for diabetic macular edema with prompt versus deferred laser treatment: 5-year randomized trial results. *Ophthalmology*. 2015;122(2):375−381. https://doi.org/10.1016/j.ophtha.2014.08.047.
5. Bressler SB, Glassman AR, Almukhtar T, et al. Five-year outcomes of ranibizumab with prompt or deferred laser versus laser or triamcinolone plus deferred ranibizumab for diabetic macular edema. *Am J Ophthalmol*. 2016;164:57−68. https://doi.org/10.1016/j.ajo.2015.12.025.

6. Diabetic Retinopathy Clinical Research Network, Wells JA, Glassman AR, et al. Aflibercept, bevacizumab, or ranibizumab for diabetic macular edema. *N Engl J Med.* 2015;372(13):1193−1203. https://doi.org/10.1056/NEJMoa1414264.

7. Wells JA, Glassman AR, Ayala AR, et al. Aflibercept, bevacizumab, or ranibizumab for diabetic macular edema: two-year results from a comparative effectiveness randomized clinical trial. *Ophthalmology.* 2016;123(6):1351−1359. https://doi.org/10.1016/j.ophtha.2016.02.022.

8. Glassman AR, Wells JA, Josic K, et al. Five-year outcomes after initial aflibercept, bevacizumab, or ranibizumab treatment for diabetic macular edema (protocol T extension study). *Ophthalmology.* 2020;127(9):1201−1210. https://doi.org/10.1016/j.ophtha.2020.03.021.

9. Writing Committee for the Diabetic Retinopathy Clinical Research Network, Gross JG, Glassman AR, et al. Panretinal photocoagulation vs intravitreous ranibizumab for proliferative diabetic retinopathy: a randomized clinical trial. *JAMA.* 2015;314(20):2137−2146. https://doi.org/10.1001/jama.2015.15217.

10. Gross JG, Glassman AR. A novel treatment for proliferative diabetic retinopathy: anti-vascular endothelial growth factor therapy. *JAMA Ophthalmol.* 2016;134(1):13−14. https://doi.org/10.1001/jamaophthalmol.2015.5079.

11. Gross JG, Glassman AR, Liu D, et al. Five-year outcomes of panretinal photocoagulation vs intravitreous ranibizumab for proliferative diabetic retinopathy: a randomized clinical trial. *JAMA Ophthalmol.* 2018;136(10):1138−1148. https://doi.org/10.1001/jamaophthalmol.2018.3255.

12. Antoszyk AN, Glassman AR, Beaulieu WT, et al. Effect of intravitreous aflibercept vs vitrectomy with panretinal photocoagulation on visual acuity in patients with vitreous hemorrhage from proliferative diabetic retinopathy: a randomized clinical trial. *JAMA.* 2020;324(23):2383−2395. https://doi.org/10.1001/jama.2020.23027.

13. Glassman AR, Beaulieu WT, Maguire MG, et al. Visual acuity, vitreous hemorrhage, and other ocular outcomes after vitrectomy vs aflibercept for vitreous hemorrhage due to diabetic retinopathy: a secondary analysis of a randomized clinical trial. *JAMA Ophthalmol.* 2021;139(7):725−733. https://doi.org/10.1001/jamaophthalmol.2021.1110.

14. Baker CW, Glassman AR, Beaulieu WT, et al. Effect of initial management with aflibercept vs laser photocoagulation vs observation on vision loss among patients with diabetic macular edema involving the center of the macula and good visual acuity: a randomized clinical trial. *JAMA.* 2019;321(19):1880−1894. https://doi.org/10.1001/jama.2019.5790.

15. Maturi RK, Glassman AR, Liu D, et al. Effect of adding dexamethasone to continued ranibizumab treatment in patients with persistent diabetic macular edema: a DRCR network phase 2 randomized clinical trial. *JAMA Ophthalmol.* 2018;136(1):29. https://doi.org/10.1001/jamaophthalmol.2017.4914.

16. Maturi RK, Glassman AR, Josic K, et al. Effect of intravitreous anti-vascular endothelial growth factor vs sham treatment for prevention of vision-threatening complications of diabetic retinopathy: the protocol W randomized clinical trial. *JAMA Ophthalmol.* 2021;139(7):701−712. https://doi.org/10.1001/jamaophthalmol.2021.0606.

17. Writing Committee, Kim JE, Glassman AR, et al. A randomized trial of photobiomodulation therapy for center-involved diabetic macular edema with good visual acuity (protocol AE). Ophthalmol Retina. Published online October 7, 2021:S2468-6530(21)00312-2. https://doi.org/10.1016/j.oret.2021.10.003.

18. Apte RS, Chen DS, Ferrara N. VEGF in signaling and disease: beyond discovery and development. *Cell.* 2019;176(6):1248−1264. https://doi.org/10.1016/j.cell.2019. 01.021.

19. Ciulla TA, Harris A, McIntyre N, Jonescu-Cuypers C. Treatment of diabetic macular edema with sustained-release glucocorticoids: intravitreal triamcinolone acetonide, dexamethasone implant, and fluocinolone acetonide implant. *Expet Opin Pharmacother.* 2014;15(7):953−959. https://doi.org/10.1517/14656566.2014.896899.

20. Rajendram R, Fraser-Bell S, Kaines A, et al. A 2-year prospective randomized controlled trial of intravitreal bevacizumab or laser therapy (BOLT) in the management of diabetic macular edema: 24-month data: report 3. *Arch Ophthalmol Chic Ill 1960.* 2012;130(8):972−979. https://doi.org/10.1001/archophthalmol.2012.393.

21. Nguyen QD, Brown DM, Marcus DM, et al. Ranibizumab for diabetic macular edema: results from 2 phase III randomized trials: RISE and RIDE. *Ophthalmology.* 2012; 119(4):789−801. https://doi.org/10.1016/j.ophtha.2011.12.039.

22. Brown DM, Schmidt-Erfurth U, Do DV, et al. Intravitreal aflibercept for diabetic macular edema: 100-week results from the VISTA and VIVID studies. *Ophthalmology.* 2015;122(10):2044−2052. https://doi.org/10.1016/j.ophtha.2015.06.017.

23. Schmidt-Erfurth U, Lang GE, Holz FG, et al. Three-year outcomes of individualized ranibizumab treatment in patients with diabetic macular edema: the RESTORE extension study. *Ophthalmology.* 2014;121(5):1045−1053. https://doi.org/10.1016/j.ophtha.2013.11.041.

24. Yorston D. Anti-VEGF drugs in the prevention of blindness. *Community Eye Health.* 2014;27(87):44−46.

25. Bressler NM, Beaulieu WT, Glassman AR, et al. Persistent macular thickening following intravitreous aflibercept, bevacizumab, or ranibizumab for central-involved diabetic macular edema with vision impairment: a secondary analysis of a randomized clinical trial. *JAMA Ophthalmol.* 2018;136(3):257−269. https://doi.org/10.1001/jamaophthalmol.2017.6565.

26. Dugel PU, Boyer DS, Antoszyk AN, et al. Phase 1 study of OPT-302 inhibition of vascular endothelial growth factors C and D for neovascular age-related macular degeneration. *Ophthalmol Retina.* 2020;4(3):250−263. https://doi.org/10.1016/j.oret.2019.10.008.

27. Boyer DS. Phase 1b/2a DME study results of OPT-302 to block VEGF-C/-D in combination with aflibercept. Presented at AAO 2020 Virtual; November 13, 2020.

28. Iglicki M, González DP, Loewenstein A, Zur D. Next-generation anti-VEGF agents for diabetic macular oedema. *Eye Lond Engl.* 2022;36(2):273−277. https://doi.org/10.1038/s41433-021-01722-8.

29. Samanta A, Aziz AA, Jhingan M, Singh SR, Khanani AM, Chhablani J. Emerging therapies in neovascular age-related macular degeneration in 2020. *Asia-Pac J Ophthalmol Phila Pa.* 2020;9(3):250−259. https://doi.org/10.1097/APO.0000000000000291.

30. Kim HM, Woo SJ. Ocular drug delivery to the retina: current innovations and future perspectives. *Pharmaceutics.* 2021;13(1):108. https://doi.org/10.3390/pharmaceutics13010108.

31. Del Amo EM, Rimpelä AK, Heikkinen E, et al. Pharmacokinetic aspects of retinal drug delivery. *Prog Retin Eye Res.* 2017;57:134−185. https://doi.org/10.1016/j.preteyeres.2016.12.001.

32. Chandrasekaran PR, Madanagopalan VG. KSI-301: antibody biopolymer conjugate in retinal disorders. *Ther Adv Ophthalmol.* 2021;13. https://doi.org/10.1177/25158414211027708, 25158414211027708.

33. Kodiak Sciences Announces Top-Line Results from its initial Phase 2b/3 Study of KSI-301 in Patients with Neovascular (Wet) Age-Related Macular Degeneration. Available Online https://ir.kodiak.com/news-releases/news-release-details/kodiak-sciences-announces-top-line-results-its-initial-phase-2b3.

34. Thomas CN, Sim DA, Lee WH, et al. Emerging therapies and their delivery for treating age-related macular degeneration. *Br J Pharmacol.* Published online March 26, 2021. doi:10.1111/bph.15459

35. Souied EH, Devin F, Mauget-Faÿsse M, et al. Treatment of exudative age-related macular degeneration with a designed ankyrin repeat protein that binds vascular endothelial growth factor: a phase I/II study. *Am J Ophthalmol.* 2014;158(4):724–732.e2. https://doi.org/10.1016/j.ajo.2014.05.037.

36. Campochiaro PA, Channa R, Berger BB, et al. Treatment of diabetic macular edema with a designed ankyrin repeat protein that binds vascular endothelial growth factor: a phase I/II study. *Am J Ophthalmol.* 2013;155(4):697–704. https://doi.org/10.1016/j.ajo.2012.09.032, 704.e1-2.

37. Krohne TU, Liu Z, Holz FG, Meyer CH. Intraocular pharmacokinetics of ranibizumab following a single intravitreal injection in humans. *Am J Ophthalmol.* 2012;154(4):682–686.e2. https://doi.org/10.1016/j.ajo.2012.03.047.

38. Callanan D, Kunimoto D, Maturi RK, et al. Double-masked, randomized, phase 2 evaluation of abicipar pegol (an anti-VEGF DARPin therapeutic) in neovascular age-related macular degeneration. *J Ocul Pharmacol Ther Off J Assoc Ocul Pharmacol Ther.* 2018;34(10):700–709. https://doi.org/10.1089/jop.2018.0062.

39. Kunimoto D, Yoon YH, Wykoff CC, et al. Efficacy and safety of abicipar in neovascular age-related macular degeneration: 52-week results of phase 3 randomized controlled study. *Ophthalmology.* 2020;127(10):1331–1344. https://doi.org/10.1016/j.ophtha.2020.03.035.

40. Khurana RN, Kunimoto D, Yoon YH, et al. Two-year results of the phase 3 randomized controlled study of abicipar in neovascular age-related macular degeneration. *Ophthalmology.* 2021;128(7):1027–1038. https://doi.org/10.1016/j.ophtha.2020.11.017.

41. Striglia E, Caccioppo A, Castellino N, Reibaldi M, Porta M. Emerging drugs for the treatment of diabetic retinopathy. *Expet Opin Emerg Drugs.* 2020;25(3):261–271. https://doi.org/10.1080/14728214.2020.1801631.

42. Biosimilars for the Treatment of Wet AMD. Available online https://www.ophthalmologymanagement.com/newsletters/amd-update/july-2020.

43. Kapur M, Nirula S, Naik MP. Future of anti-VEGF: biosimilars and biobetters. *Int J Retina Vitr.* 2022;8(1):2. https://doi.org/10.1186/s40942-021-00343-3.

44. Sharma A, Hafeez Faridi M, Kumar N, et al. Immunogenicity and efficacy after switching from original Ranibizumab to a Ranibizumab biosimilar: real-world data. *Eye Lond Engl.* 2020;34(6):1008–1009. https://doi.org/10.1038/s41433-019-0745-z.

45. Biological products products. Available online https://www.fda.gov/media/108557/download.

46. Sharma A, Reddy P, Kuppermann BD, Bandello F, Lowenstein A. Biosimilars in ophthalmology: "Is there a big change on the horizon?". *Clin Ophthalmol Auckl NZ.* 2018;12:2137–2143. https://doi.org/10.2147/OPTH.S180393.

47. Sharma A, Kumar N, Bandello F, Loewenstein A, Kuppermann BD. Need of education on biosimilars amongst ophthalmologists: combating the nocebo effect. *Eye Lond Engl.* 2020;34(6):1006−1007. https://doi.org/10.1038/s41433-019-0722-6.

48. Sharma A, Kumar N, Kuppermann BD, Francesco B, Lowenstein A. Ophthalmic biosimilars: lessons from India. *Indian J Ophthalmol.* 2019;67(8):1384−1385. https://doi.org/10.4103/ijo.IJO_430_19.

49. Kumar A, Agarwal D, Kumar A. Commentary: use of biosimilars for retinal diseases in India: challenges and concerns. *Indian J Ophthalmol.* 2021;69(2):357. https://doi.org/10.4103/ijo.IJO_39_21.

50. FDA Approves First Biosimilar to Treat Macular Degeneration Disease and Other Eye Conditions. Available online https://www.fda.gov/news-events/press-announcements/fda-approves-first-biosimilar-treat-macular-degeneration-disease-and-other-eye-conditions.

51. Sharma A, Kumar N, Parachuri N, Bandello F, Kuppermann BD, Loewenstein A. Biosimilars for retinal diseases: an update. *Am J Ophthalmol.* 2021;224:36−42. https://doi.org/10.1016/j.ajo.2020.11.017.

52. Catrina SB, Zheng X. Hypoxia and hypoxia-inducible factors in diabetes and its complications. *Diabetologia.* 2021;64(4):709−716. https://doi.org/10.1007/s00125-021-05380-z.

53. Loukovaara S, Koivunen P, Inglés M, Escobar J, Vento M, Andersson S. Elevated protein carbonyl and HIF-1α levels in eyes with proliferative diabetic retinopathy. *Acta Ophthalmol.* 2014;92(4):323−327. https://doi.org/10.1111/aos.12186.

54. Lim JI, Spee C, Hinton DR. A comparison of hypoxia-inducible factor-α in surgically excised neovascular membranes of patients with diabetes compared with idiopathic epiretinal membranes in nondiabetic patients. *Retina.* 2010;30(9):1472−1478. https://doi.org/10.1097/IAE.0b013e3181d6df09.

55. Wang X, Wang G, Wang Y. Intravitreous vascular endothelial growth factor and hypoxia-inducible factor 1a in patients with proliferative diabetic retinopathy. *Am J Ophthalmol.* 2009;148(6):883−889. https://doi.org/10.1016/j.ajo.2009.07.007.

56. Li W. Basic and clinical studies of AMD in future: questions more than answers. In: *Age-Related Macular Degeneration.* Elsevier; 2022:261−272. https://doi.org/10.1016/B978-0-12-822061-0.00008-6.

57. Vadlapatla R, Vadlapudi A, Mitra A. Hypoxia-inducible factor-1 (HIF-1): a potential target for intervention in ocular neovascular diseases. *Curr Drug Targets.* 2013;14(8):919−935. https://doi.org/10.2174/13894501113149990015.

58. Jiang J, Xia XB, Xu HZ, et al. Inhibition of retinal neovascularization by gene transfer of small interfering RNA targeting HIF-1alpha and VEGF. *J Cell Physiol.* 2009;218(1):66−74. https://doi.org/10.1002/jcp.21566.

59. Greenberger LM, Horak ID, Filpula D, et al. A RNA antagonist of hypoxia-inducible factor-1α, EZN-2968, inhibits tumor cell growth. *Mol Cancer Therapeut.* 2008;7(11):3598−3608. https://doi.org/10.1158/1535-7163.MCT-08-0510.

60. Jeong W, Rapisarda A, Park SR, et al. Pilot trial of EZN-2968, an antisense oligonucleotide inhibitor of hypoxia-inducible factor-1 alpha (HIF-1α), in patients with refractory solid tumors. *Cancer Chemother Pharmacol.* 2014;73(2):343−348. https://doi.org/10.1007/s00280-013-2362-z.

61. Zhang H, Qian DZ, Tan YS, et al. Digoxin and other cardiac glycosides inhibit HIF-1 synthesis and block tumor growth. *Proc Natl Acad Sci USA.* 2008;105(50):19579−19586. https://doi.org/10.1073/pnas.0809763105.

62. Wang D, Wang L, Gu J, et al. Scutellarin inhibits high glucose−induced and hypoxia-mimetic agent−induced angiogenic effects in human retinal endothelial cells through reactive oxygen species/hypoxia-inducible factor-1α/vascular endothelial growth factor pathway. *J Cardiovasc Pharmacol*. 2014;64(3):218−227. https://doi.org/10.1097/FJC.0000000000000109.

63. Kim WY, Oh SH, Woo JK, Hong WK, Lee HY. Targeting heat shock protein 90 overrides the resistance of lung cancer cells by blocking radiation-induced stabilization of hypoxia-inducible factor-1α. *Cancer Res*. 2009;69(4):1624−1632. https://doi.org/10.1158/0008-5472.CAN-08-0505.

64. Park SW, Kim JH, Kim K, et al. Beta-lapachone inhibits pathological retinal neovascularization in oxygen-induced retinopathy *via* regulation of HIF -1α. *J Cell Mol Med*. 2014;18(5):875−884. https://doi.org/10.1111/jcmm.12235.

65. Zeng M, Shen J, Liu Y, et al. The HIF-1 antagonist acriflavine: visualization in retina and suppression of ocular neovascularization. *J Mol Med*. 2017;95(4):417−429. https://doi.org/10.1007/s00109-016-1498-9.

66. Olenyuk BZ, Zhang GJ, Klco JM, Nickols NG, Kaelin WG, Dervan PB. Inhibition of vascular endothelial growth factor with a sequence-specific hypoxia response element antagonist. *Proc Natl Acad Sci USA*. 2004;101(48):16768−16773. https://doi.org/10.1073/pnas.0407617101.

67. Lee K, Qian DZ, Rey S, Wei H, Liu JO, Semenza GL. Anthracycline chemotherapy inhibits HIF-1 transcriptional activity and tumor-induced mobilization of circulating angiogenic cells. *Proc Natl Acad Sci USA*. 2009;106(7):2353−2358. https://doi.org/10.1073/pnas.0812801106.

68. Iwase T, Fu J, Yoshida T, et al. Sustained delivery of a HIF-1 antagonist for ocular neovascularization. *J Controlled Release*. 2013;172(3):625−633. https://doi.org/10.1016/j.jconrel.2013.10.008.

69. Yoshida T, Zhang H, Iwase T, Shen J, Semenza GL, Campochiaro PA. Digoxin inhibits retinal ischemia-induced HIF-1α expression and ocular neovascularization. *FASEB J*. 2010;24(6):1759−1767. https://doi.org/10.1096/fj.09-145664.

70. Zhang JS, Da Wang J, An Y, et al. Cedilanid inhibits retinal neovascularization in a mouse model of oxygen-induced retinopathy. *Mol Vis*. 2017;23:346−355.

71. Lee K, Zhang H, Qian DZ, Rey S, Liu JO, Semenza GL. Acriflavine inhibits HIF-1 dimerization, tumor growth, and vascularization. *Proc Natl Acad Sci USA*. 2009;106(42):17910−17915. https://doi.org/10.1073/pnas.0909353106.

72. Atzori MG, Tentori L, Ruffini F, et al. The anti-vascular endothelial growth factor receptor-1 monoclonal antibody D16F7 inhibits glioma growth and angiogenesis in vivo. *J Pharmacol Exp Therapeut*. 2018;364(1):77−86. https://doi.org/10.1124/jpet.117.244434.

73. Lee SH. Tanibirumab (TTAC-0001): a fully human monoclonal antibody targets vascular endothelial growth factor receptor 2 (VEGFR-2). *Arch Pharm Res (Seoul)*. 2011;34(8):1223−1226. https://doi.org/10.1007/s12272-011-0821-9.

74. Poole RM, Vaidya A. Ramucirumab: first global approval. *Drugs*. 2014;74(9):1047−1058. https://doi.org/10.1007/s40265-014-0244-2.

75. Di Stasi R, De Rosa L, Diana D, Fattorusso R, D'Andrea LD. Human recombinant VEGFR2D4 biochemical characterization to investigate novel anti-VEGFR2D4 antibodies for allosteric targeting of VEGFR2. *Mol Biotechnol*. 2019;61(7):513−520. https://doi.org/10.1007/s12033-019-00181-7.

76. Bhargava P, Robinson MO. Development of second-generation VEGFR tyrosine kinase inhibitors: current status. *Curr Oncol Rep*. 2011;13(2):103−111. https://doi.org/10.1007/s11912-011-0154-3.

77. Lee WS, Shim SR, Lee SY, Yoo JS, Cho SK. Preclinical pharmacokinetics, interspecies scaling, and pharmacokinetics of a Phase I clinical trial of TTAC-0001, a fully human monoclonal antibody against vascular endothelial growth factor 2. *Drug Des Dev Ther*. 2018;12:495−504. https://doi.org/10.2147/DDDT.S150241.

78. Hyde CAC, Giese A, Stuttfeld E, et al. Targeting extracellular domains D4 and D7 of vascular endothelial growth factor receptor 2 reveals allosteric receptor regulatory sites. *Mol Cell Biol*. 2012;32(19):3802−3813. https://doi.org/10.1128/MCB.06787-11.

79. Uemura A, Fruttiger M, D'Amore PA, et al. VEGFR1 signaling in retinal angiogenesis and microinflammation. *Prog Retin Eye Res*. 2021;84:100954. https://doi.org/10.1016/j.preteyeres.2021.100954.

80. Shibuya M. VEGF-VEGFR system as a target for suppressing inflammation and other diseases. *Endocr, Metab Immune Disord: Drug Targets*. 2015;15(2):135−144. https://doi.org/10.2174/1871530315666150316121956.

81. Al-Khersan H, Hussain RM, Ciulla TA, Dugel PU. Innovative therapies for neovascular age-related macular degeneration. *Expet Opin Pharmacother*. 2019;20(15):1879−1891. https://doi.org/10.1080/14656566.2019.1636031.

82. Hussain RM, Shaukat BA, Ciulla LM, Berrocal AM, Sridhar J. Vascular endothelial growth factor Antagonists: promising players in the treatment of neovascular age-related macular degeneration. *Drug Des Dev Ther*. 2021;15:2653−2665. https://doi.org/10.2147/DDDT.S295223.

83. https://graybug.com/graybug-vision-presents-top-line-results-of-phase-1-2a-adagio-study-at-hawaiian-eye-retina-2019/.

84. Jackson TL, Boyer D, Brown DM, et al. Oral tyrosine kinase inhibitor for neovascular age-related macular degeneration: a phase 1 dose-escalation study. *JAMA Ophthalmol*. 2017;135(7):761−767. https://doi.org/10.1001/jamaophthalmol.2017.1571.

85. Csaky KG, Dugel PU, Pierce AJ, et al. Clinical evaluation of pazopanib eye drops versus ranibizumab intravitreal injections in subjects with neovascular age-related macular degeneration. *Ophthalmology*. 2015;122(3):579−588. https://doi.org/10.1016/j.ophtha.2014.09.036.

86. Patnaik A, LoRusso PM, Messersmith WA, et al. A Phase Ib study evaluating MNRP1685A, a fully human anti-NRP1 monoclonal antibody, in combination with bevacizumab and paclitaxel in patients with advanced solid tumors. *Cancer Chemother Pharmacol*. 2014;73(5):951−960. https://doi.org/10.1007/s00280-014-2426-8.

87. Weekes CD, Beeram M, Tolcher AW, et al. A phase I study of the human monoclonal anti-NRP1 antibody MNRP1685A in patients with advanced solid tumors. *Invest N Drugs*. 2014;32(4):653−660. https://doi.org/10.1007/s10637-014-0071-z.

88. Barczyk M, Carracedo S, Gullberg D. Integrins. *Cell Tissue Res*. 2010;339(1):269−280. https://doi.org/10.1007/s00441-009-0834-6.

89. Bhatwadekar AD, Kansara V, Luo Q, Ciulla T. Anti-integrin therapy for retinovascular diseases. *Expet Opin Invest Drugs*. 2020;29(9):935−945. https://doi.org/10.1080/13543784.2020.1795639.

90. Friedlander M, Theesfeld CL, Sugita M, et al. Involvement of integrins alpha v beta 3 and alpha v beta 5 in ocular neovascular diseases. *Proc Natl Acad Sci U S A*. 1996;93(18):9764−9769. https://doi.org/10.1073/pnas.93.18.9764.

91. Ramakrishnan V, Bhaskar V, Law DA, et al. Preclinical evaluation of an anti-alpha5-beta1 integrin antibody as a novel anti-angiogenic agent. *J Exp Therapeut Oncol.* 2006;5(4):273−286.

92. Joussen AM, Murata T, Tsujikawa A, Kirchhof B, Bursell SE, Adamis AP. Leukocyte-mediated endothelial cell injury and death in the diabetic retina. *Am J Pathol.* 2001; 158(1):147−152. https://doi.org/10.1016/S0002-9440(10)63952-1.

93. Miyamoto K, Khosrof S, Bursell SE, et al. Prevention of leukostasis and vascular leakage in streptozotocin-induced diabetic retinopathy via intercellular adhesion molecule-1 inhibition. *Proc Natl Acad Sci U S A.* 1999;96(19):10836−10841. https://doi.org/10.1073/pnas.96.19.10836.

94. Barouch FC, Miyamoto K, Allport JR, et al. Integrin-mediated neutrophil adhesion and retinal leukostasis in diabetes. *Invest Ophthalmol Vis Sci.* 2000;41(5):1153−1158.

95. Allegro Ophthalmics L Risuteganib (LUMINATE®). Potential para- digm shift in the treatment of oxidative stress-induced DME. In: *Ophthalmic Innovations Symposium.* 2018. Chicago (IL).

96. Oxurion NV. *Expert Presentation of Positive Topline Data from a Phase 1 Study Evaluating THR-687 for the Treatment of DME, at Angiogenesis, Exudation, and Degeneration 2020 Conference.* 2020. Miami, FL.

97. cited 2020 Jun 26. *A Phase 1 Study of THR 687: An Integrin Antagonist for the Treatment of Diabetic Macular Edema (DME)*; 2020. Available from: https://www.oxurion.com/content/phase-1-study-thr-687-integrin-	antagonist-treatment-diabetic-macular-edema-dme.

98. http://www.scifluor.com/media-center/docs/SciFluor_SF0166-Phase-I_IIDME-results-9-27-2017-Final.pdf - Google search. 2020 [cited 2020 Jun 4]. Available from: http://www.scifluor.com/media-center/docs/SciFluor_SF0166-Phase-I_II%20DME-results-9-27-2017-Final.pdf.

99. Wilkinson-Berka JL, Jones D, Taylor G, et al. SB-267268, a nonpeptidic antagonist of alpha(v)beta3 and alpha(v)beta5 integrins, reduces angiogenesis and VEGF expression in a mouse model of retinopathy of prematurity. *Invest Ophthalmol Vis Sci.* 2006;47(4): 1600−1605. https://doi.org/10.1167/iovs.05-1314.

100. Mirando AC, Shen J, Silva RLE, et al. A collagen IV-derived peptide disrupts α5β1 integrin and potentiates Ang2/Tie2 signaling. *JCI Insight.* 2019;4(4):122043. https://doi.org/10.1172/jci.insight.122043.

101. Santulli RJ, Kinney WA, Ghosh S, et al. Studies with an orally bioavailable alpha V integrin antagonist in animal models of ocular vasculopathy: retinal neovascularization in mice and retinal vascular permeability in diabetic rats. *J Pharmacol Exp Therapeut.* 2008;324(3):894−901. https://doi.org/10.1124/jpet.107.131656.

102. Kobayashi Y, Yoshida S, Zhou Y, et al. Tenascin-C secreted by transdifferentiated retinal pigment epithelial cells promotes choroidal neovascularization via integrin αV. *Lab Investig J Tech Methods Pathol.* 2016;96(11):1178−1188. https://doi.org/10.1038/labinvest.2016.99.

103. Montassar F, Darche M, Blaizot A, et al. Lebecetin, a C-type lectin, inhibits choroidal and retinal neovascularization. *FASEB J Off Publ Fed Am Soc Exp Biol.* 2017;31(3): 1107−1119. https://doi.org/10.1096/fj.201600351R.

104. Oliveira LB, Meyer CH, Kumar J, et al. RGD peptide-assisted vitrectomy to facilitate induction of a posterior vitreous detachment: a new principle in pharmacological vitreolysis. *Curr Eye Res.* 2002;25(6):333−340. https://doi.org/10.1076/ceyr.25.6.333.14234.

105. Yasukawa T, Hoffmann S, Eichler W, Friedrichs U, Wang YS, Wiedemann P. Inhibition of experimental choroidal neovascularization in rats by an alpha(v)-integrin antagonist. *Curr Eye Res*. 2004;28(5):359−366. https://doi.org/10.1076/ceyr.28.5.359.28678.

106. Shaw LT, Mackin A, Shah R, et al. Risuteganib-a novel integrin inhibitor for the treatment of non-exudative (dry) age-related macular degeneration and diabetic macular edema. *Expet Opin Invest Drugs*. 2020;29(6):547−554. https://doi.org/10.1080/13543784.2020.1763953.

107. Fachinger G, Deutsch U, Risau W. Functional interaction of vascular endothelial-protein-tyrosine phosphatase with the angiopoietin receptor Tie-2. *Oncogene*. 1999;18(43):5948−5953. https://doi.org/10.1038/sj.onc.1202992.

108. Hussain RM, Neiweem AE, Kansara V, Harris A, Ciulla TA. Tie-2/Angiopoietin pathway modulation as a therapeutic strategy for retinal disease. *Expet Opin Invest Drugs*. 2019;28(10):861−869. https://doi.org/10.1080/13543784.2019.1667333.

109. Campochiaro PA, Peters KG. Targeting Tie2 for treatment of diabetic retinopathy and diabetic macular edema. *Curr Diabetes Rep*. 2016;16(12):126. https://doi.org/10.1007/s11892-016-0816-5.

110. Campochiaro PA, Khanani A, Singer M, et al. Enhanced benefit in diabetic macular edema from AKB-9778 Tie2 activation combined with vascular endothelial growth factor suppression. *Ophthalmology*. 2016;123(8):1722−1730. https://doi.org/10.1016/j.ophtha.2016.04.025.

111. Wykoff CC, Abreu F, Adamis AP, et al. Efficacy, durability, and safety of intravitreal faricimab with extended dosing up to every 16 weeks in patients with diabetic macular oedema (YOSEMITE and RHINE): two randomised, double-masked, phase 3 trials. Published online January 21 *Lancet Lond Engl*. 2022. https://doi.org/10.1016/S0140-6736(22)00018-6. S0140-6736(22)00018-6.

112. Grisanti S, Canbek S, Kaiserling E, et al. Expression of endoglin in choroidal neovascularization. *Exp Eye Res*. 2004;78(2):207−213. https://doi.org/10.1016/j.exer.2003.11.008.

113. Korenfeld MS, Silverstein SM, Cooke DL, Vogel R, Crockett RS. Difluprednate ophthalmic emulsion 0.05% (durezol) study group. Difluprednate ophthalmic emulsion 0.05% for postoperative inflammation and pain. *J Cataract Refract Surg*. 2009;35(1):26−34. https://doi.org/10.1016/j.jcrs.2008.09.024.

114. Foster CS, Davanzo R, Flynn TE, McLeod K, Vogel R, Crockett RS. Durezol (Difluprednate Ophthalmic Emulsion 0.05%) compared with Pred Forte 1% ophthalmic suspension in the treatment of endogenous anterior uveitis. *J Ocul Pharmacol Ther Off J Assoc Ocul Pharmacol Ther*. 2010;26(5):475−483. https://doi.org/10.1089/jop.2010.0059.

115. Nakano S, Yamamoto T, Kirii E, Abe S, Yamashita H. Steroid eye drop treatment (difluprednate ophthalmic emulsion) is effective in reducing refractory diabetic macular edema. *Graefes Arch Clin Exp Ophthalmol Albrecht Von Graefes Arch Klin Exp Ophthalmol*. 2010;248(6):805−810. https://doi.org/10.1007/s00417-010-1316-y.

116. Nakano Goto S, Yamamoto T, Kirii E, Abe S, Yamashita H. Treatment of diffuse diabetic macular oedema using steroid eye drops. *Acta Ophthalmol*. 2012;90(7):628−632. https://doi.org/10.1111/j.1755-3768.2010.02066.x.

117. Kaur S, Yangzes S, Singh S, Sachdev N. Efficacy and safety of topical difluprednate in persistent diabetic macular edema. *Int Ophthalmol*. 2016;36(3):335−340. https://doi.org/10.1007/s10792-015-0121-3.

118. Tanito M, Hara K, Takai Y, et al. Topical dexamethasone-cyclodextrin microparticle eye drops for diabetic macular edema. *Invest Ophthalmol Vis Sci*. 2011;52(11): 7944−7948. https://doi.org/10.1167/iovs.11-8178.

119. Ohira A, Hara K, Jóhannesson G, et al. Topical dexamethasone γ-cyclodextrin nanoparticle eye drops increase visual acuity and decrease macular thickness in diabetic macular oedema. *Acta Ophthalmol*. 2015;93(7):610−615. https://doi.org/10.1111/aos.12803.

120. Rao P, Knaus EE. Evolution of nonsteroidal anti-inflammatory drugs (NSAIDs): cyclooxygenase (COX) inhibition and beyond. *J Pharm Pharm Sci Publ Can Soc Pharm Sci Soc Can Sci Pharm*. 2008;11(2):81s−110s. https://doi.org/10.18433/j3t886.

121. Jones J, Francis P. Ophthalmic utility of topical bromfenac, a twice-daily nonsteroidal anti-inflammatory agent. *Expet Opin Pharmacother*. 2009;10(14):2379−2385. https://doi.org/10.1517/14656560903188425.

122. Gaynes BI, Onyekwuluje A. Topical ophthalmic NSAIDs: a discussion with focus on nepafenac ophthalmic suspension. *Clin Ophthalmol Auckl NZ*. 2008;2(2):355−368. https://doi.org/10.2147/opth.s1067.

123. Pinna A, Blasetti F, Ricci GD, Boscia F. Bromfenac eyedrops in the treatment of diabetic macular edema: a pilot study. *Eur J Ophthalmol*. 2017;27(3):326−330. https://doi.org/10.5301/ejo.5000888.

124. Callanan D, Williams P. Topical nepafenac in the treatment of diabetic macular edema. *Clin Ophthalmol Auckl NZ*. 2008;2(4):689−692. https://doi.org/10.2147/opth.s3965.

125. Evliyaoğlu F, Akpolat Ç, Kurt MM, Çekiç O, Nuri Elçioğlu M. Retinal vascular caliber changes after topical nepafenac treatment for diabetic macular edema. *Curr Eye Res*. 2018;43(3):357−361. https://doi.org/10.1080/02713683.2017.1399425.

126. Howaidy A, Eldaly ZH, Anis M, Othman TM. Prophylaxis of macular edema after cataract surgery in diabetic patients, topical Nepafenac versus intravitreal Ranibizumab. *Eur J Ophthalmol*. 2022;32(1):205−212. https://doi.org/10.1177/11206721211001275.

127. Noda K, Nakao S, Zandi S, Engelstädter V, Mashima Y, Hafezi-Moghadam A. Vascular adhesion protein-1 regulates leukocyte transmigration rate in the retina during diabetes. *Exp Eye Res*. 2009;89(5):774−781. https://doi.org/10.1016/j.exer.2009.07.010.

128. Singh AD, Kulkarni YA. Vascular adhesion protein-1 and microvascular diabetic complications. *Pharmacol Rep*. 2022;74(1):40−46. https://doi.org/10.1007/s43440-021-00343-y.

129. Murata M, Noda K, Fukuhara J, et al. Soluble vascular adhesion protein-1 accumulates in proliferative diabetic retinopathy. *Investig Opthalmology Vis Sci*. 2012;53(7):4055. https://doi.org/10.1167/iovs.12-9857.

130. Salmi M, Jalkanen S. Vascular adhesion protein-1: a cell surface amine oxidase in translation. *Antioxidants Redox Signal*. 2019;30(3):314−332. https://doi.org/10.1089/ars.2017.7418.

131. Stolen CM, Marttila-Ichihara F, Koskinen K, et al. Absence of the endothelial oxidase AOC3 leads to abnormal leukocyte traffic in vivo. *Immunity*. 2005;22(1):105−115. https://doi.org/10.1016/j.immuni.2004.12.006.

132. Yoshikawa N, Noda K, Ozawa Y, Tsubota K, Mashima Y, Ishida S. Blockade of vascular adhesion protein-1 attenuates choroidal neovascularization. *Mol Vis*. 2012; 18:593−600.

133. Matsuda T, Noda K, Murata M, et al. Vascular adhesion protein-1 blockade suppresses ocular inflammation after retinal laser photocoagulation in mice. *Invest Ophthalmol Vis Sci*. 2017;58(7):3254−3261. https://doi.org/10.1167/iovs.17-21555.

134. Tékus V, Horváth ÁI, Csekő K, et al. Protective effects of the novel amine-oxidase inhibitor multi-target drug SZV 1287 on streptozotocin-induced beta cell damage and diabetic complications in rats. *Biomed Pharmacother.* 2021;134:111105. https://doi.org/10.1016/j.biopha.2020.111105.

135. Nguyen QD, Sepah YJ, Berger B, et al. Primary outcomes of the VIDI study: phase 2, double-masked, randomized, active-controlled study of ASP8232 for diabetic macular edema. *Int J Retina Vitr.* 2019;5:28. https://doi.org/10.1186/s40942-019-0178-7.

136. *Business Wire. R-Tech Ueno: Announcement on Completion of the Phase I Single-Dose Clinical Trial for the Novel VAP-1 Inhibitor RTU-1096*; 2015. https://www.businesswire.com/news/home/20150524005057/en/R-Tech-Ueno-Announcement-Completion-Phase-Single-Dose-Clinical. Accessed January 25, 2021.

137. Schilter HC, Collison A, Russo RC, et al. Effects of an anti-inflammatory VAP-1/SSAO inhibitor, PXS-4728A, on pulmonary neutrophil migration. *Respir Res.* 2015;16:42. https://doi.org/10.1186/s12931-015-0200-z.

138. Jarnicki AG, Schilter H, Liu G, et al. The inhibitor of semicarbazide-sensitive amine oxidase, PXS-4728A, ameliorates key features of chronic obstructive pulmonary disease in a mouse model. *Br J Pharmacol.* 2016;173(22):3161–3175. https://doi.org/10.1111/bph.13573.

139. NCT03238963. A randomized, double-masked, placebo-controlled exploratory study to evaluate safety, tolerability, pharmacodynamics and pharmacokinetics of orally administered BI 1467335 for 12 weeks with a 12 week follow up period in patients with non-proliferative diabetic retinopathy without center-involved diabetic macular edema (ROBIN Study). https://clinicaltrials.gov/ct2/show/NCT03238963. Accessed 25 Jan 2021.

140. Boehringer Ingelheim. *Boehringer Ingelheim Discontinues Development of BI 1467335 for Diabetic Retinopathy*; 2020. https://www.boehringer-ingelheim.com/press-release/discontinuation-bi-1467335-diabetic-retinopathy. Accessed January 25, 2021.

141. Yao Y, Li R, Du J, Long L, Li X, Luo N. Interleukin-6 and diabetic retinopathy: a systematic review and meta-analysis. *Curr Eye Res.* 2019;44(5):564–574. https://doi.org/10.1080/02713683.2019.1570274.

142. Shimizu E. Plasma level of interleukin-6 is an indicator for predicting diabetic macular edema. *Jpn J Ophthalmol.* 2002;46(1):78–83. https://doi.org/10.1016/S0021-5155(01)00452-X.

143. Mocan MC, Kadayifcilar S, Eldem B. Elevated intravitreal interleukin-6 levels in patients with proliferative diabetic retinopathy. *Can J Ophthalmol.* 2006;41(6):747–752. https://doi.org/10.3129/i06-070.

144. Hou T, Tieu B, Ray S, et al. Roles of IL-6-gp130 signaling in vascular inflammation. *Curr Cardiol Rev.* 2008;4(3):179–192. https://doi.org/10.2174/157340308785160570.

145. Koleva-Georgieva DN, Sivkova NP, Terzieva D. Serum inflammatory cytokines IL-1β, IL-6, TNF-α and VEGF have influence on the development of diabetic retinopathy. *Folia Med (Plovdiv).* 2011;53(2). https://doi.org/10.2478/v10153-010-0036-8.

146. Gustavsson C, Agardh CD, Agardh E. Profile of intraocular tumour necrosis factor-α and interleukin-6 in diabetic subjects with different degrees of diabetic retinopathy. *Acta Ophthalmol.* 2013;91(5):445–452. https://doi.org/10.1111/j.1755-3768.2012.02430.x.

147. Mesquida M, Drawnel F, Lait PJ, et al. Modelling macular edema: the effect of IL-6 and IL-6R blockade on human blood–retinal barrier integrity in vitro. *Transl Vis Sci Technol.* 2019;8(5):32. https://doi.org/10.1167/tvst.8.5.32.

148. Valle ML, Dworshak J, Sharma A, Ibrahim AS, Al-Shabrawey M, Sharma S. Inhibition of interleukin-6 trans-signaling prevents inflammation and endothelial barrier disruption in retinal endothelial cells. *Exp Eye Res*. 2019;178:27−36. https://doi.org/10.1016/j.exer.2018.09.009.

149. Jo DH, Yun JH, Cho CS, Kim JH, Kim JH, Cho CH. Interaction between microglia and retinal pigment epithelial cells determines the integrity of outer blood-retinal barrier in diabetic retinopathy. *Glia*. 2019;67(2):321−331. https://doi.org/10.1002/glia.23542.

150. Barnes TC, Anderson ME, Moots RJ. The many faces of interleukin-6: the role of IL-6 in inflammation, vasculopathy, and fibrosis in systemic sclerosis. *Int J Rheumatol*. 2011;2011:1−6. https://doi.org/10.1155/2011/721608.

151. Rose-John S. IL-6 trans-signaling via the soluble IL-6 receptor: importance for the pro-inflammatory activities of IL-6. *Int J Biol Sci*. 2012;8(9):1237−1247. https://doi.org/10.7150/ijbs.4989.

152. Robinson R., Srinivasan M., Shanmugam A., et al. Interleukin-6 trans-signaling inhibition prevents oxidative stress in a mouse model of early diabetic retinopathy. Redox Biol. 2020;34:101574. https://doi.org/10.1016/j.redox.2020.101574.

153. Ebihara N, Matsuda A, Nakamura S, Matsuda H, Murakami A. Role of the IL-6 classic- and trans-signaling pathways in corneal sterile inflammation and wound healing. *Investig Opthalmology Vis Sci*. 2011;52(12):8549. https://doi.org/10.1167/iovs.11-7956.

154. Scheller J, Chalaris A, Schmidt-Arras D, Rose-John S. The pro- and anti-inflammatory properties of the cytokine interleukin-6. *Biochim Biophys Acta BBA Mol Cell Res*. 2011;1813(5):878−888. https://doi.org/10.1016/j.bbamcr.2011.01.034.

155. Reeh H, Rudolph N, Billing U, et al. Response to IL-6 trans- and IL-6 classic signalling is determined by the ratio of the IL-6 receptor α to gp130 expression: fusing experimental insights and dynamic modelling. *Cell Commun Signal*. 2019;17(1):46. https://doi.org/10.1186/s12964-019-0356-0.

156. Sharma S. Interleukin-6 trans-signaling: a pathway with therapeutic potential for diabetic retinopathy. *Front Physiol*. 2021;12:689429. https://doi.org/10.3389/fphys.2021.689429.

157. Ohsugi Y, Kishimoto T. The recombinant humanized anti-IL-6 receptor antibody tocilizumab, an innovative drug for the treatment of rheumatoid arthritis. *Expet Opin Biol Ther*. 2008;8(5):669−681. https://doi.org/10.1517/14712598.8.5.669.

158. Deuchler S, Schubert R, Singh P, et al. Vitreous expression of cytokines and growth factors in patients with diabetic retinopathy-An investigation of their expression based on clinical diabetic retinopathy grade. *PLoS One*. 2021;16(5):e0248439. https://doi.org/10.1371/journal.pone.0248439.

159. Mitoma H, Horiuchi T, Tsukamoto H, Ueda N. Molecular mechanisms of action of anti-TNF-α agents - comparison among therapeutic TNF-α antagonists. *Cytokine*. 2018;101:56−63. https://doi.org/10.1016/j.cyto.2016.08.014.

160. Shanmuganathan S, Angayarkanni N. Chebulagic acid Chebulinic acid and Gallic acid, the active principles of Triphala, inhibit TNFα induced pro-angiogenic and pro-inflammatory activities in retinal capillary endothelial cells by inhibiting p38, ERK and NFkB phosphorylation. *Vasc Pharmacol*. 2018;108:23−35. https://doi.org/10.1016/j.vph.2018.04.005.

161. Xiao A, Zhong H, Xiong L, et al. Sequential and dynamic variations of IL-6, CD18, ICAM, TNF-α, and microstructure in the early stage of diabetic retinopathy. *Dis Markers*. 2022;2022:1946104. https://doi.org/10.1155/2022/1946104.

162. Lee MY, Park S, Song JY, Ra H, Baek JU, Baek J. Inflammatory cytokines and retinal nonperfusion area in quiescent proliferative diabetic retinopathy. *Cytokine*. 2022;154: 155774. https://doi.org/10.1016/j.cyto.2021.155774.

163. Hagbi-Levi S, Tiosano L, Rinsky B, et al. Anti-tumor necrosis factor alpha reduces the proangiogenic effects of activated macrophages derived from patients with age-related macular degeneration. *Mol Vis*. 2021;27:622−631.

164. Feng S, Yu H, Yu Y, et al. Levels of inflammatory cytokines IL-1β, IL-6, IL-8, IL-17A, and TNF-α in aqueous humour of patients with diabetic retinopathy. *J Diabetes Res*. 2018;2018:8546423. https://doi.org/10.1155/2018/8546423.

165. Wu F, Phone A, Lamy R, et al. Correlation of aqueous, vitreous, and plasma cytokine levels in patients with proliferative diabetic retinopathy. *Invest Ophthalmol Vis Sci*. 2020;61(2):26. https://doi.org/10.1167/iovs.61.2.26.

166. Storti F, Pulley J, Kuner P, Abt M, Luhmann UFO. Circulating biomarkers of inflammation and endothelial activation in diabetic retinopathy. *Transl Vis Sci Technol*. 2021;10(12):8. https://doi.org/10.1167/tvst.10.12.8.

167. Sfikakis PP, Markomichelakis N, Theodossiadis GP, Grigoropoulos V, Katsilambros N, Theodossiadis PG. Regression of sight-threatening macular edema in type 2 diabetes following treatment with the anti-tumor necrosis factor monoclonal antibody infliximab. *Diabetes Care*. 2005;28(2):445−447. https://doi.org/10.2337/ diacare.28.2.445.

168. Yrjänheikki J, Tikka T, Keinänen R, Goldsteins G, Chan PH, Koistinaho J. A tetracycline derivative, minocycline, reduces inflammation and protects against focal cerebral ischemia with a wide therapeutic window. *Proc Natl Acad Sci U S A*. 1999; 96(23):13496−13500. https://doi.org/10.1073/pnas.96.23.13496.

169. Scholz R, Sobotka M, Caramoy A, Stempfl T, Moehle C, Langmann T. Minocycline counter-regulates pro-inflammatory microglia responses in the retina and protects from degeneration. *J Neuroinflammation*. 2015;12:209. https://doi.org/10.1186/ s12974-015-0431-4.

170. Zhang C, Lei B, Lam TT, Yang F, Sinha D, Tso MOM. Neuroprotection of photoreceptors by minocycline in light-induced retinal degeneration. *Invest Ophthalmol Vis Sci*. 2004;45(8):2753−2759. https://doi.org/10.1167/iovs.03-1344.

171. Tikka T, Fiebich BL, Goldsteins G, Keinanen R, Koistinaho J. Minocycline, a tetracycline derivative, is neuroprotective against excitotoxicity by inhibiting activation and proliferation of microglia. *J Neurosci Off J Soc Neurosci*. 2001;21(8):2580−2588.

172. Krady JK, Basu A, Allen CM, et al. Minocycline reduces proinflammatory cytokine expression, microglial activation, and caspase-3 activation in a rodent model of diabetic retinopathy. *Diabetes*. 2005;54(5):1559−1565. https://doi.org/10.2337/ diabetes.54.5.1559.

173. Chen M, Ona VO, Li M, et al. Minocycline inhibits caspase-1 and caspase-3 expression and delays mortality in a transgenic mouse model of Huntington disease. *Nat Med*. 2000;6(7):797−801. https://doi.org/10.1038/77528.

174. Teng YD, Choi H, Onario RC, et al. Minocycline inhibits contusion-triggered mitochondrial cytochrome *c* release and mitigates functional deficits after spinal cord injury. *Proc Natl Acad Sci U S A*. 2004;101(9):3071−3076. https://doi.org/10.1073/ pnas.0306239101.

175. Cukras CA, Petrou P, Chew EY, Meyerle CB, Wong WT. Oral minocycline for the treatment of diabetic macular edema (DME): results of a phase I/II clinical study. *Invest Ophthalmol Vis Sci*. 2012;53(7):3865−3874. https://doi.org/10.1167/iovs.11-9413.

176. Zhang J, Wu Y, Jin Y, et al. Intravitreal injection of erythropoietin protects both retinal vascular and neuronal cells in early diabetes. *Invest Ophthalmol Vis Sci.* 2008;49(2): 732−742. https://doi.org/10.1167/iovs.07-0721.

177. Wang Q, Pfister F, Dorn-Beineke A, et al. Low-dose erythropoietin inhibits oxidative stress and early vascular changes in the experimental diabetic retina. *Diabetologia.* 2010;53(6):1227−1238. https://doi.org/10.1007/s00125-010-1727-7.

178. Zhu B, Wang W, Gu Q, Xu X. Erythropoietin protects retinal neurons and glial cells in early-stage streptozotocin-induced diabetic rats. *Exp Eye Res.* 2008;86(2):375−382. https://doi.org/10.1016/j.exer.2007.11.010.

179. Liu X, Zhu B, Zou H, et al. Carbamylated erythropoietin mediates retinal neuroprotection in streptozotocin-induced early-stage diabetic rats. *Graefes Arch Clin Exp Ophthalmol Albrecht Von Graefes Arch Klin Exp Ophthalmol.* 2015;253(8):1263−1272. https://doi.org/10.1007/s00417-015-2969-3.

180. Mitsuhashi J, Morikawa S, Shimizu K, Ezaki T, Yasuda Y, Hori S. Intravitreal injection of erythropoietin protects against retinal vascular regression at the early stage of diabetic retinopathy in streptozotocin-induced diabetic rats. *Exp Eye Res.* 2013;106: 64−73. https://doi.org/10.1016/j.exer.2012.11.001.

181. Shen J, Wu Y, Xu JY, et al. ERK- and Akt-dependent neuroprotection by erythropoietin (EPO) against glyoxal-AGEs via modulation of Bcl-xL, Bax, and BAD. *Invest Ophthalmol Vis Sci.* 2010;51(1):35−46. https://doi.org/10.1167/iovs.09-3544.

182. Hu LM, Luo Y, Zhang J, et al. EPO reduces reactive gliosis and stimulates neurotrophin expression in Muller cells. *Front Biosci Elite Ed.* 2011;3:1541−1555. https://doi.org/10.2741/e355.

183. Zhang J, Hu LM, Xu G, et al. Anti-VEGF effects of intravitreal erythropoietin in early diabetic retinopathy. *Front Biosci Elite Ed.* 2010;2:912−927. https://doi.org/10.2741/e151.

184. Lei X, Zhang J, Shen J, et al. EPO attenuates inflammatory cytokines by Muller cells in diabetic retinopathy. *Front Biosci Elite Ed.* 2011;3:201−211. https://doi.org/10.2741/e234.

185. Xu G, Kang D, Zhang C, et al. Erythropoietin protects retinal cells in diabetic rats through upregulating ZnT8 via activating ERK pathway and inhibiting HIF-1α expression. *Invest Ophthalmol Vis Sci.* 2015;56(13):8166−8178. https://doi.org/10.1167/iovs.15-18093.

186. Gu L, Xu H, Wang F, et al. Erythropoietin exerts a neuroprotective function against glutamate neurotoxicity in experimental diabetic retina. *Invest Ophthalmol Vis Sci.* 2014;55(12):8208−8222. https://doi.org/10.1167/iovs.14-14435.

187. Liu D, Xu H, Zhang C, et al. Erythropoietin maintains VE-cadherin expression and barrier function in experimental diabetic retinopathy via inhibiting VEGF/VEGFR2/Src signaling pathway. *Life Sci.* 2020;259:118273. https://doi.org/10.1016/j.lfs.2020.118273.

188. Zhang C, Xie H, Yang Q, et al. Erythropoietin protects outer blood-retinal barrier in experimental diabetic retinopathy by up-regulating ZO-1 and occludin. *Clin Exp Ophthalmol.* 2019;47(9):1182−1197. https://doi.org/10.1111/ceo.13619.

189. Xie H, Zhang C, Liu D, et al. Erythropoietin protects the inner blood-retinal barrier by inhibiting microglia phagocytosis via Src/Akt/cofilin signalling in experimental diabetic retinopathy. *Diabetologia.* 2021;64(1):211−225. https://doi.org/10.1007/s00125-020-05299-x.

190. Li W, Sinclair SH, Xu GT. Effects of intravitreal erythropoietin therapy for patients with chronic and progressive diabetic macular edema. *Ophthalmic Surg Lasers Imaging Off J Int Soc Imaging Eye*. 2010;41(1):18−25. https://doi.org/10.3928/15428877-20091230-03.

191. Ahmet I, Tae HJ, Juhaszova M, et al. A small nonerythropoietic helix B surface peptide based upon erythropoietin structure is cardioprotective against ischemic myocardial damage. *Mol Med*. 2011;17(3−4):194−200. https://doi.org/10.2119/molmed.2010.00235.

192. Brines M, Patel NSA, Villa P, et al. Nonerythropoietic, tissue-protective peptides derived from the tertiary structure of erythropoietin. *Proc Natl Acad Sci USA*. 2008; 105(31):10925−10930. https://doi.org/10.1073/pnas.0805594105.

193. McVicar CM, Hamilton R, Colhoun LM, et al. Intervention with an erythropoietin-derived peptide protects against neuroglial and vascular degeneration during diabetic retinopathy. *Diabetes*. 2011;60(11):2995−3005. https://doi.org/10.2337/db11-0026.

194. Collino M, Benetti E, Rogazzo M, et al. A non-erythropoietic peptide derivative of erythropoietin decreases susceptibility to diet-induced insulin resistance in mice: EPO derivative effects on insulin resistance. *Br J Pharmacol*. 2014;171(24): 5802−5815. https://doi.org/10.1111/bph.12888.

195. Brines M, Dunne AN, van Velzen M, et al. ARA 290, a nonerythropoietic peptide engineered from erythropoietin, improves metabolic control and neuropathic symptoms in patients with type 2 diabetes. *Mol Med*. 2014;20(1):658−666. https://doi.org/10.2119/molmed.2014.00215.

196. Hernández C, García-Ramírez M, Corraliza L, et al. Topical administration of somatostatin prevents retinal neurodegeneration in experimental diabetes. *Diabetes*. 2013; 62(7):2569−2578. https://doi.org/10.2337/db12-0926.

197. Saylor M, McLoon LK, Harrison AR, Lee MS. Experimental and clinical evidence for brimonidine as an optic nerve and retinal neuroprotective agent: an evidence-based review. *Arch Ophthalmol Chic Ill 1960*. 2009;127(4):402−406. https://doi.org/10.1001/archophthalmol.2009.9.

198. Simó R, Hernández C, Porta M, et al. Effects of topically administered neuroprotective drugs in early stages of diabetic retinopathy: results of the EUROCONDOR clinical trial. *Diabetes*. 2019;68(2):457−463. https://doi.org/10.2337/db18-0682.

199. Grauslund J, Frydkjaer-Olsen U, Peto T, et al. Topical treatment with brimonidine and somatostatin causes retinal vascular dilation in patients with early diabetic retinopathy from the EUROCONDOR. *Invest Ophthalmol Vis Sci*. 2019;60(6):2257−2262. https://doi.org/10.1167/iovs.18-26487.

200. Naftali Ben Haim L, Moisseiev E. Drug delivery via the suprachoroidal space for the treatment of retinal diseases. *Pharmaceutics*. 2021;13(7):967. https://doi.org/10.3390/pharmaceutics13070967.

201. Barar J, Aghanejad A, Fathi M, Omidi Y. Advanced drug delivery and targeting technologies for the ocular diseases. *BioImpacts BI*. 2016;6(1):49−67. https://doi.org/10.15171/bi.2016.07.

202. Del Amo EM, Urtti A. Current and future ophthalmic drug delivery systems. A shift to the posterior segment. *Drug Discov Today*. 2008;13(3−4):135−143. https://doi.org/10.1016/j.drudis.2007.11.002.

203. Khanani AM, Aziz AA, Weng CY, et al. Port delivery system: a novel drug delivery platform to treat retinal diseases. *Expet Opin Drug Deliv*. 2021;18(11):1571−1576. https://doi.org/10.1080/17425247.2021.1968826.

204. Campochiaro PA, Marcus DM, Awh CC, et al. The port delivery system with ranibizumab for neovascular age-related macular degeneration: results from the randomized phase 2 ladder clinical trial. *Ophthalmology.* 2019;126(8):1141−1154. https://doi.org/10.1016/j.ophtha.2019.03.036.

205. Holekamp NM, Campochiaro PA, Chang MA, et al. Archway randomized phase 3 trial of the port delivery system with ranibizumab for neovascular age-related macular degeneration. Ophthalmology. Published online September 29, 2021:S0161-6420(21)00734-X. doi:10.1016/j.ophtha.2021.09.016

206. Ranta VP, Mannermaa E, Lummepuro K, et al. Barrier analysis of periocular drug delivery to the posterior segment. *J Control Release Off J Control Release Soc.* 2010;148(1):42−48. https://doi.org/10.1016/j.jconrel.2010.08.028.

207. Robinson MR, Lee SS, Kim H, et al. A rabbit model for assessing the ocular barriers to the transscleral delivery of triamcinolone acetonide. *Exp Eye Res.* 2006;82(3):479−487. https://doi.org/10.1016/j.exer.2005.08.007.

208. Wykoff CC, Khurana RN, Lampen SIR, et al. Suprachoroidal triamcinolone acetonide for diabetic macular edema: the HULK trial. *Ophthalmol Retina.* 2018;2(8):874−877. https://doi.org/10.1016/j.oret.2018.03.008.

209. Lampen SIR, Khurana RN, Noronha G, Brown DM, Wykoff CC. Suprachoroidal space alterations following delivery of triamcinolone acetonide: post-hoc analysis of the phase 1/2 HULK study of patients with diabetic macular edema. *Ophthalmic Surg Lasers Imaging Retina.* 2018;49(9):692−697. https://doi.org/10.3928/23258160-20180831-07.

210. Barakat MR, Wykoff CC, Gonzalez V, et al. Suprachoroidal CLS-TA plus intravitreal aflibercept for diabetic macular edema: a randomized, double-masked, parallel-design, controlled study. *Ophthalmol Retina.* 2021;5(1):60−70. https://doi.org/10.1016/j.oret.2020.08.007.

211. PAN-90806: Once-daily topical anti-VEGF eye drop for wet AMD and other neovascular eye disease. Available online https://www.panopticapharma.com/wp-content/uploads/2019/10/PAN-90806-Data-at-OIS@AAO.pdf.

212. Pedersen KS, Grierson PM, Picus J, et al. Vorolanib (X-82), an oral anti-VEGFR/PDGFR/CSF1R tyrosine kinase inhibitor, with everolimus in solid tumors: results of a phase I study. *Invest N Drugs.* 2021;39(5):1298−1305. https://doi.org/10.1007/s10637-021-01093-7.

213. Shen J, Frye M, Lee BL, et al. Targeting VE-PTP activates TIE2 and stabilizes the ocular vasculature. *J Clin Invest.* 2014;124(10):4564−4576. https://doi.org/10.1172/JCI74527.

214. Campochiaro PA, Sophie R, Tolentino M, et al. Treatment of diabetic macular edema with an inhibitor of vascular endothelial-protein tyrosine phosphatase that activates Tie2. *Ophthalmology.* 2015;122(3):545−554. https://doi.org/10.1016/j.ophtha.2014.09.023.

215. Kim HM, Park YJ, Lee S, et al. Intraocular pharmacokinetics of 10-fold intravitreal ranibizumab injection dose in rabbits. *Transl Vis Sci Technol.* 2020;9(4):7. https://doi.org/10.1167/tvst.9.4.7.

216. Sepah YJ, Sadiq MA, Boyer D, et al. Twenty-four-Month outcomes of the ranibizumab for edema of the macula in diabetes - protocol 3 with high dose (READ-3) study. *Ophthalmology.* 2016;123(12):2581−2587. https://doi.org/10.1016/j.ophtha.2016.08.040.

217. Jaffe GJ, McCallum RM, Branchaud B, Skalak C, Butuner Z, Ashton P. Long-term follow-up results of a pilot trial of a fluocinolone acetonide implant to treat posterior uveitis. *Ophthalmology.* 2005;112(7):1192−1198. https://doi.org/10.1016/j.ophtha.2005.03.013.

218. Kuppermann BD, Blumenkranz MS, Haller JA, et al. Randomized controlled study of an intravitreous dexamethasone drug delivery system in patients with persistent macular edema. *Arch Ophthalmol Chic Ill 1960.* 2007;125(3):309−317. https://doi.org/10.1001/archopht.125.3.309.

219. Kane FE, Burdan J, Cutino A, Green KE. Iluvien: a new sustained delivery technology for posterior eye disease. *Expet Opin Drug Deliv.* 2008;5(9):1039−1046. https://doi.org/10.1517/17425247.5.9.1039.

220. Boyer DS, Yoon YH, Belfort R, et al. Three-year, randomized, sham-controlled trial of dexamethasone intravitreal implant in patients with diabetic macular edema. *Ophthalmology.* 2014;121(10):1904−1914. https://doi.org/10.1016/j.ophtha.2014.04.024.

221. Campochiaro PA, Brown DM, Pearson A, et al. Sustained delivery fluocinolone acetonide vitreous inserts provide benefit for at least 3 years in patients with diabetic macular edema. *Ophthalmology.* 2012;119(10):2125−2132. https://doi.org/10.1016/j.ophtha.2012.04.030.

222. Cunha-Vaz J, Ashton P, Iezzi R, et al. Sustained delivery fluocinolone acetonide vitreous implants: long-term benefit in patients with chronic diabetic macular edema. *Ophthalmology.* 2014;121(10):1892−1903. https://doi.org/10.1016/j.ophtha.2014.04.019.

223. Darrow JJ. Luxturna: FDA documents reveal the value of a costly gene therapy. *Drug Discov Today.* 2019;24(4):949−954. https://doi.org/10.1016/j.drudis.2019.01.019.

224. Russell S, Bennett J, Wellman JA, et al. Efficacy and safety of voretigene neparvovec (AAV2-hRPE65v2) in patients with RPE65-mediated inherited retinal dystrophy: a randomised, controlled, open-label, phase 3 trial. *Lancet Lond Engl.* 2017;390(10097):849−860. https://doi.org/10.1016/S0140-6736(17)31868-8.

225. Liu Y, Fortmann SD, Shen J, et al. AAV8-antiVEGFfab ocular gene transfer for neovascular age-related macular degeneration. *Mol Ther J Am Soc Gene Ther.* 2018;26(2):542−549. https://doi.org/10.1016/j.ymthe.2017.12.002.

226. Ding K, Shen J, Hafiz Z, et al. AAV8-vectored suprachoroidal gene transfer produces widespread ocular transgene expression. *J Clin Invest.* 2019;129(11):4901−4911. https://doi.org/10.1172/JCI129085.

227. Chung SH, Frick SL, Yiu G. Targeting vascular endothelial growth factor using retinal gene therapy. *Ann Transl Med.* 2021;9(15):1277. https://doi.org/10.21037/atm-20-4417.

228. REGENXBIO Presents Positive Initial Data from Phase II ALTITUDETM Trial of RGX-314 for the Treatment of Diabetic Retinopathy Using Suprachoroidal Delivery at American Society of Retina Specialists Annual Meeting. Available Online Https pipelinereviewcomindexphp2021101079376DNA-RNA–CellsREGENXBIO-Presents-Posit-Initial-Data–Phase-II-Alt-Trial–RGX-314—Treat–Diabet-Retin-Using-Suprachoroidal-Deliv–Am-Sochtml.

229. Grishanin R, Vuillemenot B, Sharma P, et al. Preclinical evaluation of ADVM-022, a novel gene therapy approach to treating wet age-related macular degeneration. *Mol Ther J Am Soc Gene Ther.* 2019;27(1):118−129. https://doi.org/10.1016/j.ymthe.2018.11.003.

230. Gelfman CM, Grishanin R, Bender KO, et al. Comprehensive preclinical assessment of ADVM-022, an intravitreal anti-VEGF gene therapy for the treatment of neovascular AMD and diabetic macular edema. *J Ocul Pharmacol Ther Off J Assoc Ocul Pharmacol Ther*. 2021;37(3):181−190. https://doi.org/10.1089/jop.2021.0001.

231. Lai CM, Estcourt MJ, Himbeck RP, et al. Preclinical safety evaluation of subretinal AAV2.sFlt-1 in non-human primates. *Gene Ther*. 2012;19(10):999−1009. https://doi.org/10.1038/gt.2011.169.

232. Rakoczy EP, Lai CM, Magno AL, et al. Gene therapy with recombinant adeno-associated vectors for neovascular age-related macular degeneration: 1 year follow-up of a phase 1 randomised clinical trial. *Lancet Lond Engl*. 2015;386(10011):2395−2403. https://doi.org/10.1016/S0140-6736(15)00345-1.

233. Constable IJ, Pierce CM, Lai CM, et al. Phase 2a randomized clinical trial: safety and post hoc analysis of subretinal rAAV.sFLT-1 for wet age-related macular degeneration. *EBioMedicine*. 2016;14:168−175. https://doi.org/10.1016/j.ebiom.2016.11.016.

234. Heier JS, Kherani S, Desai S, et al. Intravitreous injection of AAV2-sFLT01 in patients with advanced neovascular age-related macular degeneration: a phase 1, open-label trial. *Lancet Lond Engl*. 2017;390(10089):50−61. https://doi.org/10.1016/S0140-6736(17)30979-0.

235. Scholz P, Altay L, Fauser S. A review of subthreshold micropulse laser for treatment of macular disorders. *Adv Ther*. 2017;34(7):1528−1555. https://doi.org/10.1007/s12325-017-0559-y.

236. Lavinsky D, Wang J, Huie P, et al. Nondamaging retinal laser therapy: rationale and applications to the macula. *Invest Ophthalmol Vis Sci*. 2016;57(6):2488−2500. https://doi.org/10.1167/iovs.15-18981.

237. Luttrull JK, Sramek C, Palanker D, Spink CJ, Musch DC. Long-term safety, high-resolution imaging, and tissue temperature modeling of subvisible diode micropulse photocoagulation for retinovascular macular edema. *Retina Phila Pa*. 2012;32(2):375−386. https://doi.org/10.1097/IAE.0b013e3182206f6c.

238. Lavinsky D, Sramek C, Wang J, et al. Subvisible retinal laser therapy: titration algorithm and tissue response. *Retina Phila Pa*. 2014;34(1):87−97. https://doi.org/10.1097/IAE.0b013e3182993edc.

239. Mainster MA. Wavelength selection in macular photocoagulation. Tissue optics, thermal effects, and laser systems. *Ophthalmology*. 1986;93(7):952−958. https://doi.org/10.1016/s0161-6420(86)33637-6.

240. Frizziero L, Calciati A, Midena G, et al. Subthreshold micropulse laser modulates retinal neuroinflammatory biomarkers in diabetic macular edema. *J Clin Med*. 2021;10(14):3134. https://doi.org/10.3390/jcm10143134.

241. Passos RM, Malerbi FK, Rocha M, Maia M, Farah ME. Real-life outcomes of subthreshold laser therapy for diabetic macular edema. *Int J Retina Vitr*. 2021;7(1):4. https://doi.org/10.1186/s40942-020-00268-3.

242. Sivaprasad S, Sandhu R, Tandon A, Sayed-Ahmed K, McHugh DA. Subthreshold micropulse diode laser photocoagulation for clinically significant diabetic macular oedema: a three-year follow up. *Clin Exp Ophthalmol*. 2007;35(7):640−644. https://doi.org/10.1111/j.1442-9071.2007.01566.x.

243. Chhablani J, Alshareef R, Kim DT, Narayanan R, Goud A, Mathai A. Comparison of different settings for yellow subthreshold laser treatment in diabetic macular edema. *BMC Ophthalmol*. 2018;18(1):168. https://doi.org/10.1186/s12886-018-0841-z.

244. Vujosevic S, Martini F, Longhin E, Convento E, Cavarzeran F, Midena E. Subthreshold micropulse yellow laser versus subthreshold micropulse infrared laser in center-involving diabetic macular edema: morphologic and functional safety. *Retina Phila Pa*. 2015;35(8):1594−1603. https://doi.org/10.1097/IAE.0000000000000521.

245. Donati MC, Murro V, Mucciolo DP, et al. Subthreshold yellow micropulse laser for treatment of diabetic macular edema: comparison between fixed and variable treatment regimen. *Eur J Ophthalmol*. 2021;31(3):1254−1260. https://doi.org/10.1177/1120672120915169.

246. El Matri L, Chebil A, El Matri K, Falfoul Y, Chebbi Z. Subthreshold micropulse laser adjuvant to bevacizumab versus bevacizumab monotherapy in treating diabetic macular edema: one- year- follow-up. *Ther Adv Ophthalmol*. 2021;13. https://doi.org/10.1177/25158414211040887, 25158414211040890.

247. Moisseiev E, Abbassi S, Thinda S, Yoon J, Yiu G, Morse LS. Subthreshold micropulse laser reduces anti-VEGF injection burden in patients with diabetic macular edema. *Eur J Ophthalmol*. 2018;28(1):68−73. https://doi.org/10.5301/ejo.5001000.

248. Antonetti DA, Klein R, Gardner TW. Diabetic retinopathy. *N Engl J Med*. 2012;366(13):1227−1239. https://doi.org/10.1056/NEJMra1005073.

249. Schreur V, Brouwers J, Van Huet RAC, et al. Long-term outcomes of vitrectomy for proliferative diabetic retinopathy. *Acta Ophthalmol*. 2021;99(1):83−89. https://doi.org/10.1111/aos.14482.

250. Nawaz IM, Rezzola S, Cancarini A, et al. Human vitreous in proliferative diabetic retinopathy: characterization and translational implications. *Prog Retin Eye Res*. 2019;72:100756. https://doi.org/10.1016/j.preteyeres.2019.03.002.

251. Muqit MMK, Stanga PE. Swept-source optical coherence tomography imaging of the cortical vitreous and the vitreoretinal interface in proliferative diabetic retinopathy: assessment of vitreoschisis, neovascularisation and the internal limiting membrane. *Br J Ophthalmol*. 2014;98(7):994−997. https://doi.org/10.1136/bjophthalmol-2013-304452.

252. de Smet MD, Castilla M. Ocriplasmin for diabetic retinopathy. *Expet Opin Biol Ther*. 2013;13(12):1741−1747. https://doi.org/10.1517/14712598.2013.853737.

253. Tamaki K, Usui-Ouchi A, Murakami A, Ebihara N. Fibrocytes and fibrovascular membrane formation in proliferative diabetic retinopathy. *Invest Ophthalmol Vis Sci*. 2016;57(11):4999−5005. https://doi.org/10.1167/iovs.16-19798.

254. Ahronovich EZ, Simaan N, Joos KM. A review of robotic and OCT-aided systems for vitreoretinal surgery. *Adv Ther*. 2021;38(5):2114−2129. https://doi.org/10.1007/s12325-021-01692-z.

255. Blinder KJ, Awh CC, Tewari A, Garg SJ, Srivastava SK, Kolesnitchenko V. Introduction to hypersonic vitrectomy. *Curr Opin Ophthalmol*. 2019;30(3):133−137. https://doi.org/10.1097/ICU.0000000000000563.

256. Rizzo S, Faraldi F. The future of small gauge vitrectomy. *Retina Today*. Published online 2014:69−71.

257. Garweg JG. Eye surgery/vitrectomy–past, present and future. *Graefes Arch Clin Exp Ophthalmol Albrecht Von Graefes Arch Klin Exp Ophthalmol*. 2004;242(8):623−624. https://doi.org/10.1007/s00417-004-0981-0.

258. Abraham JR, Srivastava SK, Le T K, et al. Intraoperative OCT-assisted retinal detachment repair in the DISCOVER study: impact and outcomes. *Ophthalmol Retina*. 2020;4(4):378−383. https://doi.org/10.1016/j.oret.2019.11.002.

Future perspectives for diabetic retinopathy management

10

Based on epidemiological forecasting, the diabetic patient population will increase in number worldwide in the coming years (see Chapter 1). Diabetic retinopathy (DR), as a retinal neurovascular disease of diabetes mellitus (DM), is a leading cause of blindness in the working-age population. To date, no permanent treatment for DR is available. Epidemiological studies suggest that the development and progression of DR are influenced by two primary risk factors: the duration of diabetes and the level of hyperglycemia (hemoglobin A_{1c}, HbA_{1c}).[1] Therefore, diabetic control is the fundamental step for DR management, both at present and in the future. Additionally, DR comprises both retinal neurodegeneration and microangiopathy. Thus, elucidation of the underlying mechanisms of the structural and functional damage to the retinal neurovascular unit (NVU) at cellular and molecular levels requires continually multidisciplinary collaboration. This chapter focuses not only on how to improve durability and efficacy of current therapy but also on how to translate ongoing research on the pathogenesis of DR to clinical application.

Multidisciplinary collaboration for DR care
Pharmacological approaches to DM

DR is a complication of DM. The most effective therapy of DR is diabetic prevention and control. DM refers to a group of systemic disorders, characterized by chronic high blood glucose levels. However, type 1 diabetes mellitus (T1DM) and type 2 diabetes mellitus (T2DM) have different etiologies that demand distinct therapeutic strategies. T1DM is an autoimmune disease that is caused by the destruction of insulin-producing β cells in the pancreas. Both genetic and undefined environmental factors work together to precipitate this disease. The high mortality and morbidity that are associated with the complications of T1DM, such as cardiovascular diseases (CVDS) and blindness due to proliferative diabetic retinopathy (PDR), emphasize the importance of preventing this chronic disorder.[2,3] Increasing data demonstrate that T1DM may be preventable because the autoimmune etiology could be detected, and the responsible T cell population might be regulated.[4,5] Traditionally, the essential treatment of T1DM is external insulin therapy that replaces the functions of pancreatic β cells in an attempt to achieve blood glucose levels in the normal range. Other treatments for T1DM consisting of immunotherapy and cell-based β-cell replacement are evolving rapidly.

T2DM is a state of disturbance in insulin sensing and signaling. Insulin resistance and β cell exhaustion develop simultaneously in a chronic process.[6] The pathophysiologic disturbances of T2DM collectively consist of eight categories, resulting in hyperglycemia (Fig. 10.1). These eight core defects are listed as follows: (1) decreased insulin secretion; (2) decreased incretin effect: incretin hormones are gut peptides that are secreted after nutrient intake and elevated glucose level to stimulate insulin secretion; (3) increased lipolysis; (4) increased glucose reabsorption; (5) decreased glucose uptake; (6) neurotransmitter dysfunction; (7) increased hepatic glucose production; and (8) increased glucagon secretion.[7] Based on these metabolic disturbances in different organs, seven classes of the Food and Drug Administration (FDA)-approved glucose lowering drugs are widely used, which comprise metformin, sulfonylureas, thiazolidinediones, glucagon-like peptide-1 receptor agonist (GLP-1RAs), dipeptidyl peptidase-4 inhibitors (DPP4is), sodium-glucose cotransporter 2 inhibitors (SGLT2is), and insulin.[8] Five other classes of approved drugs are less widely used, that is, meglitinides, α-glucosidase inhibitors, amylinomimetics, bile acid

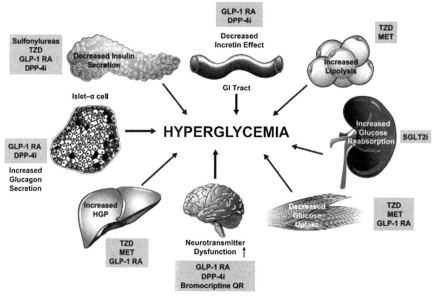

FIGURE 10.1

Key mechanisms and sites of action of glucose-lowering medications based on pathophysiologic targets present in T2DM. Abbreviations: DPP-4i, dipeptidyl peptidase-4 inhibitor; GI, gastrointestinal; GLP-1RA, glucagon-like peptide-1 receptor agonist; HGP, hepatic glucose production; MET, metformin; QR, quick release; SGLT2i, sodium-glucose cotransporter 2 inhibitor; T2DMs, type 2 diabetes mellitus; TZD, thiazolidinedione.

Modified from Thrasher, 2017.[7]

sequestrants, and bromocriptine (a D2/D3 dopaminergic agonist) (Fig. 10.1). New classes of glucose-lowering medications are on the horizon.[8]

The goal of glycemic control is to prevent both macro- and microvascular complications in diabetic patients.[8,9] Regarding DR prevention, the benefits of intensive glycemic control for microvascular complications of T1DM were reported by the Diabetes Control and Complications Trial (DCCT) in 1993.[10] DCCT is a randomized clinical trial demonstrating reduced progression of microvascular complications including retinopathy, nephropathy, and neuropathy with the intensive treatment as compared with the conventional treatment group. Participants in a 10-year follow-up study, namely the Epidemiology of Diabetes Interventions and Complications (EDIC) study, showed 50% risk reduction of retinopathy progression in the original intensive treatment group.[11] Similar to the findings in the DCCT and EDIC, patients with T2DM and tight glycemic control group in another clinical trial, that is, the United Kingdom Prospective Diabetes Study (UKPDS), showed a significant reduction in risk for microvascular complications as compared to the conventional treatment group.[12] Most importantly, patients with either T1DM or T2DM, who received intensive glycemic treatment early in the disease, present a prolonged beneficial effects on microvascular complications. This phenomenon, termed "metabolic memory," has been discussed in Chapter 2. Although the underlying mechanism of "metabolic memory" is not completely understood, keeping blood glucose levels as normal as possible is a fundamental strategy for patients after diagnosis of diabetes.

Side effects of glycemic control

Undesirable effects related to glycemic control for patients with diabetes do exist, specifically, hypoglycemia and transient worsening of DR after tight glycemic control. Hypoglycemia is a common side effect of standard management of DM, creating a hurdle to achieving adequate dosing of glucose lowering drugs such as insulin for patients with T1DM, or sulfonylureas for T2DM patients, as well as a cause of morbidity and mortality of diabetic patients. The global Hypoglycemia Assessment Tool study showed that up to 97.4% of T1DM patients and 95% of T2DM patients have at least one episode of hypoglycemia in a period of 4 weeks.[13] For T1DM, accumulating data showed that insulin pump therapy (IPT) could reduce frequency of severe hypoglycemic events, especially when IPT was coupled with continuous glucose monitoring.[14] Despite improvement in insulin delivery systems, hypoglycemia is still a considerable complication of insulin therapy. Therefore, promotion of hypoglycemia awareness and comanagement of hypoglycemia with insulin therapy are required.[15] For example, fast acting glucagon obtained approval from FDA for severe hypoglycemia in children and adults in the 2010s. The injectable formulations, a stable nonaqueous glucagon solution and the glucagon analog dasiglucagon were developed, showing an efficacy similar to traditional glucagon, and were approved in the United States in 2021 for severe hypoglycemia in adults and in children.[16] Glucagon is secreted by pancreatic alpha cells and regulated by the combination of blood glucose and ambient insulin levels. When the blood glucose is below 70 mg/dL, the glucagon-release system in alpha cells starts to activate.[17,18] The pathophysiology underlying glucagon-release theory has been translated into preclinical trials. For instance, neuronostatin, a somatostatin-derived peptide discovered through a bioinformative approach, is capable of forming a ligand-receptor system directly acting on alpha cells.[15] It is proposed that by using disinhibition of alpha cell glucagon release, protection against hypoglycemia in insulin therapy may be achieved. Thus, a glucagon-release system minimizing hypoglycemic events may provide therapeutic advantages over insulin monotherapy. Among T2DM patients, a potentially modifiable risk factor for hypoglycemia is the choice of glucose lowering therapy because it is known that insulin and insulin secretagogues (e.g., sulfonylureas and meglitinides) pose the highest risk. In the Outcome Reduction with an Initial Glargine Intervention trial, the risk of severe hypoglycemia increased twofold with sulfonylureas and 4.5-fold with insulin.[19,20]

A paradoxical worsening of DR after tight blood glucose control was first reported approximately 30 years ago in patients with an uncontrolled T1DM.[21] This kind of aggravation of DR called "early worsening of diabetic retinopathy" (EWDR) has been found in both T1DM and T2DM patients. Of the DCCT patients with T1DM, EWDR was observed at 3 months in 11% (21/197) with intensive therapy and 3.6% (7/192) with conventional therapy. In the long run, the beneficial effects of tight glycemic control override the problem of early worsening, resulting in the reduction of DR progression when compared to patients with poor glycemic control. The risk factors for EWDR patients with long-term diabetes include high baseline DR severity and poor glycemic control as reflected by high HbA_{1c} levels. The current management of EWDR has been introduced in Chapter 1. The detailed mechanism behind EWDR is not completely elucidated.[22,23] In order to minimize this side effect of tight glycemic control, understanding the mechanisms of EWDR is required. For example, Thangarajah et al. reported that both isolated fibroblasts from patients with T2DM and fibroblasts cultured in high concentrations of glucose lost their capacity to upregulate vascular endothelial growth factor (VEGF) in response to hypoxia.[24] Based on this finding, it is postulated that hypoxia-inducible factor-1α (HIF-1α)/VEGF axis is blunted in the ischemic diabetic retina when the ambient glucose levels are high. If glucose levels are rapidly normalized, the expression of VEGF is restimulated. Therefore, although glycemic control is achieved, the downstream effects of upregulated VEGF may lead to blood—retinal barrier (BRB) breakdown and activation of angiogenesis, resulting in worsening of DR.

The report of the Action to Control Cardiovascular Risk in Diabetes Follow-on Research Group in 2016 showed again the persistent effects of intensive glycemic control on reducing the risk of DR.[25] This result confirms the findings from 1983 by the DCCT to the observational EDIC study in 2013 in patients with T1DM.[26] Based on the UKPDS, the beneficial effects of intensive therapy for microvascular complications such as DR are similar in patients with T2DM. The effects of intensive glycemic control on macrovascular complication such as CVD event rates in patients with T2DM were studied by the Action to Control Cardiovascular Risk in

Diabetes (ACCORD).[27] In the glycemic control arm of the ACCORD study, after 3.5-year follow-up, the intensive treatment arm was discontinued due to significant increase in all-cause mortality, particularly the risk of mortality by CVD (increased by 35%).[28] However, the beneficial effects of intensive therapy on microvascular complications in the participants whose intensive therapy was discontinued in ACCORD still persisted. It is worth mentioning that the discrepancy in effects of intensive therapy on microvascular and macrovascular complications by ACCORD is not in agreement with the data obtained from DCCT for T1DM and UKPDS for T2DM.[29] A crucial point for future study is that: while follow-up for DCCT and UKPDS was 20 years, the ACCORD Study follow-up was only 3 years. The long-term and longitudinal follow-up of these studies are extremely valuable. It is also important to consider that for diabetic patients who have high risk of CVD, adequate control rather than strict control of HbA_{1c} is a more sensible goal because the latter may need diabetes polypharmacy.[9]

Hypertension as a systemic risk factor of DR

In addition to hyperglycemia, the other systemic risk factors of DR are mainly hypertension and dyslipidemia.[30] Because the association of DR with dyslipidemia is controversial, only hypertension as a systemic risk factor is discussed in this section.[31] It is postulated that hypertension aggravates DR through increased blood flow and cyclic stretch to vascular endothelial cells, resulting in release of VEGF.[32] Based on longitudinal cohort studies, every 10 mmHg increase in systolic blood pressure (SBP) is associated with 3%–20% higher risk of early DR and a 15% higher risk of PDR after adjustments for age, sex, and albumin excretion rate.[33,34] The beneficial effects of blood pressure (BP) control in reducing the risk of DR have been documented in numerous clinical trials. A recent Asian population-based study further clarified the association of hypertension control with DR. This study showed that higher levels of SBP and pulse pressure are associated with early DR and vision-threating DR. For patients with diabetes and hypertension, tight control of BP may help prevent DR.[35]

It is important to know that the association of hypertension with DR may also include other contributing factors. For instance, angiotensin-converting enzyme inhibitors (ACEIs) have shown a reduction in the progression of retinopathy in patients with T1DM even in normotensive state, as well as in T2DM patients.[36–38] These studies suggest that these drugs may have benefits on the retina independent of their anti-hypertensive mechanisms. The possibility that ACEIs may affect local production of angiotensin-converting enzyme (ACE) by retinal vascular endothelial cells has been discussed in Chapter 2.[39]

Oxidative stress as a unifying mechanism and key therapeutic target for DR

Chronic hyperglycemia generates oxidative stress and nitrosative stress via several major metabolic pathways. These pathways, such as glycolysis, the polyol pathway, hexosamine biosynthetic pathway (HBP), protein kinase C (PKC) activation, renin—angiotensin—aldosterone system (RAAS), and increased accumulation of advanced glycation end products (AGEs), have been identified as prooxidative processes and are usually upregulated in DR (see Fig. 2.1 in Chapter 2). The hyperglycemia-activated biochemical pathways sequentially activate poly(ADP-ribose) polymerase (PARP) through increased oxidative stress. Notably, these activated pathways can be blocked at the step of PARP. For example, activation of PARP1 leads to inhibition of glyceraldehyde-3-phosphate dehydrogenase (GAPDH) by poly-ADP-ribosylation. The inhibition of GAPDH leads to the accumulation of its substrate, glyceraldehyde-3-P, which appears to be the center of diabetes-associated oxidative stress. The increased level of glyceraldehyde-3-P further activates two major prooxidative pathways in diabetes, that is, the AGEs pathway in which methylglyoxal is synthesized from nonenzymatic dephosphorylation of the triose phosphates, and the PKC pathway by promoting the synthesis of diacylglycerol. In addition, it causes the accumulation of glycolytic metabolites upstream, which leads to excessive stimulation of other prooxidative pathways such as HBP and the polyol pathway. Therefore, a unifying mechanism is summarized in Fig. 10.2.

Targeting interactions of oxidative stress with six key metabolic abnormalities

Under physiological conditions, the production of free radicals, mainly reactive nitrogen species (RNS) and reactive oxygen species (ROS), is normal and essential for signal transduction. In contrast, the high levels of RNS and ROS in diabetic retina, resulting from excessive production of free radicals and repressed antioxidant defense systems, is defined as oxidative stress. The hyperglycemia-induced oxidative stress can be implicated in pathogenic pathways that contribute to retinal cell damage and DR development and progression. First, hyperglycemia directly induces oxidative stress through abnormal glycolysis (Fig. 2.1 in Chapter 2). Second, six major metabolic abnormalities induced by hyperglycemia trigger oxidative stress (Fig. 2.1 in Chapter 2). Of the six major abnormalities, four of them are classical sources of oxidative stress, that is, polyol pathway, HBP, increased AGEs, and PKC activation. The other two, that is, RAAS and low-grade inflammation, also contribute to the molecular events of oxidative stress.

Since these six metabolic abnormalities amplify oxidative stress, suppression of excessive oxidative stress may serve as therapeutic targets. First, hyperglycemia, high blood glucose per se through glycolysis causes excessive production of superoxide anion radical (O_2), which suppresses the antioxidant systems, resulting in oxidative stress.[40] Second, in addition to the direct role of glycolysis pathway, hyperglycemia-induced increase in electron transfer donors, that is, reduced nicotinamide adenine dinucleotide and flavan adenine dinucleotide (FADH2) increase electron flux through the mitochondrial electron transport chain.[41,42] Third, an abnormal increase in glycolytic flux generates large amounts of intermediate metabolites that can be shunted into different pathways including the four classical pathways that is,

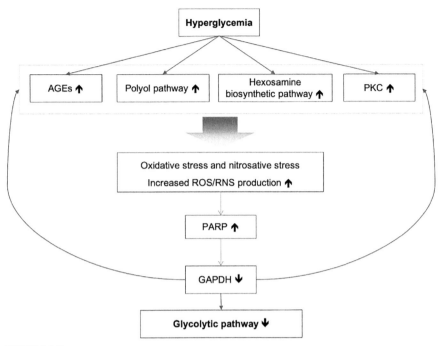

FIGURE 10.2

Biochemical aberrations of glucose metabolism in diabetes by a unifying mechanism. Hyperglycemia stimulates the production of AGEs, activates PKC, and enhances the polyol pathway and HBP. These biochemical pathways augment ROS and RNS generation and subsequently facilitate oxidative stress and nitrosative stress in the retina. ROS/RNS causes DNA breaks and PARP activation. PARP activation depletes its substrate, NAD$^+$, slowing the rate of glycolysis, electron transport, and ATP formation, resulting in inhibition of GAPDH by poly-ADP-ribosylation. The reduced GAPDH activity further aggravates hyperglycemia-activated biochemical pathways, forming the vicious cycle. Oxidative stress and nitrosative stress potentiate the abnormalities of these metabolic pathways, which cause mitochondrial damage, DNA damage, retinal cell apoptosis, lipid peroxidation, and irregular epigenetic modification on genes of antioxidant defense system in the retina. Abbreviations: AGEs, advanced glycation end products; ADP, adenosine diphosphate; ATP, adenosine triphosphate; DNA, deoxyribonucleic acid; GAPDH, glyceraldehyde-3-P dehydrogenase; HBP, hexosamine biosynthetic pathway; NAD, nicotinamide adenine dinucleotide; PARP, poly(ADP-ribose) polymerase; PKC, protein kinase C; RAAS, renin–angiotensin–aldosterone system; RNSs, reactive nitrogen species; ROS, reactive oxygen species.

polyol, HBP, PKC, and AGEs, and other metabolic processes such as RAAS and inflammation which involve nuclear factor kappa B (NF-κB), prostaglandins, cyclooxygenase-2 (COX-2), and nicotinamide adenine dinucleotide phosphate (NADPH) oxidases (NOXs).[42,43] In diabetic retina, ROS produced through RAAS is derived from NOXs, in which a NADPH oxidase catalytic subunit NOX2 within the retinal vessels is increased.[44] It has been documented in a diabetic animal model that NOX inhibition or a deficiency of NOX2 reduced retinal inflammation, intercellular adhesion molecule 1 (ICAM-1) expression, and vascular leakage of diabetic animal model.[45] Therefore, RAAS activation that contributes to the ROS production in diabetic retina vasculature can be considered as a therapeutic target (see Chapter 5).

Inflammatory responses in the retinal microvascular cells can be triggered by hyperglycemia (Fig. 2.1 of Chapter 2). The innate immune system recognizes endogenous stress signals, known as damage-associated molecular patterns (DAMPs). Through Toll-like receptors,[46] DAMPs induce intracellular signaling pathways that promote the expression of proinflammatory cytokines,[47] including tumor necrosis factor α (TNF-α), interleukin (IL)-1β, IL-6, and monocyte chemoattractant protein-1 (MCP-1).[48] Based on current understanding, the following therapeutic approaches against inflammation and oxidative stress are summarized in Table 10.1, including (1) the nonsteroidal anti-inflammatory drugs; (2) blockage of inflammatory molecules and inflammatory growth factors; (3) specific blockade of the RAAS with the angiotensin II receptor type 1 blocker, such as Losartan and Candesartan, or ACEIs such as Enalapril; and (4) tetracyclines. In addition, photobiomodulation (PBM) is promising.[48] PBM refers to low-level laser therapy or far-red to near-infrared light therapy. Specific wavelengths of light (600–1,000 nm) can promote the activation of some signaling pathways. It has been shown that PBM effectively inhibits increased superoxide production, leukostasis, and ICAM-1 expression in diabetic rat retinas.[67] The safety and efficacy of PBM has been demonstrated in a pilot case series. Future randomized clinical trials with large sample size are required to prove the applicability of PBM for DR treatment. The benefit of PBM therapy is not limited to retinal microvasculature. Since retinal neurons, including photoreceptors, are the major source of ROS and local inflammation in diabetic retina, PBM exerts effects on multiple cell types, including neurons, glia, and their communication.[48,68]

Antioxidants for early DR

Since oxidative stress is considered to be a unifying mechanism by which DR develops, antioxidative stress is a key therapeutic strategy in the current and future treatment of early DR. This translational approach is summarized in Table 10.1.[69]

Regulation of apoptotic pathways as therapeutic strategy

Cell death appears to be a prominent feature in the development and progression of diabetic retinal neurodegeneration as well as in microangiopathy (see Chapter 4). In the study of molecular mechanisms of cell death, it is notable that there are overlapping cell death pathways and mechanisms for neurons, glia, and vascular cells in the

Table 10.1 Antioxidative stress as potential treatment of DR.

Treatment category and newly discovered agents	Mechanisms of action	Status of translational research including references
Systemic glycemic control: SGLT2 inhibitor GLP-1 agonist DPP-4 inhibitor New GLP-1RAs: Liraglutide Semaglutide	• Restoration of insulin sensing and signaling • Antioxidative effects and possible neuroprotection • Long acting glucagon-like peptide-1 (GLP-1)	Basic and clinical studies on molecular mechanisms of insulin generation and storage[49] Preclinical studies[50] Clinical trials for GLP-1-based therapy[51,52]
Aldose reductase inhibitors: Synthetic aldose reductase differential inhibitors (ARDIs)	• Suppression of polyol pathway and inflammation	Preclinical study for ARDIs[53]
AGE inhibitors: Pyridoxamine RAGE blocker: TTP448 EPS-ZM1	• Inhibition of AGE formation, restoring functions of antioxidant enzymes, transcription factors, and mitochondrial proteins • Blocking AGE-RAGE pathway mediated proin-flammatory signaling	Preclinical study[54] Clinical trials[55]
Hexosamine biosynthesis inhibitor: Azaserine	• Inhibition of hexosamine pathway • Glutamine: F-6-P amido-transferase inhibitor, neuroprotection	Preclinical study[56]
Protein kinase C (PKC) inhibitor: PKCβ inhibitor	• Inhibition of PKC activation induced by high glucose due to an increased DAG level. • Suppression of overproduction of growth hormone and IGF	Clinical trial[57]
RAAS inhibitor: Angiotensin II receptor type 1 (AT1R) blocker Angiotensin-converting enzyme inhibitor (ACEI)	• Inhibition of RAAS pathway • Neuroprotection due to suppressed retinal inflammation	Clinical trial[48] Clinical trial[58]
PARP inhibitor: 1,5-lisoquinolinediol	• Inhibition of NADPH oxidase-derived oxidative stress	Preclinical study[59,60]
Anti-inflammatory drugs: Glucocorticoid	• Glucocorticoid signaling anti-inflammation	Clinical trials[61]

Continued

Table 10.1 Antioxidative stress as potential treatment of DR.—*cont'd*

Treatment category and newly discovered agents	Mechanisms of action	Status of translational research including references
NSAIDs Biologics: IL-6 inhibitor EBI-031 IL-6 receptor inhibitor Tocilizumab Integrin inhibitor Luminate		
Antioxidants: Polyphenols Lutein Astaxanthin Zeaxanthin Lipoic acid Vitamins Polyphenols	• Antioxidative stress	Clinical trials[62]
Activation of antioxidant defence system: Sulforaphane Ferriprotoporphyrin IX Mycophenolate mofetil (MMF), dimethylfumarate (DMF)	• Reactivating suppressed Nrf2 activity by hyperglycemia because Nrf2 upregulates various detoxifying and antioxidant defence genes	Clinical trials[62,63]
Inhibitors or activators for epigenetic modification: Nrf2 activator Bardoxolone methyl therapy BG-12	• Histone modification • DNA methylation • Nucleosome remodeling • Target oxidative stress-related genes	Clinical trials[62,64]
miRNA Long noncoding RNAs (lncRNAs)	• Binding target mRNAs to suppress posttranscription governing gene expressions	Pre- and clinical studies[62]
Sirtuin 1 (Sirt 1) activator: Resveratrol	• Inhibition of NF-κB pathways and exerting protective effects on mitochondria	Pre- and clinical studies[65,66]

Abbreviations: AGEs, advanced glycation end-products; DAG, diacylglycerol; DR, diabetic retinopathy; DPP-4, dipeptidyl peptidase 4; F-6-P, fructose-6-phosphate; GLP-1, glucagon-like peptide-1; GLP-1RAs, GLP-1 receptor agonists; IGF, insulin-like growth factor; miRNA, microRNA; Nrf 2, nuclear factor erythroid 2-related factor 2; PARP, poly ADP-ribose polymerase; RAAS, renin—angiotensin—aldosterone system; RAGEs, receptor of AGEs; SGLT2, sodium-glucose cotransporter 2.

NVU. In addition to apoptosis, various retinal cells may undergo different modes of cell death under diabetic conditions. In the study of apoptosis of different retinal cell types, oxidative stress is considered as the initiating factor because it appears to be interrelated with other biochemical imbalances. These biochemical imbalances lead to structural and functional changes, accelerating loss of retinal cells. Under physiological conditions, a balance exists between the production of ROS and their neutralization. In diabetic condition, this balance is disturbed, resulting in oxidative stress on retinal cells.

Growing evidence demonstrates that apoptosis can be categorized into extrinsic and intrinsic pathways. For instance, under oxidative stress, ROS triggers different cytotoxic stimuli that induce cell surface death receptors.[70] The extrinsic cell death pathway is initiated upon ligand–receptor interactions (Fig. 10.3). The death receptor signaling pathways involve cross-talk with the mitochondrial pathway, that is, intrinsic pathway and can in some cases be influenced by mitochondrial membrane potential changes. The intrinsic cell death pathway is initiated from the mitochondria/endoplasmic reticulum (ER). Mitochondria are the major endogenous source of ROS.[72,73] ROS can trigger mitochondria to release cytochrome c and damage mitochondrial membrane integrity, transmembrane potential, and the respiratory chain, and consequently accelerate ROS production. The ROS may activate either mitochondria-independent mechanisms such as effector mitogen-activated protein kinase,[74] or mitochondria-dependent mechanisms such as an imbalance between pro- and anti-apoptotic factors, for example, B cell lymphoma 2 (Bcl2) family proteins,[75] resulting in pore formation in the outer or inner mitochondrial membranes (Fig. 10.3). This releases mitochondrial apoptogenic factors which ultimately induce apoptosis in caspase-dependent or caspase-independent manner.[70] For instance, in the diabetic condition, evidence indicates that vascular cells and retinal neurons undergo mitochondria-dependent apoptotic pathways.[76,77]

Under oxidative stress, retinal neurons such as retinal ganglion cells (RGCs) can undergo either extrinsic or intrinsic apoptotic pathways. For example, RGC death can be induced by intravitreal injection of the excitotoxin, N-methyl-D-aspartate (NMDA), into mice who are deficient in apoptotic machinery including tumor necrosis factor (TNF) signaling, c-Jun N-terminal kinase (JNK) activation, and ER stress. In fact, absence of TNF or its canonical downstream mediator, BH3 interacting-domain death agonist (BID), does not confer short- or long-term protection to RGCs. Attenuation of JNK signaling does not prevent RGCs death after excitotoxic insult. Furthermore, deficiency of the ER stress, which is involved in RGCs death, does not lessen NMDA-induced RGCs death. These experimental results point out that the drivers of excitotoxic injury remain unclear. It appears to have multiple cell death pathways that are activated in response to injury.[78] Since various extrinsic and intrinsic apoptotic pathways are involved in the death of different retinal cell types, the common final apoptotic pathway should be targeted in DR therapy. In fact, neurotrophic or cytoprotective strategies aimed at blocking or regulating the final apoptotic pathway for treating DR have been studied as outlined below.[71,79]

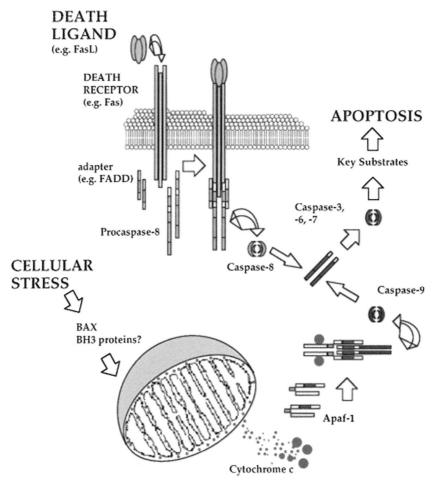

FIGURE 10.3

Two pathways of caspase activation and apoptosis. Two independent apoptosis pathways (extrinsic and intrinsic) are presented that classically converge through the activation of "downstream" caspases (−3, −6, −7), key substrate cleavage, and apoptotic death. The first involves ligation of death receptors by their ligands, resulting in the recruitment of adaptor proteins and procaspase molecules. The complex is an "apoptosome" in which the aggregated procaspase transactivates. The active caspase (e.g., caspase-8) then acts to cleave and activate the downstream caspases. In the second pathway, various forms of cellular stress trigger mitochondrial release of cytochrome *c*, which binds to apoptotic protease-activating factor 1 (Apaf1), which in turn self-associates and binds procaspase-9, resulting in an apoptosome. Transactivation of the complexed procaspase-9 to active caspase-9 follows, and the caspase then cleaves and activates downstream caspases.

Modified from Green 1998.[71]

Peroxisome proliferator-activated receptor γ agonist

The peroxisome proliferator-activated receptors (PPARs) are a subfamily of ligand-inducible transcription factors, which belong to the superfamily of nuclear hormone receptors. In mammals, the PPARs subfamily consists of three members: PPARα, PPARβ/δ, and PPARγ. PPARγ agonists regulate insulin signaling. Pioglitazone, an extensively studied PPARγ agonist, is capable of restoring insulin signal transduction through reduction of TNF-α and suppression of cytokine signaling 3 (SOCS3) pathways in retinal endothelial cells and Müller cells in vitro and in a type 2 diabetic rat model. These functions of PPARγ agonist could protect these types of retinal cells from apoptosis by blocking the extrinsic pathway as well as the common apoptotic pathway via caspase 3 inhibition.[80] Moreover, a PPARγ agonist, Saroglitazar was utilized to treat DR in a rat model. The treatment ameliorated serum triglyceride level, retinal vascular permeability, and leukostasis, indicating that PPARγ agonists possess multiple mechanisms of action and potential benefits for patients with DR. Translating anti-apoptotic strategy into clinical practice for DR using PPARγ agonists is rapidly advancing.[81]

RAAS blockers

In Chapter 2 and the early part of this chapter, we discussed how dysfunction of RAAS contributes to the pathogenesis of DR. ACEIs have also been shown to have a beneficial effect on retinopathy development in patients with diabetes independent of their reduction in BP, although discrepancies were found in the cell protective effects of ACEIs after systematic review and metaanalysis.[82] For instance, Aliskiren blocks the activity of renin, a key rate-limiting enzyme in the first step of the RAAS cascade. Batenburg et al. reported that when Aliskiren was administered subcutaneously to *Ren2* transgenic diabetic rats, apoptotic cell death was significantly reduced in the retina, resulting in the reduction of acellular capillaries.[83] Therefore, large-scale randomized controlled trials are needed to further clarify the effect of RAAS inhibitors on retinopathy in diabetes. Meanwhile, the anti-apoptotic effects of ACEIs on DR also need further study.

Apoptosis repressor with caspase recruitment domain

Apoptosis repressor with caspase recruitment domain (ARC) is a highly potent and multifunctional inhibitor of apoptosis that is physiologically expressed predominantly in postmitotic cells such as cardiomyocytes, skeletal muscle cells, smooth muscle cells, and neurons.[84,85] ARC is an endogenous inhibitor of apoptosis, which antagonizes both the extrinsic (death receptor) and intrinsic (mitochondria/ER) apoptosis pathways.[84] Multiple studies have demonstrated a strong correlation between β-cell apoptosis and T2DM in humans. The pathogenic role of ARC on diabetes currently focuses on how to promote β-cells survival.[73] Since ARC is expressed in both neurons and vascular smooth muscle cells, which are equivalent to retinal neurons and vascular pericytes, translational research on ARC contribution to cell survival in diabetic retina should be pursued.

Erythropoietin, a neurotrophic and anti-apoptotic factor

Erythropoietin (EPO) is a hematopoietic glycoprotein produced in the fetal liver and adult kidney. EPO has been known to promote hematopoiesis and used routinely for the treatment of anemia in clinical practice. In addition, angiogenic, anti-inflammatory, and endothelial cell stabilization effects of systemic EPO have shown neuroprotective and neurotrophic activities in central nervous system (CNS) cells.[86] EPO has both neuroprotective and vascular protective functions in the retina because all components of the retinal NVU express the EPO receptor (EpoR). EPO and EpoR are found to be expressed in the human CNS.[87,88] EPO promotes neural outgrowth from RGCs in a dose-dependent manner and preserves their survival after axotomy.[89] Hypoxia-induced retinal EPO expression appears to protect retinal neurons from transient global ischemia and reperfusion injury through an anti-apoptotic pathway.[90]

The anti-apoptotic function of EPO was utilized in a diabetic rat model with early DR by our research team. At the onset of diabetes, a single intravitreal injection of EPO (0.05–200 ng/eye) was administered. In the diabetic rats, BRB breakdown was detected soon after the onset of diabetes, peaked at 2 weeks, and plateaued from 2–4 weeks. The number of TUNEL-positive cells increased in the neurosensory retina after diabetes onset and reached a peak at 4–6 weeks. The retinal thickness and the number of cells in the outer nuclear layer were reduced significantly. Electron microscopy observations demonstrated vascular and photoreceptor cell death starting soon after the onset of diabetes. All these changes were largely prevented by EPO treatment. Upregulation of EpoR in the neurosensory retina was detected at both the transcriptional and protein levels 4–8 weeks after the onset of diabetes, whereas the EPO levels of neurosensory retinas were essentially unchanged during the same period. In EPO-treated diabetic groups, EpoR expression remained at upregulated levels. These data demonstrate that apoptosis is a major mode of neuronal cell death in the early course of DR. The upregulation of EpoR may be a compensatory response of retinal cells and tissue to diabetic stress. The EPO/EpoR system appears to be a maintenance-survival mechanism of retinal neurons responding to the insults of early diabetes. Exogenous EPO administration by intravitreal injection in early diabetes can prevent retinal cell death and protect BRB integrity.[87] Our group reported a small cohort study using intravitreal EPO for patients with intractable diabetic macular edema (DME). Five eyes of five patients had progressive vision loss and persistent or worsening edema with prior multimodal treatment. These eyes received injections of recombinant human EPO alpha. EPO (5 U/50 μL) was injected intravitreally every 6 weeks for three doses and followed for an additional 6 weeks as the primary end point. The best corrected visual acuity of all patients was subjectively improved, by three or more Early Treatment Diabetic Retinopathy Study lines in three eyes and one line in two eyes. Visual acuity improved to a larger extent than anatomic improvement by optical coherence tomography (OCT). Clearing of hard exudates but only minor improvement in leakage on fluorescein angiography was observed. Improvement in vision occurred within 1 week after the first injection and was maintained until the end point of the current case series (at 18 weeks after the first injection). This case series seems to show a short-term positive response to EPO for a specific group of patients with chronic DME who were unresponsive to currently available therapies.[91]

Based on preclinical studies and this clinical case series, intravitreal EPO for DR and DME seems safe and efficacious. We understand there are some theoretical and practical hurdles in EPO application for clinical DR. First, in a genotyping study, the T allele of single nucleotide polymorphism (SNP) rs1617640 in the promoter of the EPO gene is significantly associated with PDR and end-stage renal disease in three European-American case-and-control groups.[92] This study found the EPO gene to be a disease risk-associated gene and the EPO/EpoR pathway to mediate severe diabetic microvascular complications. Second, a clinical cohort study showed that the EPO level in human vitreous was 12.7-fold higher in PDR patients than in subjects without diabetes.[93] This indicates that EPO is an ischemia-induced angiogenic factor in PDR. Interestingly, the vitreous EPO level of patients with DME was found to be as high as that of PDR patients, suggesting other factors apart from ischemia are involved in the overexpression of EPO in DR.[94] As described, the increase in endogenous EPO in diabetic eyes is either associated with promoter polymorphism of EPO gene or proliferative stage, that is, severe ischemic retina. Under these conditions, the high exogenous EPO administered in the diabetic eye might aggravate ischemia-induced angiogenic functions. However, the relationship between EPO and retinal ischemia is complex. The versatile functions of EPO are disease-context dependent. For instance, in different clinical phases or stages of retinopathy of prematurity (ROP) and DR, the therapeutic potential of EPO may vary. ROP has two distinct phases in which hypoxia-induced angiogenic factors are involved.[95] In phase 1, suppressed growth factors and loss of the maternal–fetal interaction result in an arrest of retinal vascularization. In phase 2, the activated metabolism and poorly vascularized retina lead to retinal hypoxia, stimulating growth factor–induced vasoproliferation.[96] Chen and Smith pointed out that EPO may act as a "double-edged sword" in eyes with ROP. The angiogenic action of EPO could be crucial in the first phase of ROP, where the appropriate concentration of EPO in eye could be neuroprotective and stimulate physiological angiogenesis. In the second phase, the angiogenic effect of EPO may aggravate abnormal neovascularization, leading to a worsening of ROP.[95,97] The "double-edged sword" functions of EPO may also apply for different stages of DR. The early, mild, and moderate nonproliferative stages of diabetic retinopathy (NPDR) are characterized by vasoregression, that is, loss of pericytes, microaneurysm formation, acellular capillary formation, and altered secreted factors. Specifically, hyperglycemia-induced angiopoietin-2 (Ang-2) upregulation results in vasoregression and failure of vasculogenesis (see Chapter 7). The neuroprotective and angiogenic action of EPO administered in these stages could slow down the apoptotic pathway and facilitate the revascularization of retinal area that lost blood supply. However, in the PDR stage, the angiogenic effect of exogenous EPO may aggravate abnormal neovascularization rather than protect vasculature. At this stage, EPO utilization may be contraindicated. The understanding of the relationship between EPO and DR remains incomplete. Future work filling the translational gap between the identification of

EPO-anti-apoptotic targets and conversion of this knowledge into effective treatment for DR is required. In that regard, it is worth noting a commentary in the journal *Neurotherapeutics*. In this article, Steinman wrote that a domain of the EPO molecule containing the anti-inflammatory and neuroprotective functions without the erythropoietic effect has been identified. Bioengineering of EPO to create new molecules with only desirable functions may be efficacious in the treatment of diabetic retina in the future.[98]

In addition to EPO, other neurotrophic factors such as pigment epithelium-derived factor (PEDF) and ciliary neurotrophic factor (CNTF) have been studied. The neurogenic potential of PEDF and CNTF might be used for the treatment of DR in the future.[99,100]

Cell-based treatment for DR

Due to the involvement of neuronal and vascular loss in the progression of DR, cell replacement via stem cell therapy is a fundamental approach. In Chapter 4, the underlying mechanisms of both neuronal and vascular cell death have been discussed. In addition to cell death, the metabolic and physiological changes in diabetes are involved in the production of proinflammatory cytokines. The inflammatory cascades aggravate neural cell damage and vascular cell dysfunction in the NVU. Current studies suggest that the endothelial damage arises from the loss of pericytes. Pericytes are known to be involved in the formation of the BRB. Pericyte dropout directly induces inflammatory responses in endothelial cells and perivascular infiltration of macrophages.[101] A complex interplay of microvascular abnormalities and neurodegeneration in diabetic retina has been implicated. Therefore, to slow DR progression, restoring BRB integrity and protecting neuroglia degeneration are essential. Embryonic or induced pluripotent stem cells (iPSCs), hematopoietic stem cells, endothelial progenitor cells (EPCs), and mesenchymal stromal cells (MSCs) have all been used in preclinical models for the treatment of DR.

In Chapter 7, we discussed how bone marrow-sourced CD34+ progenitor cells (EPCs) are able to move toward the ischemic field and contribute to microvascular repair. Therefore, improving diabetes-induced compromised functions of EPCs induced by diabetes such as reduced mobility to the damaged area and decreased regenerative capability is the target of future EPC research. In human clinical trials, iPSCs have been shown to be a promising source of retinal stem cells to replace neurons and RPE cells.[102] iPSCs are differentiated from somatic cells to cells possessing pluripotent qualities by forced expression of specific transcription factors including Oct4, Sox2, plus (Myc, Klf4 or Nanog, Lin28).[102] In some trials, adipose or bone marrow−derived stem cells (ADSCs or BMSCs) were directly transplanted into the subretinal space to repair retinal damage in patients with age-related macular degeneration and other blinding disorders.[102] Ongoing clinical studies are exemplified by intravitreal injections of CD34+ bone marrow MSCs to patients with irreversible vision loss from retinal degenerative diseases or retinal vascular disease, including DR. In DR, it has also been observed that iPSCs are able to generate endothelial cells and pericytes in areas with capillary degeneration.[102] iPSC technology producing retinal organoids is another novel approach. This is called "retina-in-a-dish." One of the limitations of retina research is that it is heavily reliant on animal models. Thereby, the clinical fidelity of the animal research is always limited. The patient-specific retinal organoids technique may help circumvent this limitation. iPSC-RPE from donor diabetic patients has decreased barrier function and attenuated autophagic capacity as compared with iPSC-RPE derived from control individuals without diabetes.[103] Based on the pilot studies, it may be proposed that iPSC-pericyte-endothelial cell preparations from patients with diabetes should be used to study inner BRB breakdown in DR. Similarly, an iPSC-derived outer BRB model, that is, iPSC RPE-choriocapillaris endothelial cells organoid, may be used to develop more patient-specific therapeutic approaches.[104]

Gene therapy combined with cell therapy

As discussed above, evidence exists that EPO is a safe and effective neuro- and vascular protectant for subjects with DR at vasoregression stage.[91] In diabetic animals, intravitreal bone marrow stem cells (BMSCs) can be used to improve visual function, indicating a neuroprotective function.[105] Our research team led by Xu conducted a stem cell therapy and a stem cell−based gene therapy for the treatment of sodium iodate (SI)−induced retinal degeneration. Three cell types, that is, rat mesenchymal stem cells (rMSCs) alone, EPO gene-modified rMSCs (EPO-rMSCs), or doxycycline-inducible EPO-expressing rMSCs (Tet-on EPO-rMSCs) by using a tetracycline-controlled Tet-off and Tet-on gene expression system,[106] were transplanted into the subretinal spaces of SI-treated rats. After 8 weeks, the visual function of rats treated with rMSCs alone or with the two types of EPO-rMSCs were all monitored by electroretinography. Following the transplantation, labeled transplanted cells that had adopted RPE morphology were observed in the subretinal space. EPO concentration in vitreous and retina of eyes receiving EPO-rMSCs or Tet-on EPO-rMSCs was markedly increased, consistent with the improvement of retinal morphology and function. These findings suggest that rMSCs transplantation, particularly with EPO gene modification, is a novel therapy for degenerative retinal diseases since the combined gene and cell therapy may protect and rescue multiple retinal cells.[107] In this regard, stem cell−based therapy is a promising alternative in treating DR at the vasoregression stage.[108]

VEGF and non-VEGF signaling pathways as therapeutic targets

Anti-VEGF therapies have been established as the first-line approach for DME and are being increasingly used as key alternatives for moderate to severe NPDR and PDR.[109] This clinical practice is based on the understanding of the central role of VEGF in retinal leakage, inflammation, and angiogenesis during DR. In order to improve the efficacy, durability, and bioavailability, novel anti-VEGF agents and new delivery routes and systems are under development. In Chapter 9, future directions for anti-VEGF therapy have been categorized as regulation of the HIF-1α pathway, VEGF family, VEGF-A and its isoforms, or VEGF receptors and coreceptors. It is an interesting phenomenon that in clinical trials, the response to anti-VEGF drugs in DME is not as robust as in PDR. Many patients with DME do not show complete resolution of fluid despite multiple injections or may show only a transitory response to anti-VEGF drugs.[110] Therefore, in addition to VEGF pathways, the role of non-VEGF signaling pathways in pathogenesis of DR and DME needs to be explored. In this section, the following essential non-VEGF pathways that have been introduced in previous chapters are revisited as alternative therapeutic approaches to DR/DME.

Ang-2/Tie2 signaling

A typical example of crosstalk between VEGF and non-VEGF pathways is the synergistic action of VEGF-A and Ang-2/Tie2 in inducing retinal neurovascular cell death, BRB breakdown, and angiogenesis. Antibodies containing two different antigen-binding sites in one molecule are bispecific. In diabetic microvasculature, upregulated Ang-2 blocks angiopoietin-1 (Ang-1), a vascular stabilizing factor, from competitive binding to the Tie2 receptor. This competitive function leads to pericyte loss, vessel destabilization, and increase in inflammatory cytokines. Most importantly, the retinal vasculature becomes sensitized to the effect of VEGF-A. Based on this molecular mechanism, faricimab, a bispecific antibody neutralizing both Ang-2 and VEGF-A has been developed (see Chapter 9). The results of two phase 3 clinical trials met the primary endpoints at 1 year with both faricimab arms producing equivalent visual gains as compared with aflibercept. In July 2021, the FDA accepted faricimab biologics license application, which received FDA approval in January 2022. In future translational research, fine-tuning of bispecific formulations is needed to produce optimal dual-target molecules that may synergistically regulate two physically linked binding specificities in diabetic retina.[111]

Anti-inflammatory therapy

The specific anti-inflammatory strategies including anti-leukostasis, regulation of activated microglia, antibodies to specific cytokines to protect BRB, and regulation of innate and adaptive immune systems as potential therapeutic targets have been introduced in Chapters 5 and 9. Among the anti-inflammatory therapies, steroid treatment is pivotal for inflammatory diseases including DR and DME. However, prolonged use may increase intraocular pressure (IOP). Therefore, modifying corticosteroid molecules to explore different routes, dosages, and durations of steroid administration is an important future goal. For instance, targeted administration of steroids into the suprachoroidal space of the posterior segment of the eye for DR and DME could minimize contact with anterior segment structures, reducing the possibility of IOP spike.[112,113] Regarding different routes and formulations of steroid administration, a topical formulation of dexamethasone with soluble nanoparticle technology, OCS-01 (1.5% ophthalmic suspension, Oculis), has met its primary endpoint in a phase 2 clinical trial for DME.[114] In addition, a bioerodible intravitreal implant manufactured using PRINT technology, AR-1105 (Aerie), releases dexamethasone to treat DME.[113] This product is an addition to the armamentarium of intraocular biodegradable steroid implants.

Kallikrein-kinin system

Preclinical studies demonstrated that activation of the intraocular kallikrein-kinin system (KKS) alters retinal vascular permeability, vasodilation, and retinal thickening. Proteomic analysis from the vitreous of eyes with DME showed that KKS and VEGF pathways are potentially independent biologic pathways. Furthermore, proteins associated with DME in the vitreous are significantly more correlated with the KKS pathway than the VEGF pathway. Preclinical experiments on diabetic animals showed that inhibition of KKS components is an effective approach to decreasing retinal vascular permeability. In this regard, clinical trials investigating plasma kallikrein inhibitors in patients with DME are in progress to serve as an initial step in the translation of scientific research into a novel clinical intervention. For instance, intravitreal injection of THR-149 (Oxurion), a plasma kallikrein inhibitor, reduced retinal thickening in a diabetic rat model, implicating KKS in the pathogenesis of DME.[115]

Anti-integrin therapy

Integrins are a family of multifunctional cell-adhesion molecules and heterodimeric receptors that connect extracellular matrix to cell cortex. Their regulatory functions including cellular adhesion, migration, proliferation, invasion, survival, and apoptosis of neurovascular cells are critical targets for treating diabetic retina. In Chapter 9, novel anti-integrin therapies that may contribute to the inflammatory, angiogenic, and fibrotic events in DR have been introduced. Since integrin-driven molecular mechanisms in diabetic retina are distinct from VEGF pathways, it is worthy of note to emphasize that anti-integrin therapy may serve as a primary therapy for some nonresponders to anti-VEGF therapy or as an adjunctive therapy to anti-VEGF agents in future.[116,117]

Genetics of DR

DR is a polygenic disorder. That genetic factors play a major role in the etiology of DM has long been appreciated due to ethnic differences in terms of onset frequency, increased familial aggregation, and a dramatically higher concordance in monozygotic than dizygotic twins.[118] However, the susceptibility genes for DR have not been firmly identified. By using an epidemiological approach, heritability has been estimated to be as high as 27% for any DR and 52% for PDR.[119] In the era of Genome-Wide Association Studies (GWAS), important epidemiologic discoveries of genetic association with T2DM have been established.[120] Although the genetic basis of diabetes is increasingly clear, the genetic effects on the development of DR are still elusive. The second-generation sequencing approach has been used to identify common and rare variants associated with DR. To date, no variants have been replicated across multiple studies.[119] This discrepancy may be attributed to the highly complex and multifactorial nature of DR.

A recent study using lymphoblastoid cell lines derived from subjects with different stages of DR analyzed gene expression by microarrays to characterize the transcriptional response to elevated glucose. One hundred and three (103) genes were found to be differentially expressed in the cell lines from participants with diabetes. Seven thousand two hundred fifty-three (7,253) SNPs that influence gene expression (eSNPs) from the 103 differential response genes are enriched for association with DR. Here, eSNP refers to SNP with expression quantitative trait loci (eQTL). Further assessment and validation of the significance of the eSNP enrichment were performed. The most significant retinopathy-associated eSNP among the set of 7,253 eSNPs tested is rs11867934, an intergenic eSNP for folliculin gene (*FLCN*). *FLCN* is expressed in multiple biologically relevant tissues including vascular and neuronal tissues. Evidence exists that FLCN is a negative regulator of AMP-activated protein kinase (AMPK). AMPK is responsible for resistance to cellular stresses via autophagy and cellular bioenergetics. Activation of the AMPK pathway resulting from loss of FLCN may lead to cell apoptosis. This work has implicated *FLCN* as a putative DR susceptibility gene. Since independent cohorts of individuals with diabetes revealed an association of FLCN eQTLs with DR, integration of genetic association with gene expression may implicate *FLCN* as a disease gene for DR.[121] The concern about this report is that the second passages of primary cell lines were used. The cultured cells receive environmental exposure which could influence gene expression.[122] Nevertheless, this report is a breakthrough in the study of genetics of DR and yields further genetic understanding of DR-susceptible genes. The future for translational research on the genetics of DR is exciting. Studies with larger populations and multiple cell lines with improved sequencing techniques will provide further insights into genetic associations with DR. In particular, studies will focus on more heritable forms of DR such as PDR. Based on these findings, genetic variants leading to DR may be modified with preventive and regenerative achievement.

A recent proteomic study of vitreous from patients with 50-year history of T1DM, but without DR, revealed an overexpressed protein that may protect the retina from DR. Under similar levels of glycemic control, this special protein is expressed much higher in no-DR or mild DR eyes than in PDR eyes. Biochemical characterization of this protein identifies it as a retinol transport protein, known as retinol-binding protein 3 (RBP3), which is mainly produced by photoreceptors. The distinctly high expression of RBP3 in the subpopulation of patients who did not develop clinical

DR indicates that RBP3 is a disease protector against DR. This paper also demonstrated that the protective benefit is partially mediated by RBP3 binding to glucose transporter 1 (GLUT1) and sequential inhibition of glucose uptake in endothelial and Müller cells, leading to decreased expression of VEGF and inflammatory cytokines. The discovery of endogenous protective factors may prove to be as important as elucidating exogenous risk factors in future translational research on DR.[123]

Application of artificial intelligence in DR
Current application of AI in DR

Artificial intelligence (AI) is a branch of computer science that aims to create intelligent machines. Advances in computational technology have enabled the application of AI for medicine.[124] AI is a fast-growing field, and its applications to diabetes can reform the approach to diagnosis and management of this chronic condition. AI can assist with image interpretation, diagnosis, multidisciplinary management, risk stratification, and prognosis assessment. Thus, AI can increase efficiency of screening, reduce barriers to healthcare access, and improve patient outcomes as a result of early detection and treatment.[125] For instance, AI techniques that are used in image segmentation, automated diagnosis, disease prediction, and prognosis can be used in aiding the management of DR.

Deep learning (DL) is a subset of machine learning, in which technology mimics the human brain by using multiple layers of artificial neural networks.[126] Connections between layers are weighted according to the predictive power of known factors and strengthen or weaken with input data, including clinical data, images, or genomic data. DL systems use a backpropagation algorithm, a method of supervised learning, to determine how machine learning should alter its parameters. In comparisons with real-time recurrent learning, after each forward pass through a network, backpropagation performs a backward pass while checking the model's parameters via weights and biases. Instead of using programmed features, DL algorithms learn features based on a large, labeled sample dataset and can extract and classify features based on the input directly.

Undiagnosed DR is one of the main causes of vision loss. Screening for DR, coupled with prompt referral and treatment, is a key strategy for blindness prevention (Fig. 10.4). Screening methods involve a variety of imaging. DL algorithms can detect DR without defining specific disease features such as microaneurysms, hard exudates, and hemorrhages. In 2018, the IDx-DR fundus camera for DR screening was approved by the FDA as the first fully autonomous AI-based DR diagnostic system in the United States.[124] This system is currently being used for patient screening and referral in the clinical setting. A model of AI in diabetic care is illustrated in Fig. 10.4.[125]

Translating AI data from bench to bedside

The use of AI and DL in ophthalmology has the potential to improve early diagnosis and longitudinal care, thereby reducing cases of preventable blindness by DR.[125]

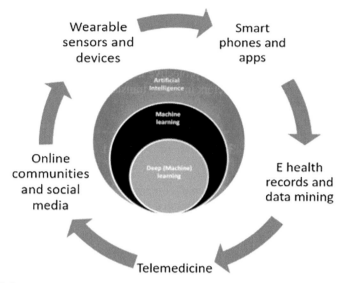

FIGURE 10.4

Application of artificial intelligence (AI) and deep learning (DL) in diabetic care including prevention and management of diabetic retinopathy.

Modified from Ellahham 2020.[125]

However, translation of AI and DL data to the real-world clinic is still not on the horizon. For example, the identification of specific abnormalities of DR by AI may miss some important ocular and systemic factors for accurate diagnosis. Challenges for clinical implementation comprise explanation of algorithm results, regulatory restrictions, and the understanding and acceptance of AI and DL by physicians and patients. Specifically, large-scale adoption of AI in healthcare is still not accepted by most physicians, who view AI and DL as "black boxes."[126] Future efforts to integrate AI and DL into clinical practice should make use of real-world ocular images from heterogeneous patient populations obtained from various imaging machines that elucidate complex pathologies. In addition, these future efforts should attempt to identify specific imaging biomarkers to open up the black box of AI and DL methodology for ophthalmology applications.

In summary, diabetes and its complications are the major chronic diseases seriously affecting quality of life. Currently, insulin and oral anti-diabetic drugs are the primary modes of therapy for diabetic patients. In order to achieve glycemic control, multidisciplinary efforts improving insulin sensing and signaling are required. Among anti-diabetic drugs, the relationship between their effects of glycemic control and DR development should be considered because the duration and intensity of hyperglycemia are determinants of DR development. For instance, newly discovered GLP-1RAs that possess excellent lowering glucose function and body weight regulation may unfortunately increase the risk of DR development in short or long term based on limited meta-analyses.[52] To validate this observation affecting the translational process from bench to bedside, future research by multidisciplinary collaboration is imperative. With clarification of the pathogenesis of DR at cellular and molecular levels, oxidative stress interacting with the six major metabolic disturbances (see Fig. 2.1 in Chapter 2) may be recognized as a unifying mechanism underlying DR. Therefore, antioxidative stress may be the key translational strategy for the treatment of DR in future. Besides improving efficacy and duration of anti-VEGF therapy, targeting alternative pathways such as apoptosis, inflammation, neurodegeneration, and non-VEGF pathways, for example, the KKS, and the Ang-2/Tie2 system will be key in translational research on DR. In the era of GWAS and improved sequencing techniques, important discoveries of genetic associations with DR provide further genetic understanding of the pathogenesis and potential therapeutic targets of DR. With the development of advanced OCT and the advent of AI, screening, diagnosis, and management of DR must be learned through multidisciplinary channels from which novel ideas and new treatment options will significantly impact future therapeutic advances for DR.

References

1. The DCCT/EDIC Research Group. Frequency of evidence-based screening for retinopathy in type 1 diabetes. *N Engl J Med.* 2017;376(16):1507–1516. https://doi.org/10.1056/NEJMoa1612836.
2. Mameli C. Explaining the increased mortality in type 1 diabetes. *WJD.* 2015;6(7):889. https://doi.org/10.4239/wjd.v6.i7.889.
3. Hainsworth DP, Bebu I, Aiello LP, et al. Risk factors for retinopathy in type 1 diabetes: the DCCT/EDIC study. *Diabetes Care.* 2019;42(5):875–882. https://doi.org/10.2337/dc18-2308.
4. Ilonen J, Lempainen J, Veijola R. The heterogeneous pathogenesis of type 1 diabetes mellitus. *Nat Rev Endocrinol.* 2019;15(11):635–650. https://doi.org/10.1038/s41574-019-0254-y.
5. Gillespie KM. Type 1 diabetes: pathogenesis and prevention. *CMAJ (Can Med Assoc J).* 2006;175(2):165–170. https://doi.org/10.1503/cmaj.060244.
6. Colberg SR, Sigal RJ, Yardley JE, et al. Physical activity/exercise and diabetes: a position statement of the American diabetes association. *Diabetes Care.* 2016;39(11):2065–2079. https://doi.org/10.2337/dc16-1728.
7. Thrasher J. Pharmacologic management of type 2 diabetes mellitus: available therapies. *Am J Med.* 2017;130(6):S4–S17. https://doi.org/10.1016/j.amjmed.2017.04.004.
8. Taylor SI, Yazdi ZS, Beitelshees AL. Pharmacological treatment of hyperglycemia in type 2 diabetes. *J Clin Invest.* 2021;131(2):e142243. https://doi.org/10.1172/JCI142243.
9. Ferris FL, Nathan DM. Preventing diabetic retinopathy progression. *Ophthalmology.* 2016;123(9):1840–1842. https://doi.org/10.1016/j.ophtha.2016.05.039.
10. Diabetes Control and Complications Trial Research Group, Nathan DM, Genuth S, et al. The effect of intensive treatment of diabetes on the development and progression of long-term complications in insulin-dependent diabetes mellitus. *N Engl J Med.* 1993;329(14):977–986. https://doi.org/10.1056/NEJM199309303291401.

11. Prolonged effect of intensive therapy on the risk of retinopathy complications in patients with type 1 diabetes mellitus: 10 years after the diabetes control and complications trial. *Arch Ophthalmol*. 2008;126(12):1707. https://doi.org/10.1001/archopht.126.12.1707.

12. Holman RR, Paul SK, Bethel MA, Matthews DR, Neil HAW. 10-Year follow-up of intensive glucose control in type 2 diabetes. *N Engl J Med*. 2008;359(15): 1577−1589. https://doi.org/10.1056/NEJMoa0806470.

13. Guzmán G, Martínez V, Yara JD, et al. Glycemic control and hypoglycemia in patients treated with insulin pump therapy: an observational study. *J Diabetes Res*. 2020;2020: 1−8. https://doi.org/10.1155/2020/1581726.

14. Freeland B. Hypoglycemia in diabetes mellitus. *Home Healthc Now*. 2017;35(8): 414−419. https://doi.org/10.1097/NHH.0000000000000584.

15. Samson WK, Stein LM, Elrick M, et al. Hypoglycemia unawareness prevention: targeting glucagon production. *Physiol Behav*. 2016;162:147−150. https://doi.org/10.1016/j.physbeh.2016.04.012.

16. La Sala L, Pontiroli AE. New fast acting glucagon for recovery from hypoglycemia, a life-threatening situation: nasal powder and injected stable solutions. *Int J Mol Sci*. 2021;22(19):10643. https://doi.org/10.3390/ijms221910643.

17. Cryer PE. Hypoglycemia, functional brain failure, and brain death. *J Clin Invest*. 2007; 117(4):868−870. https://doi.org/10.1172/JCI31669.

18. Unger RH, Cherrington AD. Glucagonocentric restructuring of diabetes: a pathophysiologic and therapeutic makeover. *J Clin Invest*. 2012;122(1):4−12. https://doi.org/10.1172/JCI60016.

19. Silbert R, Salcido-Montenegro A, Rodriguez-Gutierrez R, Katabi A, McCoy RG. Hypoglycemia among patients with type 2 diabetes: epidemiology, risk factors, and prevention strategies. *Curr Diabetes Rep*. 2018;18(8):53. https://doi.org/10.1007/s11892-018-1018-0.

20. ORIGIN Trial Investigators. Predictors of nonsevere and severe hypoglycemia during glucose-lowering treatment with insulin glargine or standard drugs in the ORIGIN trial. *Diabetes Care*. 2015;38(1):22−28. https://doi.org/10.2337/dc14-1329.

21. Hooymans JM, Ballegooie EV, Schweitzer NM, Doorebos H, Reitsma WD, Slutter WJ. Worsening of diabetic retinopathy with strict control of blood sugar. *Lancet*. 1982; 2(8295):438. https://doi.org/10.1016/s0140-6736(82)90464-0.

22. Feldman-Billard S, Larger É, Massin P. Standards for screeningand surveillance of ocular complications in people with diabetes SFD study group. Early worsening of diabetic retinopathy after rapid improvement of blood glucose control in patients with diabetes. *Diabetes Metab*. 2018;44(1):4−14. https://doi.org/10.1016/j.diabet.2017.10.014.

23. Bain SC, Klufas MA, Ho A, Matthews DR. Worsening of diabetic retinopathy with rapid improvement in systemic glucose control: a review. *Diabetes Obes Metabol*. 2019;21(3):454−466. https://doi.org/10.1111/dom.13538.

24. Thangarajah H, Yao D, Chang EI, et al. The molecular basis for impaired hypoxia-induced VEGF expression in diabetic tissues. *Proc Natl Acad Sci USA*. 2009; 106(32):13505−13510. https://doi.org/10.1073/pnas.0906670106.

25. Action to control cardiovascular risk in diabetes follow-on (ACCORDION) eye study group and the action to control cardiovascular risk in diabetes follow-on (ACCORDION) study group. Persistent effects of intensive glycemic control on retinopathy in type 2 diabetes in the action to control cardiovascular risk in diabetes (ACCORD)

follow-on study. *Diabetes Care*. 2016;39(7):1089−1100. https://doi.org/10.2337/dc16-0024.

26. Nathan DM, Bayless M, Cleary P, et al. Diabetes control and complications trial/epidemiology of diabetes Interventions and complications study at 30 years: advances and contributions. *Diabetes*. 2013;62(12):3976−3986. https://doi.org/10.2337/db13-1093.

27. Buse JB. Action to control cardiovascular risk in diabetes (ACCORD) trial: design and methods. *Am J Cardiol*. 2007;99(12):S21−S33. https://doi.org/10.1016/j.amjcard.2007.03.003.

28. Effects of intensive glucose lowering in type 2 diabetes. *N Engl J Med*. 2008;358(24):2545−2559. https://doi.org/10.1056/NEJMoa0802743.

29. Intensive diabetes treatment and cardiovascular disease in patients with type 1 diabetes. *N Engl J Med*. 2005;353(25):2643−2653. https://doi.org/10.1056/NEJMoa052187.

30. Cheung N, Mitchell P, Wong TY. Diabetic retinopathy. *Lancet*. 2010;376(9735):124−136. https://doi.org/10.1016/S0140-6736(09)62124-3.

31. Zhou Y, Wang C, Shi K, Yin X. Relationship between dyslipidemia and diabetic retinopathy: a systematic review and meta-analysis. *Medicine (Baltim)*. 2018;97(36):e12283. https://doi.org/10.1097/MD.0000000000012283.

32. Suzuma I, Hata Y, Clermont A, et al. Cyclic stretch and hypertension induce retinal expression of vascular endothelial growth factor and vascular endothelial growth factor receptor-2: potential mechanisms for exacerbation of diabetic retinopathy by hypertension. *Diabetes*. 2001;50(2):444−454. https://doi.org/10.2337/diabetes.50.2.444.

33. Klein R, Knudtson MD, Lee KE, Gangnon R, Klein BEK. The Wisconsin Epidemiologic Study of Diabetic Retinopathy: XXII the twenty-five-year progression of retinopathy in persons with type 1 diabetes. *Ophthalmology*. 2008;115(11):1859−1868. https://doi.org/10.1016/j.ophtha.2008.08.023.

34. Gallego PH, Craig ME, Hing S, Donaghue KC. Role of blood pressure in development of early retinopathy in adolescents with type 1 diabetes: prospective cohort study. *BMJ*. 2008;337:a918. https://doi.org/10.1136/bmj.a918.

35. Liu L, Quang ND, Banu R, et al. Hypertension, blood pressure control and diabetic retinopathy in a large population-based study. *PLoS One*. 2020;15(3):e0229665. https://doi.org/10.1371/journal.pone.0229665.

36. Chaturvedi N, Sjolie AK, Stephenson JM, et al. Effect of lisinopril on progression of retinopathy in normotensive people with type 1 diabetes. The EUCLID study group. EURODIAB controlled trial of lisinopril in insulin-dependent diabetes mellitus. *Lancet*. 1998;351(9095):28−31. https://doi.org/10.1016/s0140-6736(97)06209-0.

37. Matthews DR, Stratton IM, Aldington SJ, Holman RR, Kohner EM, UK Prospective Diabetes Study Group. Risks of progression of retinopathy and vision loss related to tight blood pressure control in type 2 diabetes mellitus: UKPDS 69. *Arch Ophthalmol*. 2004;122(11):1631−1640. https://doi.org/10.1001/archopht.122.11.1631.

38. Patel A, ADVANCE Collaborative Group, MacMahon S, et al. Effects of a fixed combination of perindopril and indapamide on macrovascular and microvascular outcomes in patients with type 2 diabetes mellitus (the ADVANCE trial): a randomised controlled trial. *Lancet*. 2007;370(9590):829−840. https://doi.org/10.1016/S0140-6736(07)61303-8.

39. Danser AH, Derkx FH, Admiraal PJ, Deinum J, de Jong PT, Schalekamp MA. Angiotensin levels in the eye. *Invest Ophthalmol Vis Sci*. 1994;35(3):1008−1018.

40. Rolo AP, Palmeira CM. Diabetes and mitochondrial function: role of hyperglycemia and oxidative stress. *Toxicol Appl Pharmacol*. 2006;212(2):167−178. https://doi.org/10.1016/j.taap.2006.01.003.

41. Du XL, Edelstein D, Rossetti L, et al. Hyperglycemia-induced mitochondrial superoxide overproduction activates the hexosamine pathway and induces plasminogen activator inhibitor-1 expression by increasing Sp1 glycosylation. *Proc Natl Acad Sci U S A*. 2000;97(22):12222−12226. https://doi.org/10.1073/pnas.97.22.12222.

42. Nebbioso M, Lambiase A, Armentano M, et al. Diabetic retinopathy, oxidative stress, and sirtuins: an in depth look in enzymatic patterns and new therapeutic horizons. *Surv Ophthalmol*. April 14, 2021. https://doi.org/10.1016/j.survophthal.2021.04.003. S0039-6257(21)00101-00106.

43. Yumnamcha T, Guerra M, Singh LP, Ibrahim AS. Metabolic dysregulation and neurovascular dysfunction in diabetic retinopathy. *Antioxidants*. 2020;9(12):1244. https://doi.org/10.3390/antiox9121244.

44. Wilkinson-Berka JL, Agrotis A, Deliyanti D. The retinal renin-angiotensin system: roles of angiotensin II and aldosterone. *Peptides*. 2012;36(1):142−150. https://doi.org/10.1016/j.peptides.2012.04.008.

45. Al-Shabrawey M, Rojas M, Sanders T, et al. Role of NADPH oxidase in retinal vascular inflammation. *Invest Ophthalmol Vis Sci*. 2008;49(7):3239−3244. https://doi.org/10.1167/iovs.08-1755.

46. Jialal I, Kaur H. The role of Toll-like receptors in diabetes-induced inflammation: implications for vascular complications. *Curr Diabetes Rep*. February 8, 2012. https://doi.org/10.1007/s11892-012-0258-7.

47. Rodríguez ML, Pérez S, Mena-Mollá S, Desco MC, Ortega ÁL. Oxidative stress and microvascular alterations in diabetic retinopathy: future therapies. *Oxid Med Cell Longev*. 2019;2019:1−18. https://doi.org/10.1155/2019/4940825.

48. Rübsam A, Parikh S, Fort PE. Role of inflammation in diabetic retinopathy. *Int J Mol Sci*. 2018;19(4):E942. https://doi.org/10.3390/ijms19040942.

49. Liu M, Huang Y, Xu X, et al. Normal and defective pathways in biogenesis and maintenance of the insulin storage pool. *J Clin Invest*. 2021;131(2):142240. https://doi.org/10.1172/JCI142240.

50. El Mouhayyar C, Riachy R, Khalil AB, Eid A, Azar S. SGLT2 inhibitors, GLP-1 agonists, and DPP-4 inhibitors in diabetes and microvascular complications: a review. *Internet J Endocrinol*. 2020;2020:1762164. https://doi.org/10.1155/2020/1762164.

51. Knudsen LB, Lau J. The discovery and development of liraglutide and semaglutide. *Front Endocrinol*. 2019;10:155. https://doi.org/10.3389/fendo.2019.00155.

52. Bethel MA, Diaz R, Castellana N, Bhattacharya I, Gerstein HC, Lakshmanan MC. HbA1c change and diabetic retinopathy during GLP-1 receptor agonist cardiovascular outcome trials: a meta-analysis and meta-regression. *Diabetes Care*. 2021;44(1):290−296. https://doi.org/10.2337/dc20-1815.

53. Quattrini L, La Motta C. Aldose reductase inhibitors: 2013-present. *Expert Opin Ther Pat*. 2019;29(3):199−213. https://doi.org/10.1080/13543776.2019.1582646.

54. Milne R, Brownstein S. Advanced glycation end products and diabetic retinopathy. *Amino Acids*. 2013;44(6):1397−1407. https://doi.org/10.1007/s00726-011-1071-3.

55. Hudson BI, Lippman ME. Targeting RAGE signaling in inflammatory disease. *Annu Rev Med*. 2018;69(1):349−364. https://doi.org/10.1146/annurev-med-041316-085215.

56. Nakamura M, Barber AJ, Antonetti DA, et al. Excessive hexosamines block the neuroprotective effect of insulin and induce apoptosis in retinal neurons. *J Biol Chem*. 2001;276(47):43748−43755. https://doi.org/10.1074/jbc.M108594200.

57. Joy SV, Scates AC, Bearelly S, et al. Ruboxistaurin, a protein kinase C beta inhibitor, as an emerging treatment for diabetes microvascular complications. *Ann Pharmacother.* 2005;39(10):1693−1699. https://doi.org/10.1345/aph.1E572.

58. McGill JB. Improving microvascular outcomes in patients with diabetes through management of hypertension. *Postgrad Med.* 2009;121(2):89−101. https://doi.org/10.3810/pgm.2009.03.1980.

59. Mohammad G, Siddiquei MM, Abu El-Asrar AM. Poly (ADP-ribose) polymerase mediates diabetes-induced retinal neuropathy. *Mediat Inflamm.* 2013;2013:1−10. https://doi.org/10.1155/2013/510451.

60. Mohammad G, Alrashed SH, Almater AI, Siddiquei MM, Abu El-Asrar AM. The poly(ADP-ribose)polymerase-1 inhibitor 1,5-isoquinolinediol attenuate diabetes-induced NADPH oxidase-derived oxidative stress in retina. *J Ocul Pharmacol Therapeut.* 2018;34(7):512−520. https://doi.org/10.1089/jop.2017.0117.

61. Wang W, Lo A. Diabetic retinopathy: pathophysiology and treatments. *Indian J Manag Sci.* 2018;19(6):1816. https://doi.org/10.3390/ijms19061816.

62. Kang Q, Yang C. Oxidative stress and diabetic retinopathy: molecular mechanisms, pathogenetic role and therapeutic implications. *Redox Biol.* 2020;37:101799. https://doi.org/10.1016/j.redox.2020.101799.

63. Zhong Q, Mishra M, Kowluru RA. Transcription factor Nrf2-mediated antioxidant defense system in the development of diabetic retinopathy. *Invest Ophthalmol Vis Sci.* 2013;54(6):3941−3948. https://doi.org/10.1167/iovs.13-11598.

64. Hybertson BM, Gao B, Bose SK, McCord JM. Oxidative stress in health and disease: the therapeutic potential of Nrf2 activation. *Mol Aspect Med.* 2011;32(4−6):234−246. https://doi.org/10.1016/j.mam.2011.10.006.

65. Zheng Z, Chen H, Li J, et al. Sirtuin 1−mediated cellular metabolic memory of high glucose via the LKB1/AMPK/ROS pathway and therapeutic effects of metformin. *Diabetes.* 2012;61(1):217−228. https://doi.org/10.2337/db11-0416.

66. Huang DD, Shi G, Jiang Y, Yao C, Zhu C. A review on the potential of resveratrol in prevention and therapy of diabetes and diabetic complications. *Biomed Pharmacother.* 2020;125:109767. https://doi.org/10.1016/j.biopha.2019.109767.

67. Tang J, Du Y, Lee CA, Talahalli R, Eells JT, Kern TS. Low-intensity far-red light inhibits early lesions that contribute to diabetic retinopathy: in vivo and in vitro. *Invest Ophthalmol Vis Sci.* 2013;54(5):3681−3690. https://doi.org/10.1167/iovs.12-11018.

68. Du Y, Veenstra A, Palczewski K, Kern TS. Photoreceptor cells are major contributors to diabetes-induced oxidative stress and local inflammation in the retina. *Proc Natl Acad Sci USA.* 2013;110(41):16586−16591. https://doi.org/10.1073/pnas.1314575110.

69. Whitehead M, Wickremasinghe S, Osborne A, Van Wijngaarden P, Martin KR. Diabetic retinopathy: a complex pathophysiology requiring novel therapeutic strategies. *Expet Opin Biol Ther.* 2018;18(12):1257−1270. https://doi.org/10.1080/14712598.2018.1545836.

70. Sinha K, Das J, Pal PB, Sil PC. Oxidative stress: the mitochondria-dependent and mitochondria-independent pathways of apoptosis. *Arch Toxicol.* 2013;87(7):1157−1180. https://doi.org/10.1007/s00204-013-1034-4.

71. Green DR. Apoptotic pathways: the roads to ruin. *Cell.* 1998;94(6):695−698. https://doi.org/10.1016/s0092-8674(00)81728-6.

72. Radi R, Cassina A, Hodara R. Nitric oxide and peroxynitrite interactions with mitochondria. *Biol Chem.* 2002;383(3−4):401−409. https://doi.org/10.1515/BC.2002.044.

73. McKimpson WM, Weinberger J, Czerski L, et al. The apoptosis inhibitor ARC alleviates the ER stress response to promote β-cell survival. *Diabetes*. 2013;62(1):183−193. https://doi.org/10.2337/db12-0504.

74. Wu C, Xu K, Liu W, et al. Protective effect of raf-1 kinase inhibitory protein on diabetic retinal neurodegeneration through P38-MAPK pathway. *Curr Eye Res*. July 26, 2021: 1−8. https://doi.org/10.1080/02713683.2021.1944644.

75. Madsen-Bouterse SA, Kowluru RA. Oxidative stress and diabetic retinopathy: pathophysiological mechanisms and treatment perspectives. *Rev Endocr Metab Disord*. 2008;9(4):315−327. https://doi.org/10.1007/s11154-008-9090-4.

76. Kowluru RA. Diabetic retinopathy: mitochondrial dysfunction and retinal capillary cell death. *Antioxidants Redox Signal*. 2005;7(11−12):1581−1587. https://doi.org/10.1089/ars.2005.7.1581.

77. Abu El-Asrar AM, Dralands L, Missotten L, Geboes K. Expression of antiapoptotic and proapoptotic molecules in diabetic retinas. *Eye (Lond)*. 2007;21(2):238−245. https://doi.org/10.1038/sj.eye.6702225.

78. Fahrenthold BK, Fernandes KA, Libby RT. Assessment of intrinsic and extrinsic signaling pathway in excitotoxic retinal ganglion cell death. *Sci Rep*. 2018;8(1):4641. https://doi.org/10.1038/s41598-018-22848-y.

79. Green DR. Apoptotic pathways: ten minutes to dead. *Cell*. 2005;121(5):671−674. https://doi.org/10.1016/j.cell.2005.05.019.

80. Jiang Y, Thakran S, Bheemreddy R, et al. Pioglitazone normalizes insulin signaling in the diabetic rat retina through reduction in tumor necrosis factor α and suppressor of cytokine signaling 3. *J Biol Chem*. 2014;289(38):26395−26405. https://doi.org/10.1074/jbc.M114.583880.

81. Joharapurkar A, Patel V, Kshirsagar S, Patel MS, Savsani H, Jain M. Effect of dual PPAR-α/γ agonist saroglitazar on diabetic retinopathy and oxygen-induced retinopathy. *Eur J Pharmacol*. 2021;899:174032. https://doi.org/10.1016/j.ejphar.2021.174032.

82. Wang B, Wang F, Zhang Y, et al. Effects of RAS inhibitors on diabetic retinopathy: a systematic review and meta-analysis. *Lancet Diabetes Endocrinol*. 2015;3(4):263−274. https://doi.org/10.1016/S2213-8587(14)70256-6.

83. Batenburg WW, Verma A, Wang Y, et al. Combined renin inhibition/(pro)renin receptor blockade in diabetic retinopathy—a study in transgenic (mREN2)27 rats. *PLoS One*. 2014;9(6):e100954. https://doi.org/10.1371/journal.pone.0100954.

84. Ludwig-Galezowska AH, Flanagan L, Rehm M. Apoptosis repressor with caspase recruitment domain, a multifunctional modulator of cell death. *J Cell Mol Med*. 2011;15(5):1044−1053. https://doi.org/10.1111/j.1582-4934.2010.01221.x.

85. Liu M, Yu T, Li M, et al. Apoptosis repressor with caspase recruitment domain promotes cell proliferation and phenotypic modulation through 14−3-3ε/YAP signaling in vascular smooth muscle cells. *J Mol Cell Cardiol*. 2020;147:35−48. https://doi.org/10.1016/j.yjmcc.2020.08.003.

86. Alural B, Duran GA, Tufekci KU, et al. EPO mediates neurotrophic, neuroprotective, anti-oxidant, and anti-apoptotic effects via downregulation of miR-451 and miR-885-5p in SH-SY5Y neuron-like cells. *Front Immunol*. 2014;5:475. https://doi.org/10.3389/fimmu.2014.00475.

87. Zhang J, Wu Y, Jin Y, et al. Intravitreal injection of erythropoietin protects both retinal vascular and neuronal cells in early diabetes. *Invest Ophthalmol Vis Sci*. 2008;49(2):732−742. https://doi.org/10.1167/iovs.07-0721.

88. Abri Aghdam K, Soltan Sanjari M, Ghasemi Falavarjani K. Erythropoietin in ophthalmology: a literature review. *Journal of Current Ophthalmology.* 2016;28(1):5−11. https://doi.org/10.1016/j.joco.2016.01.008.

89. Böcker-Meffert S, Rosenstiel P, Röhl C, et al. Erythropoietin and VEGF promote neural outgrowth from retinal explants in postnatal rats. *Invest Ophthalmol Vis Sci.* 2002;43(6): 2021−2026.

90. Junk AK, Mammis A, Savitz SI, et al. Erythropoietin administration protects retinal neurons from acute ischemia-reperfusion injury. *Proc Natl Acad Sci U S A.* 2002; 99(16):10659−10664. https://doi.org/10.1073/pnas.152321399.

91. Li W, Sinclair SH, Xu GT. Effects of intravitreal erythropoietin therapy for patients with chronic and progressive diabetic macular edema. *Ophthalmic Surg Laser Imag.* 2010; 41(1):18−25. https://doi.org/10.3928/15428877-20091230-03.

92. Tong Z, Yang Z, Patel S, et al. Promoter polymorphism of the erythropoietin gene in severe diabetic eye and kidney complications. *Proc Natl Acad Sci U S A.* 2008; 105(19):6998−7003. https://doi.org/10.1073/pnas.0800454105.

93. Watanabe D, Suzuma K, Matsui S, et al. Erythropoietin as a retinal angiogenic factor in proliferative diabetic retinopathy. *N Engl J Med.* 2005;353(8):782−792. https://doi.org/10.1056/NEJMoa041773.

94. Hernández C, Fonollosa A, García-Ramírez M, et al. Erythropoietin is expressed in the human retina and it is highly elevated in the vitreous fluid of patients with diabetic macular edema. *Diabetes Care.* 2006;29(9):2028−2033. https://doi.org/10.2337/dc06-0556.

95. Romagnoli C, Tesfagabir MG, Giannantonio C, Papacci P. Erythropoietin and retinopathy of prematurity. *Early Hum Dev.* 2011;87:S39−S42. https://doi.org/10.1016/j.earlhumdev.2011.01.027.

96. Hellström A, Smith LEH, Dammann O. Retinopathy of prematurity. *Lancet.* 2013; 382(9902):1445−1457. https://doi.org/10.1016/S0140-6736(13)60178-6.

97. Chen J, Smith LEH. A double-edged sword: erythropoietin eyed in retinopathy of prematurity. *J Am Assoc Pediatr Ophthalmol Strabismus.* 2008;12(3):221−222. https://doi.org/10.1016/j.jaapos.2008.02.001.

98. Steinman L. Parsing physiological functions of erythropoietin one domain at a time. *Neurotherapeutics.* 2015;12(4):848−849. https://doi.org/10.1007/s13311-015-0384-4.

99. Brook N, Brook E, Dharmarajan A, Chan A, Dass CR. Pigment epithelium-derived factor regulation of neuronal and stem cell fate. *Exp Cell Res.* 2020;389(2):111891. https://doi.org/10.1016/j.yexcr.2020.111891.

100. Sieving PA, Caruso RC, Tao W, et al. Ciliary neurotrophic factor (CNTF) for human retinal degeneration: phase I trial of CNTF delivered by encapsulated cell intraocular implants. *Proc Natl Acad Sci U S A.* 2006;103(10):3896−3901. https://doi.org/10.1073/pnas.0600236103.

101. Ogura S, Kurata K, Hattori Y, et al. Sustained inflammation after pericyte depletion induces irreversible blood-retina barrier breakdown. *JCI Insight.* 2017;2(3). https://doi.org/10.1172/jci.insight.90905.

102. Bhattacharya S, Gangaraju R, Chaum E. Recent advances in retinal stem cell therapy. *Curr Mol Biol Rep.* 2017;3(3):172−182. https://doi.org/10.1007/s40610-017-0069-3.

103. Kiamehr M, Klettner A, Richert E, et al. Compromised barrier function in human induced pluripotent stem-cell-derived retinal pigment epithelial cells from type 2 diabetic patients. *Int J Mol Sci.* 2019;20(15):E3773. https://doi.org/10.3390/ijms20153773.

104. Antonetti DA, Silva PS, Stitt AW. Current understanding of the molecular and cellular pathology of diabetic retinopathy. *Nat Rev Endocrinol.* 2021;17(4):195–206. https://doi.org/10.1038/s41574-020-00451-4.

105. Çerman E, Akkoç T, Eraslan M, et al. Retinal electrophysiological effects of intravitreal bone marrow derived mesenchymal stem cells in streptozotocin induced diabetic rats. *PLoS One.* 2016;11(6):e0156495. https://doi.org/10.1371/journal.pone.0156495.

106. Das AT, Tenenbaum L, Berkhout B. Tet-on systems for doxycycline-inducible gene expression. *Curr Gene Ther.* 2016;16(3):156–167. https://doi.org/10.2174/1566523216666160524144041.

107. Guan Y, Cui L, Qu Z, et al. Subretinal transplantation of rat MSCs and erythropoietin gene modified rat MSCs for protecting and rescuing degenerative retina in rats. *Curr Mol Med.* 2013;13(9):1419–1431. https://doi.org/10.2174/15665240113139990071.

108. Kutlutürk Karagöz I, Allahverdiyev A, Bağırova M, Abamor EŞ, Dinparvar S. Current approaches in treatment of diabetic retinopathy and future perspectives. *J Ocul Pharmacol Therapeut.* 2020;36(7):487–496. https://doi.org/10.1089/jop.2019.0137.

109. Brown DM, Emanuelli A, Bandello F, et al. KESTREL and KITE: 52-week results from two Phase III pivotal trials of brolucizumab for diabetic macular edema. *Am J Ophthalmol.* January 2022. https://doi.org/10.1016/j.ajo.2022.01.004. S000293942200006X.

110. Elman MJ, Aiello LP, Beck RW, et al. Randomized trial evaluating ranibizumab plus prompt or deferred laser or triamcinolone plus prompt laser for diabetic macular edema. *Ophthalmology.* 2010;117(6):1064–1077.e35. https://doi.org/10.1016/j.ophtha.2010.02.031.

111. Lim SI. Fine-tuning bispecific therapeutics. *Pharmacol Ther.* 2020;212:107582. https://doi.org/10.1016/j.pharmthera.2020.107582.

112. Patel SR, Berezovsky DE, McCarey BE, Zarnitsyn V, Edelhauser HF, Prausnitz MR. Targeted administration into the suprachoroidal space using a microneedle for drug delivery to the posterior segment of the eye. *Invest Ophthalmol Vis Sci.* 2012;53(8):4433–4441. https://doi.org/10.1167/iovs.12-9872.

113. Roberti G, Oddone F, Agnifili L, et al. Steroid-induced glaucoma: Epidemiology, pathophysiology, and clinical management. *Surv Ophthalmol.* 2020;65(4):458–472. https://doi.org/10.1016/j.survophthal.2020.01.002.

114. Chen X. *The Diabetic Eye Disease Pipeline in 2021.* 2021:20–22.

115. Van Bergen T, Hu TT, Little K, et al. Targeting plasma kallikrein with a novel bicyclic peptide inhibitor (THR-149) reduces retinal thickening in a diabetic rat model. *Invest Ophthalmol Vis Sci.* 2021;62(13):18. https://doi.org/10.1167/iovs.62.13.18.

116. Bhatwadekar AD, Kansara V, Luo Q, Ciulla T. Anti-integrin therapy for retinovascular diseases. *Expet Opin Invest Drugs.* 2020;29(9):935–945. https://doi.org/10.1080/13543784.2020.1795639.

117. Park SW, Yun JH, Kim JH, Kim KW, Cho CH, Kim JH. Angiopoietin 2 induces pericyte apoptosis via α3β1 integrin signaling in diabetic retinopathy. *Diabetes.* 2014;63(9):3057–3068. https://doi.org/10.2337/db13-1942.

118. Kuo JZ, Wong TY, Rotter JI. Challenges in elucidating the genetics of diabetic retinopathy. *JAMA Ophthalmol.* 2014;132(1):96. https://doi.org/10.1001/jamaophthalmol.2013.5024.

119. Han J, Lando L, Skowronska-Krawczyk D, Chao DL. Genetics of diabetic retinopathy. *Curr Diabetes Rep.* 2019;19(9):67. https://doi.org/10.1007/s11892-019-1186-6.

120. Billings LK, Florez JC. The genetics of type 2 diabetes: what have we learned from GWAS?: genetics of type 2 diabetes. *Ann N Y Acad Sci*. 2010;1212(1):59–77. https://doi.org/10.1111/j.1749-6632.2010.05838.x.

121. Skol AD, Jung SC, Sokovic AM, et al. Integration of genomics and transcriptomics predicts diabetic retinopathy susceptibility genes. *Elife*. 2020;9:e59980. https://doi.org/10.7554/eLife.59980.

122. Wright FA, Sullivan PF, Brooks AI, et al. Heritability and genomics of gene expression in peripheral blood. *Nat Genet*. 2014;46(5):430–437. https://doi.org/10.1038/ng.2951.

123. Yokomizo H, Maeda Y, Park K, et al. Retinol binding protein 3 is increased in the retina of patients with diabetes resistant to diabetic retinopathy. *Sci Transl Med*. 2019; 11(499):eaau6627. https://doi.org/10.1126/scitranslmed.aau6627.

124. Schmidt-Erfurth U, Sadeghipour A, Gerendas BS, Waldstein SM, Bogunović H. Artificial intelligence in retina. *Prog Retin Eye Res*. 2018;67:1–29. https://doi.org/10.1016/j.preteyeres.2018.07.004.

125. Ellahham S. Artificial intelligence: the future for diabetes care. *Am J Med*. 2020;133(8): 895–900. https://doi.org/10.1016/j.amjmed.2020.03.033.

126. Ting DSW, Pasquale LR, Peng L, et al. Artificial intelligence and deep learning in ophthalmology. *Br J Ophthalmol*. 2019;103(2):167–175. https://doi.org/10.1136/bjophthalmol-2018-313173.

Index